Essential Immuno

KU-300-940

Caroline x

Essential Immunology

IVAN M. ROITT

MA, DSc(Oxon), FRCPath, FRS
Professor and Head of
Department of Immunology
Middlesex Hospital Medical School
London W1

FIFTH EDITION

Blackwell Scientific Publications

OXFORD LONDON EDINBURGH

BOSTON PALO ALTO MELBOURNE

To my family

© 1971, 1974, 1977, 1980, 1984 by
Blackwell Scientific Publications
Editorial offices:
Osney Mead, Oxford, OX2 0EL
8 John Street, London, WC1N 2ES
9 Forrest Road, Edinburgh, EH1 2QH
52 Beacon Street, Boston
  Massachusetts 02108, USA
706 Cowper Street, Palo Alto
  California 94301, USA
99 Barry Street, Carlton
  Victoria 3053, Australia

All rights reserved. No part of this
publication may be reproduced, stored in a
retrieval system, or transmitted, in any
form or by any means, electronic,
mechanical, photocopying, recording or
otherwise without the prior permission of
the copyright owner

First published 1971
Reprinted 1972 (twice), 1973 (twice)
Second edition 1974
Reprinted 1975
Third edition 1977
Reprinted 1978, 1979
Fourth edition 1980
Reprinted, 1982, 1983
Fifth edition 1984

Spanish editions 1972, 1975, 1978
Italian editions 1973, 1975, 1979
Portuguese editions 1973, 1976
French editions 1975, 1979
Dutch editions 1975, 1978, 1982
Japanese editions 1976, 1978, 1982
German edition 1977
Polish edition 1977
Greek edition 1978
Slovak edition 1981
ELBS editions 1978, 1982

Set by Santype International Ltd
Salisbury, Wiltshire
Printed and bound in Great Britain by
Butler & Tanner Ltd
Frome, Somerset

DISTRIBUTORS

USA
  Blackwell Mosby Book Distributors
  11830 Westline Industrial Drive
  St Louis, Missouri 63141

Canada
  Blackwell Mosby Book Distributors
  120 Melford Drive, Scarborough
  Ontario, M1B 2X4

Australia
  Blackwell Scientific Book Distributors
  31 Advantage Road, Highett
  Victoria 3190

British Library
Cataloguing in Publication Data

Roitt, Ivan M.
  Essential immunology.—5th ed.
  1. Immunology
  I. Title
  616.07'9   QR181

  ISBN 0-632-01239-0

Contents

Preface

In the four years since the appearance of the last edition, immunologists have shown little restraint in their appetite for new discoveries. Accordingly, several major changes and additions have been necessary. Many new diagrams are included and many others revised. The section on idiotype networks and the opportunities they afford for intervention is considerably extended. There is increased emphasis on the role of growth factors, interleukins, etc. Attention is drawn to the increased complexity of HLA-D loci and newer work on the structures of class I and II major histocompatibility molecules and their biological roles. I have expanded the section on monoclonal antibodies and their applications including the detection of human T-cell markers. The exciting developments in our belated understanding of the nature of the T-cell receptor are discussed, illustrating the important influence which molecular biological techniques are having on immunology. This includes our further awareness of the mechanisms generating immunoglobulin diversity and class-switching.

Additions to the subject of microbial immunity have made it more convenient to split the chapter into two; in the second I have expanded the discussion of modern vaccine development and inevitably included an account of acquired immunodeficiency syndrome (AIDS), the disease which has done more to educate the public about modern immunology than any other! The increased importance of the novel immunosuppressive drug, Cyclosporin A, is acknowledged, while recent technical developments such as Western ('immuno-') blotting and the use of phycoerythrins for double immunofluorescent staining are introduced. I have amplified the discussion of heritable factors in atopic allergy and of mast cell degranulation and the mediators this gives rise to. Factors underlying the development of autoimmunity are re-analyzed and consideration given to the roles of derepression of genes encoding class II MHC molecules and the controversial contrasuppressor cells. The increasing importance of autoimmunity to hormone receptors is documented and the contribution of thyroid growth antibodies to the spectrum of thyroid autoimmune disease given some prominence.

I finish with the fond hope that the reader will find immunology both enjoyable and exciting.

I believe the appearance of the book has been made more attractive by updating the printing format, introducing colour into the diagrams and adding more colour plates.

Acknowledgements

First edition

While not wishing to saddle my colleagues with responsibility for some of the wilder views expressed in this book it would be ungrateful of me not to acknowledge with pleasure the helpful discussions I have had with Jonathan Brostoff, George Dick, Deborah Doniach, Frank Hay, Leslie Hudson, Gerald Jones and John Playfair. I would like to express my appreciation to my secretary, Gladys Stead, who helped to prepare and assemble the manuscript with her usual impeccable expertise and who always encouraged me when my authorship seemed to be faltering. I also wish to acknowledge my debt to Valerie Petts for her excellent help with the photographs. My thanks also to the many people who supplied material for the illustrations; they are acknowledged at the appropriate place in the text. In particular, Bill Weigle kindly let me have unpublished information. Finally let me say that the pain of converting blank paper to written manuscript at home was made bearable by the loving support and understanding of my wife and family.

Second edition

The necessity for a second edition has been dictated by the breakneck increase in immunological knowledge since this book was first written—clearly the subject has too many adherents! My colleagues will know how much I have appreciated their invaluable discussions; particularly I must mention Ita Askonas, Jonathan Brostoff, Deborah Doniach, Arnold Greenberg, Hilliard Festenstein, Frank Hay, M. Hobart, Leslie Hudson, D. L. Brown, John Playfair and Mac Turner. Once again I would have been lost without the admirable help of my secretary, Gladys Stead. Even the publishers have been nice!

Third edition

The indecent speed at which we lurch forward has necessitated radical revision of many sections in this new edition. The anatomical basis of the immune response, immunity to infection and the biological significance of the major histocompatibility complex have all been given fuller treatment. A summary has been added to the end of each chapter which should be a help to those poor souls for whom circumstances make revision essential. The index has received serious attention and I hope it will be of greater value. I am most grateful to the many colleagues whose wisdom I have sought: Franco Bottazzo, Jonathan Brostoff, Peter Campbell, Deborah Doniach, Hilliard Festenstein, Peter Gould, Frank Hay, Peter Lachman, Ian McConnell, John Playfair and Martin Raff. Finally, my thanks are due to Miss Christine Meats for her most able and cheerful secretarial assistance.

Fourth edition

I am indebted for their invaluable knowledge and wisdom to my colleagues, Franco Bottazzo, Jonathan Brostoff, Anne Cooke, Deborah Doniach, Frank Hay, Peter Lydyard, Ian McConnell, Philip Penfold and John Playfair. As ever, my gratitude is due to Christine Meats for her help with secretarial and administrative matters.

Fifth edition

It is a pleasure to acknowledge my gratitude to R. Batchelor, G. F. Bottazzo, J. Brostoff, A. Cooke, D. Doniach, F. C. Hay, P. M. Lydyard, D. K. Male and J. H. L. Playfair for invaluable discussions, and Rochelle and Kurt Hirschhorn for sending a manuscript of their review on immunodeficiency. I am indebted also to my co-editors, D. K. Male and J. Brostoff, the publishers Gower Medical Publishing Ltd and the following individuals for permission to utilize or modify their Figures which will be appearing in *Immunology Illustrated* and a *Slide Atlas of Immunology*: D. K. Male and D. L. Brown for Figs. 6.24 and 6.26, G. Rook for Figs. 7.7, 7.11 and 7.15, J. Taverne for Figs. 7.13, 7.18, 7.20 and Table 7.3, J. Brostoff and T. Hall for Figs. 9.7 and 9.8, F. C. Hay for Fig. 9.17 and M. Owen and M. Crumpton for Fig. 10.3. Figure 7.1 owes much to John Playfair's *Immunology at a Glance*, while Fig. 9.12 is reproduced by courtesy of Anne Cooke.

Miss Alison Richards of Blackwell Scientific Publications has been outstanding and it was a pleasure to work with her. John Robson and his colleagues have greatly improved the appearance of the book. I am particularly grateful to my secretary, Christine Meats, for her unstinting help.

1 Introduction

The essential function of the immune system is defence against infection. Babies born with a defect in a critical part of this system suffer continued infections and in many cases may die if recourse to advanced medical technology is not available. Lower animal forms possess so-called *innate* or *non-specific* immune mechanisms such as phagocytosis of bacteria by specialized cells. Additionally, higher animals have evolved an *adaptive* or *acquired immune response* which provides a flexible, *specific* and more effective reaction to different infections.

At the heart of the adaptive immune response lie three important features, memory, specificity and the recognition of 'non-self'. Our experience of the subsequent protection (*immunity*) afforded by exposure to many infectious illnesses can in fact lead us to this view.

We rarely suffer twice from such diseases as measles, mumps, chicken-pox, whooping cough and so forth. The first contact with an infectious organism clearly imprints some information, imparts some *memory*, so that the body is effectively prepared to repel any later invasion by that organism. This protection is provided by the adaptive immune response evoked as a reaction to the infectious agent behaving as an antigen (figure 1.1). One of the agents of the immune response is antibody which combines with antigen to cause its elimination.

By following the production of antibody on the first and second contacts with antigen we can see the basis for the development of immunity. For example, when we inject a bacterial product such as staphylococcal toxoid into a rabbit, several days elapse before antibodies can be detected in the blood; these reach a peak and then fall (figure 1.2). If we now allow the animal to rest and then give a second injection of toxoid, the course of events is dramatically altered. Within two to three days the antibody level in the blood rises steeply to reach much higher values than were observed in the *primary response*. This *secondary response* then is characterized by a more rapid and more abundant production of antibody resulting from the 'tuning up' or priming of the

1

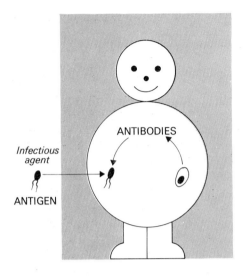

Figure 1.1. Antibodies (*anti*-foreign *bodies*) are produced by host white cells on contact with the invading micro-organism which is acting as an antigen (i.e. *gen*erates *anti*bodies). The individual may then be immune to further attacks.

antibody-forming system to provide a population of memory cells after first exposure to antigen.

Vaccination utilizes this principle by employing a relatively harmless form of the antigen (e.g. a killed virus) as the primary stimulus to imprint 'memory'. The body's defences are thereby alerted and any subsequent contact with the virulent form of the organism will lead to a secondary response with an early and explosive production of antibody which will usually prevent the infection from taking hold.

Specificity was mentioned earlier as a fundamental feature of the adaptive immunological response. The establishment of memory or immunity by one organism does not confer protection against another unrelated organism. After an attack of measles we are immune to further infection but are susceptible to other agents such as the polio or mumps

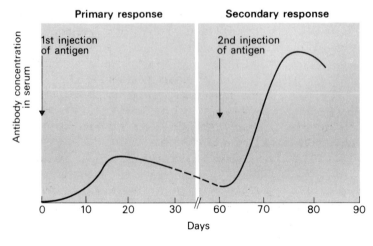

Figure 1.2. *Primary and secondary response.* A rabbit is injected on two separate occasions with staphylococcal toxoid. The antibody response on the second contact with antigen is more rapid and more intense (see also figure 4.4).

viruses. The body can, in fact, differentiate specifically between the two organisms.

This ability to recognize one antigen and distinguish it from another goes even further. The individual must also recognize what is foreign, i.e. what is '*non-self*'. The failure to discriminate between 'self' and 'non-self' could lead to the synthesis of antibodies directed against components of the subject's own body (*autoantibodies*) which in principle could prove to be highly embarrassing. On purely theoretical grounds it seemed to Burnet and Fenner that the body must develop some mechanism whereby 'self' and 'non-self' could be distinguished, and they postulated that those circulating body components which were able to reach the developing lymphoid system in the perinatal period could in some way be 'learnt' as 'self'. A permanent unresponsiveness or tolerance would then be created so that as immunological maturity was reached there would normally be an inability to respond to 'self' components. As we shall see later, these predictions have been amply verified.

The non-specific immunity mechanisms, such as the uptake of bacteria by phagocytic cells which we mentioned earlier, are not heightened by subsequent infections and in this respect differ fundamentally from the adaptive immune response. Clearly this has evolved to provide more effective defence in that the small fraction of immunological cells, which are capable of recognizing the particular agents infecting the body at any one time, increase in number and synthesize antibodies which greatly speed up the disposal of these organisms by facilitating their adherence to phagocytic cells (see chapter 7). In other words, the specific adaptive immune response operates to a considerable extent by increasing the efficiency of the non-specific immunity systems.

Some historical perspectives

Space does not allow more than a cursory survey of some of the outstanding contributions to the early development of immunology.

India and China (Ancient times)—Practice of 'variolation' in which protection against smallpox was obtained by inoculating live organisms from disease pustules (dangerous!).

Jenner (1798)—Protective effect of vaccination with non-virulent cowpox against smallpox infection (noting the pretty pox-free skin of the milkmaids).

Pasteur (1881)—Vaccine for anthrax using attenuated organisms.

Metchnikoff (1883)—Role of phagocytes in immunity.

von Behring (1890)—Recognized antibodies in serum to diphtheria toxin.

Denys & Leclef (1895)—Phagocytosis greatly enhanced by immunization—innate response amplified by adaptive.

Ehrlich (1897)—Side-chain receptor theory of antibody synthesis.

Bordet (1899)—Lysis of cells by antibody requires co-operation of serum factors now collectively termed complement.

Landsteiner (1900)—Human ABO groups and natural iso-haemagglutinins.

Richet & Portier (1902)—Anaphylaxis (opposite of prophylaxis).

Wright (1903)—Relation of opsonic activity to phago-cytosis. (Basis for Sir Colenso Ridgeon's assertion in Shaw's *The Doctor's Dilemma* that vaccines stimulate antibodies (opsonins) which 'butter' the germs for ingestion by phago-cytes, in contrast with 'B.B.'s' resonant belief that any anti-toxin would non-specifically 'stimulate the phagocytes'.)

von Pirquet & Schick (1905)—Description of serum sick-ness following injection of foreign serum.

von Pirquet (1906)—Relation of immunity and hypersensi-tivity.

Fleming (1922)—Lysozyme.

Zinsser (1925)—Contrast between immediate and delayed-type hypersensitivity.

Heidelberger & Kendall (1930–35)—Quantitative precipi-tin studies on antigen–antibody interactions.

Let us examine the work of Heidelberger and Kendall and its implications in more detail and with some benefit.

The classical precipitin reaction

When an antigen solution is mixed in correct proportions with a potent antiserum, a precipitate is formed. Quantitative analysis of this interaction by the method shown in figure 1.3 gives both the antibody content of the immune serum and also an indication of the valency of the antigen, i.e. the effec-tive number of combining sites. This can vary enormously depending on the antigen, its size, and the species making the antibody. With rabbit antisera, ovalbumin may have a valency of 10 and human thyroglobulin as many as 40 com-bining sites on its surface. By splitting antigens into large fragments with proteolytic enzymes it has become clear that the separate combining areas on the surface of a given protein (called antigenic *determinants* or *epitopes*) are by no means identical.

It will be noted from the precipitin curve in figure 1.3 that as more and more antigen is added, an optimum is reached after which consistently less precipitate is formed. At this stage the supernatant can be shown to contain soluble com-

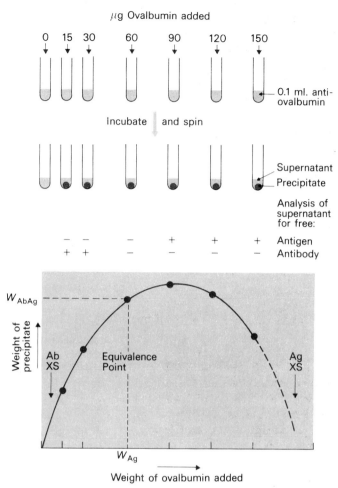

μg Ovalbumin added

0 15 30   60   90   120   150

Incubate | and spin

0.1 ml. anti-ovalbumin

Supernatant
Precipitate

Analysis of
supernatant
for free:

−	−		−	+	+	+	Antigen
+	+		−	−	−	−	Antibody

W_{AbAg}

Weight of precipitate

Ab
XS

Equivalence
Point

Ag
XS

W_{Ag}

Weight of ovalbumin added

Figure 1.3. Quantitative precipitin reaction between rabbit anti-ovalbumin and ovalbumin (after Heidelberger & Kendall). Increasing amounts of ovalbumin are added to a constant volume of the antiserum placed in a number of tubes. After incubation the precipitates formed are spun down and weighed. Each supernatant is split into two halves: by adding antigen to one and antigen to the other, the presence of reactive antibody or antigen respectively can be demonstrated. The antibody content of the serum can be calculated from the equivalence point where no antigen or antibody is present in the supernatant. All the antigen added is therefore complexed in the precipitate with all the antibody available and the antibody content in 0.1 ml of serum would therefore be given by $(W_{AgAb}-W_{Ag})$. Analysis of the precipitate formed in antibody excess (AbXS), where the antigen-combining sites are largely saturated, gives a measure of the molar ratio of antibody to antigen in the complex and hence an estimate of the antigen valency.

plexes of antigen (Ag) and antibody (Ab), many of composition Ag_4Ab_3, Ag_3Ab_2 and Ag_2Ab. In extreme antigen excess (AgXS, figure 1.3) ultracentrifugal analysis reveals the complexes to be mainly of the form Ag_2Ab, suggesting that the rabbit antibodies studied are bivalent (figure 1.4; see also figures 2.5 and 2.6). Between these extremes the cross-linking of antigen and antibody will generally give rise to

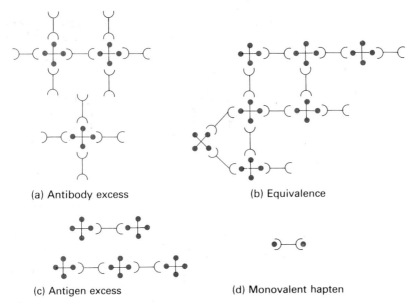

(a) Antibody excess

(b) Equivalence

(c) Antigen excess

(d) Monovalent hapten

Figure 1.4. Diagrammatic representation of complexes formed between a hypothetical tetravalent antigen ( ) and bivalent antibody ()──() mixed in different proportions. In practice, the antigen valencies are unlikely to lie in the same plane or to be formed by identical determinants as suggested in the figure.

(a) In extreme antibody excess, the antigen valencies are saturated and the molar ratio Ab:Ag approximates to the valency of the antigen.

(b) At equivalence, large lattices are formed which aggregate to form a typical immune precipitate. This secondary aggregation, and hence precipitation tends to be inhibited by high salt concentration.

(c) In extreme antigen excess where the two valencies of each antibody molecule become rapidly saturated, the complex Ag_2Ab tends to predominate.

(d) A monovalent hapten binds but is unable to cross-link antibody molecules.

three-dimensional lattice structures, as suggested by Marrack, which coalesce to form large precipitating aggregates.

The basis of specificity

Much of our understanding of the factors governing antigen specificity has come from the studies of Landsteiner and of Pauling and their colleagues on the interaction of antibody with small chemically defined groupings termed *haptens*, a typical example being *m*-aminobenzene sulphonate (figure 1.5). Whereas an antigen will both evoke antibody formation and combine with the resulting antibody, *a hapten is defined as a small molecule which by itself cannot stimulate antibody synthesis but will combine with antibody once formed.*

The problem of how to produce these antibodies was solved by injecting the haptens coupled to proteins which

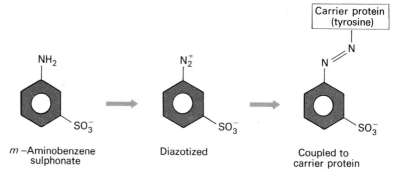

Figure 1.5. Coupling of hapten to carrier protein by diazotization to make it antigenic.

acted as 'carriers' (figure 1.5). It then became possible to relate variations in the chemical structure of a hapten to its ability to bind to a given antibody. In one experiment, antibodies raised to *m*-aminobenzene sulphonate were tested for their ability to combine with *ortho, meta* and *para* isomers of the hapten and related molecules in which the sulphonate group was substituted by arsonate or carboxylate (table 1.1). The hapten with the sulphonate group in the *ortho* position combines somewhat less well with the antibody than the original *meta* isomer, but the *para*-substituted compound (chemically similar to the *ortho*) shows very poor reactivity. The substitution of arsonate for sulphonate leads to weaker combination with the antibody; both groups are negatively charged and have a tetrahedral structure but the arsonate group is larger in size and has an extra H atom. The aminobenzoates in which the sulphonate is substituted by the negatively charged but planar carboxylate group show even less affinity for the antibody. It would appear that the overall *configuration* of the hapten is even more important than its *chemical* nature, i.e. the hapten is recognized by the overall three-dimensional shape of its outer electron cloud as distinct from its chemical reactivity. The production of antibodies against such strange moieties as benzene sulphonate and arsonate becomes more comprehensible if they are thought to be directed against a particular electron-cloud shape rather than a specific chemical structure. This view is consistent with the nature of antigen–antibody binding which is known not to involve covalent linkages.

THE FORCES BINDING ANTIGEN TO ANTIBODY

It should be stressed immediately that the forces which hold antigen and antibody together are in essence no different from the so-called 'non-specific' protein–protein inter-

Table 1.1. Effect of variations in hapten structure on strength of binding to antibodies raised against *m*-aminobenzene sulphonate.

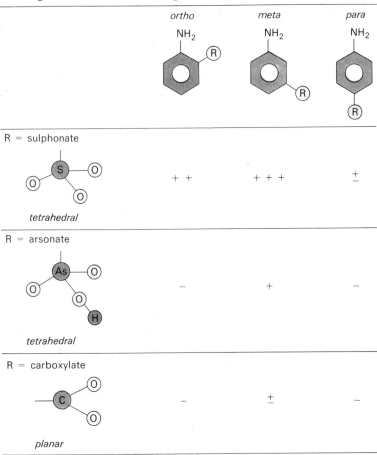

	ortho	*meta*	*para*
R = sulphonate (tetrahedral)	+ +	+ + +	±
R = arsonate (tetrahedral)	−	+	−
R = carboxylate (planar)	−	±	−

(from Landsteiner K. & van der Scheer J. (1936) *J.Exp.Med.* **63**, 325).

actions which occur between any two unrelated proteins (or other macromolecules) as, for example, human serum albumin and human transferrin. These intermolecular forces may be classified under four headings:

(a) *Electrostatic*

These are due to the attraction between oppositely charged ionic groups on the two protein side-chains as, for example, an ionized amino group (NH_3^+) on a lysine of one protein and an ionized carboxyl group ($-COO^-$) of, say, aspartate on the other (figure 1.6a). The force of attraction (F) is inversely proportional to the square of the distance (d) between the charges, i.e.

$$F \propto 1/d^2$$

Thus as the charges come closer together, the attractive force increases considerably: if we halve the distance apart, we quadruple the attraction. Dipoles on antigen and antibody can also attract each other. In addition, electrostatic forces may be generated by charge transfer reactions between antibody and antigen; for example, an electron-donating protein residue such as tryptophan could part with an electron to a group such as dinitrophenyl which is electron-accepting, thereby creating an effective $+1$ charge on the antibody and -1 on the antigen.

(b) *Hydrogen bonding*

The formation of the relatively weak and reversible hydrogen bridges between hydrophilic groups such as $\cdot OH$, $\cdot NH_2$ and $\cdot COOH$ depends very much upon the close approach of the two molecules carrying these groups (figure 1.6b).

(c) *Hydrophobic*

In the same way that oil droplets in water merge to form a single large drop, so non-polar, hydrophobic groups such as the side-chains of valine, leucine and phenylalanine, tend to associate in an aqueous environment. The driving force for this hydrophobic bonding derives from the fact that water in contact with hydrophobic molecules, with which it cannot H-bond, will associate with other water molecules but the number of configurations which allow H-bonds to form will not be as great as that occurring when they are surrounded completely by other water molecules, i.e. the entropy is lower. The greater the area of contact between water and hydrophobic surfaces, the lower the entropy and the higher the energy state. Thus if hydrophobic groups on two proteins come together so as to exclude water molecules between them, the net surface in contact with water is reduced (figure 1.6c) and the proteins take up a lower energy state than when they are separated (in other words, there is a force of attraction between them). It has been estimated that hydrophobic forces may contribute up to 50% of the total strength of the antigen–antibody bond.

(d) *Van der Waals*

These are the forces between molecules which depend upon interaction between the external 'electron clouds'. The deviation of gaseous molecules of say nitrogen or hydrogen from 'ideal' behaviour according to the kinetic theory is attributable to the Van der Waals attractions between them. The nature of this interaction is difficult to describe in non-

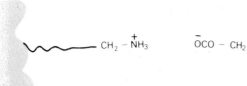

Lysine
side – chain

Aspartate
side – chain

(a)

CH_2 —O—H ---- O = C
NH
CH

(b)

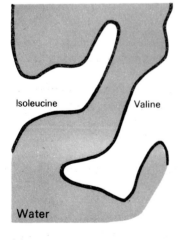

Isoleucine   Valine

Water

Isoleucine   Valine

Water

(c)

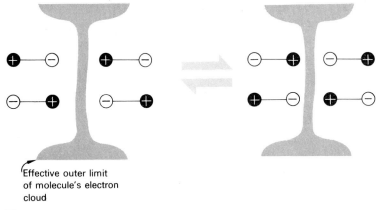

Effective outer limit
of molecule's electron
cloud

(d)

Figure 1.6. Protein–protein interactions.

(a) Coulombic attraction between oppositely charged ionic groupings.

(b) Hydrogen bonding between two proteins: the example shows an H-bond between a serine or threonine side-chain on one protein and a peptide carbonyl group on the other.

(c) Hydrophobic bonding: the region in which the water molecules are in contact with the hydrophobic groups (indicated by the thickened line) is considerably reduced when the hydrophobic groups on two proteins are in contact with each other and the lower free-energy of this system makes this a more probable state than separation of the hydrophobic groups.

(d) Van der Waals forces: the interaction between the electrons in the external orbitals of two different macromolecules may be envisaged (for simplicity!) as the attraction between induced oscillating dipoles in the two electron clouds.

mathematical terms but it has been likened to a temporary perturbation of electrons in one molecule effectively forming a dipole which induces a dipolar perturbation in the other molecule, the two dipoles then having a force of attraction between them; as the displaced electrons swing back through the equilibrium position and beyond, the dipoles oscillate (figure 1.6d). The force of attraction is inversely proportional to the seventh power of the distance, i.e.

$$F \propto 1/d^7$$

and as a result this rises very rapidly as the interacting molecules come closer together.

This last point underlines one essential feature common to all four types of force—they depend upon the close approach of both molecules before the forces become of significant magnitude. And this is at the heart of the combination of antigen and antibody. By having *complementary* electron-cloud shapes on the combining site of the antibody and the surface determinant of the antigen, the two molecules can fit snugly together like a lock and key (cf. figure 1.8a). The intermolecular distance becomes very small and the 'non-specific protein interaction forces' are considerably increased; the greater the areas of antigen and antibody which fit together, the greater the force of attraction, particu-

11

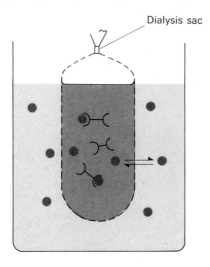

Dialysis sac

Figure 1.7. Antibody affinity determined by studying the equilibrium between antibody (◯—◯) and hapten (●). Within the dialysis sac the hapten is partly in the free form and partly bound to antibody according to the affinity of the antibody. Only hapten can diffuse through the dialysis membrane and the external concentration then will equal the concentration of unbound hapten within the sac. Measurement of total hapten in the dialysis sac then enables the amount bound to antibody to be calculated. By repeating this at different concentrations of hapten, one can calculate the average affinity constant (K) as described in the text. Constant renewal of the external buffer will lead to total dissociation and loss of hapten from inside the dialysis sac showing the reversible nature of the antigen–antibody bond.

larly if there is apposition of opposite charges and hydrophobic groupings.

By contrast, when the electron clouds of the two molecules effectively overlap, powerful repulsive forces are generated (figure 1.8b).

ANTIBODY AFFINITY

The combination of antibody with the surface determinant of an antigen or a monovalent hapten molecule (cf. figure 1.4d) is reversible and the complex may readily dissociate, depending upon the strength of binding. This can be defined through the equilibrium constant (K) of the reaction:

Ab + Hp ⇌ AbHp

(◯—◯) (●) (◯—●)

given by the mass action equation,

$$K = \frac{[AbHp]}{[Ab][Hp]}$$

where [Ab] is the concentration of free antibody combining sites and [Hp] the concentration of free hapten. If the antibody and hapten fit together very closely, the equilibrium will lie well over to the right; we refer to such antibodies which bind strongly to the hapten as *high affinity antibodies*. At a certain *free* hapten concentration $[Hp_c]$ where half of the antibody sites are bound, $[AbHp] = [Ab]$ and $K = 1/[Hp_c]$, i.e. K is equal to the reciprocal of the concentration of free hapten at the equilibrium point where half the antibody sites are in the bound form. In other words, when an antibody has a high affinity constant and binds hapten

12

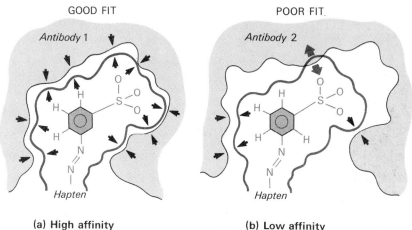

GOOD FIT

Antibody 1

Hapten

(a) High affinity

POOR FIT

Antibody 2

Hapten

(b) Low affinity

Figure 1.8. High and low affinity antibodies present in the same antiserum raised against the hapten *m*-aminobenzene sulphonate coupled to a carrier protein (cf. figure 1.5 and table 1.1). (a) Antibody 1 electron clouds fit closely to those of the hapten (outlined in red) and the strong forces of attraction (➤ ◄) *high affinity* binding. (b) In contrast, Antibody 2 fits very poorly and even overlaps in one site giving rise to a strong repulsion force (◀ ▶) the net effect being weak binding and *low affinity*. Only a portion of the antibody combining site is shown.

strongly, it only needs a low hapten concentration to half-saturate the antibody. Affinity constants, which can be determined by methods such as that shown in figure 1.7, may reach values as high as 10^{11} litres/mol.

Analysis of the binding at different hapten concentrations generally shows a heterogeneity which indicates that most antisera, even those raised against antigens with a simple structure, contain a variety of different antibodies with a range of binding affinities which depend upon the area of contact between the antibody and the antigenic determinant, the closeness of fit, repulsion due to electron cloud overlap (figure 1.8) and the distribution of charged and hydrophobic groups. If we bear in mind that antigen determinants are not two-dimensional as represented in the figures, but have a three-dimensional electron-cloud shape, one can realize that antibodies are confronted with very many different configurations even in a single determinant, depending upon the direction from which the antibody molecule approaches.

AVIDITY AND THE BONUS EFFECT OF
MULTIVALENT BINDING

The strength of the interaction of antibody with a monovalent hapten or a single antigen determinant we have labelled antibody affinity. In most practical situations we are concerned with the interaction of an antiserum with a mul-

Antigen

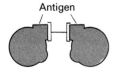 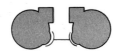 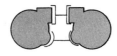

(a) Moderate   (b) Moderate   (c) Very strong

Figure 1.9. The 'bonus' effect of multivalent attachment on binding strength. The force binding the two antigen molecules in (c) with two antibody bridges is often at least 10 times greater than (a + b) where only single antibody molecules provide the link. The effect varies with K values; the weaker the affinity the more the bonus.

tivalent antigen molecule and the term employed to express this binding,

$$nAb + mAg \rightleftharpoons Ab_n Ag_m$$

is *avidity*. The factors which contribute to avidity are complicated. Not only must we contend with the heterogeneity of antibodies in a given serum which are directed against each determinant on the antigen, but we must also recognize that the differing amino acid sequences on different parts of a protein surface, for example, lead to the formation of a number of antigenic patches or determinants on a single molecule, each with its distinct shape and specificity.

The multivalence of most antigens leads to an interesting 'bonus' effect in which the binding of two antigen molecules by antibody is always greater, usually many-fold greater, than the arithmetic sum of the individual antibody links. This is illustrated in figure 1.9. The mechanism of this effect may be interpreted by considering an analogy. Let us fabricate an unheard of disease in which we cannot stop our hands opening and closing continuously. If we now try to hold an object in *one* hand it will fall the moment we open that hand. However, if we use *both* hands to hold the object, provided we open and close our hands at different times, there is much less chance of the object falling. The reversible combination of antigen and antibody is like the opening and closing of the hand; the more valencies holding the antigen the less likely it is to be lost when the complex dissociates at any one binding site (figure 1.10).

SPECIFICITY AND CROSS-REACTIONS

An antiserum raised against a given antigen can cross-react with a partially related antigen which bears one or more identical or similar determinants. In figure 1.11 it can be seen that an antiserum to antigen$_1$ will react less strongly with antigen$_2$ which bears just one identical determinant because only certain of the antibodies in the serum can bind.

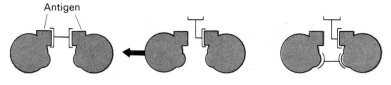

Antigen

(a) Single antibody bridge   (b) Separation   (c) No separation

Figure 1.10. The mechanism of the bonus effect. Each antigen–antibody bond is reversible and with a single antibody bridge between two antigen molecules (a), dissociation of either bond could enable an antigen molecule to 'escape' as in (b). If there are two antibody bridges, even when one dissociates the other prevents the antigen molecule from escaping and holds it in position ready to reform the broken bond.

Antigen$_3$ which possesses a similar but not identical determinant will not fit as well with the antibody and the binding is even weaker. Antigen$_4$ which has no structural similarity at all will not react significantly with the antibody.* Thus, based upon stereochemical considerations, we can see why the avidity of the antiserum for antigens$_{2+3}$ is less than for the homologous antigen, while for the unrelated antigen$_4$ it is negligible. It is in this way that the *specificity* of an antiserum is expressed.

THE ANTIBODY SITE AND ANTIGEN
DETERMINANTS

The forces which bind antigen to antibody are largely similar to those binding enzyme to substrate. The elucidation of the three-dimensional structures of certain enzymes such as lysozyme by X-ray crystallography has shown that the substrate lies within a long cleft in the surface of the molecule. Similar studies on homogeneous antibody preparations indicate that the combining site is of the order of 1.5–2.0 nm long and 1.5 nm wide and may be envisaged as a 'valley' bound on each side by 3 little 'peaks' (cf. figure 2.10).

* If the antigenic determinant is appreciably smaller than the antibody site, there could be a cross-reaction with an unrelated antigen which bound fortuitously to the remainder of the site.

Figure 1.11. Specificity and cross-reaction. The avidity of the serum antibodies ($\vdash$, $\succ\!\!\!-\!\!($) for Ag$_1$ > Ag$_2$ > Ag$_3$ ≫ Ag$_4$ so that the serum shows specificity, particularly for the original antigen.

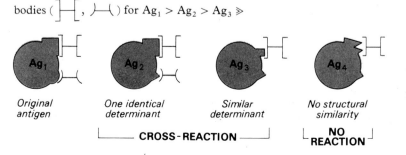

Original antigen	One identical determinant	Similar determinant	No structural similarity

CROSS-REACTION   NO REACTION

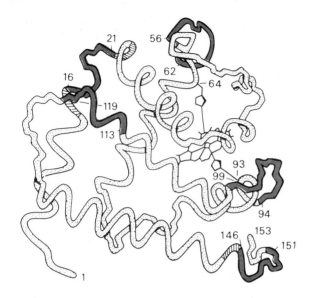

Figure 1.12. The antigenic determinants on a globular protein, myoglobin. The five independent determinants (shown in red) each consist of five to seven amino acid residues, all exposed at the surface of the molecule and localized at the corners that separate the helical region (from Attasi M.Z. (1975) *Immunochemistry* **12**, 423).

These dimensions are consistent with studies using *linear* haptens formed from repeating units of sugar molecules (Kabat) or amino acids (Sela) which have indicated that the site probably accommodates roughly six such units. Of these units, the terminal one usually shows the highest binding energy to the antibody and may be termed the 'immunodominant' group; successive units contribute progressively less to the overall binding.

So far we have discussed the interaction of linear antigens with the antibody combining site. A different situation arises with globular proteins. Studies with synthetic antigens have shown that antibodies are formed against determinants accessible on the surface and not against residues buried within the molecule. This is so with globular proteins such as myoglobin (figure 1.12) and staphylococcal nuclease, where the main antigenic determinants are located on those portions of the surface polypeptide chain which protrude as angular bends capable of lying within an antibody cleft. The linear *sequence* of amino acids in the peptide chain is clearly important for specificity but the overall *conformation* of the peptide makes a very significant contribution to the energy of binding with antibody. Lysozyme provides a case in point: this protein has an intrachain-disulphide bond which forms a loop in the peptide chain. As Arnon has shown, the loop peptide loses its ability to react with antibody when reduced to form a linear chain (figure 1.13) even though the primary amino acid sequence is unchanged.

It is worth emphasizing that our analysis has been concerned with the interaction of an antigenic determinant or a hapten with antibody but several further factors govern the

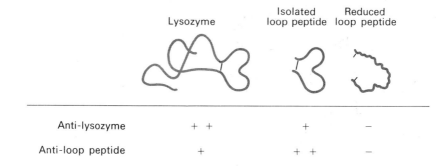

	Lysozyme	Isolated loop peptide	Reduced loop peptide
Anti-lysozyme	+ +	+	−
Anti-loop peptide	+	+ +	−

Figure 1.13. Specificity and three-dimensional configuration in a globular protein, lysozyme. Antibodies to the whole molecule and to the isolated loop peptide do not react with the peptide after reduction of its disulphide bond, showing that the linear reduced peptide has lost the antigenic configuration it had when held as a loop even though the amino acid sequence was unchanged (from Maron E., Shiowa C., Arnon R. & Sela M. (1971) *Biochemistry* **10**, 763).

ability of a given substance to act as an *antigen*, i.e. to stimulate the antigen-reactive cells in the host animal to produce antibody. These include the content of polymeric repeating structures, the rate of catabolism, the size, the degree of 'foreignness'—i.e. dissimilarity from self—and the ability of the body to recognize the substance (see Chapter 3, p. 68).

Summary

The purpose of the immune response is to defend the host against infection. 'Non-specific' immune mechanisms (e.g. phagocytosis) are enhanced by the development of *adaptive* immunity characterized by memory, specificity and the recognition of non-self. The more rapid and intense antibody response which occurs on the second contact with antigen explains the protection afforded by a primary infection against subsequent disease and provides the rationale for the immunological education of the body by vaccination.

Antigens bind to antibodies reversibly by non-covalent molecular interactions including electrostatic, hydrogen-bonding, hydrophobic and Van der Waals forces which become significant when complementarity of shape between antigen and antibody allows them to approach each other closely ('lock and key' fit like enzyme and substrate).

The binding strength of an antibody for a single determinant or hapten is measured by *affinity*. The term *avidity* describes the binding of an antiserum for the whole antigen molecule, this being influenced relative to affinity, by the bonus effect of multivalency. Antibodies discriminate between two antigens, i.e. show *specificity*, by their greater avidity for one rather than the other. Where some determinants (epitopes) on two antigens are identical or similar, they will give cross-reactions directly dependent upon their relative binding strengths to the antibodies.

The antigenic determinant must optimally be capable of lying within the 'hill-bound valley' forming the antibody combining site. With linear antigens, primary structure is crucially important for the formation of a determinant but in the case of globular molecules, tertiary conformation is usually of even greater significance.

Further reading

Original publications

Karush F. (1976) Multivalent binding and functional affinity. In *Contemporary Topics in Molecular Immunology*. F.P. Inman (ed.). Vol. 5, p. 217. Plenum Press, New York. (Bonus effect of multivalency.)

Nisonoff A. & Pressman D. (1957) Closeness of fit and forces involved in the reactions of antibody homologous to the p-(p'azophenylazo)-benzoate ion group. *J. Amer. Chem. Soc.* **79**, 1616.

Poljak R.J. *et al.* (1973) Three-dimensional structure of the Fab' fragment of a human immunoglobulin at 2.8 Å resolution. *Proc. Nat. Acad. Sci.* **70**, 3305.

Richards F.F., Konigsberg W.H. & Rosenstein R.W. (1975) On the specificity of antibodies: biochemical and biophysical evidence indicates the existence of polyfunctional antibody combining regions. *Science* **187**, 130.

Werblin T.P. & Siskind G.W. (1972) Distribution of antibody affinities: technique of measurement. *Immunochemistry* **9**, 987.

General textbooks

Fudenberg H.H., Stites D.P., Caldwell J.L. & Wells J.V. (1978) *Basic and Clinical Immunology*, 2nd edn. Lange Medical Publications, Los Altos, California.

Glynn L.E. & Steward M.W. (eds) (1977) *Immunochemistry: an Advanced Textbook*. John Wiley & Sons, Chichester.

Golub E.S. (1981) *The Cellular Basis of the Immune Response*. Sinauer Associates, Massachusetts.

Humphrey J.H. & White R.G. (1970) *Immunology for Students of Medicine*, 3rd edn. Blackwell Scientific Publications, Oxford. (Dated but scholarly.)

Kabat E.A. (1976) *Structural Concepts in Immunology and Immunochemistry*. Holt, Rinehart & Winston, New York.

McConnell I., Munro A. & Waldmann H. (1981) *The Immune System: a Course on the Molecular and Cellular Basis of Immunity*, 2nd edn. Blackwell Scientific Publications, Oxford. (An excellent text for further study of fundamental immunological principles.)

Nisonoff A. (1982) *Introduction to Molecular Immunology*. Sinauer Associates, Massachusetts.

Playfair J.H.L. (1982) *Immunology at a Glance*, 2nd edn. Blackwell Scientific Publications, Oxford. (Very useful for revision.)

Thaler M.S., Klausner R.D. & Cohen H.J. (1977) *Medical Immunology*. Lippincott, Philadelphia.

Historical

Landsteiner K. (1946) *The Specificity of Serological Reactions.* Harvard University Press (reprinted 1962 by Dover Publications, New York).

Metchnikoff E. (1893) *Comparative Pathology of Inflammation.* Transl. F.A. & E.H. Starling. Kegan Paul, Trench, Trübner & Co., London.

Parish H.J. (1968) *Victory with Vaccines.* Churchill Livingstone, Edinburgh.

Series for the advanced student

* *Advances in Immunology* (Annual). Academic Press, London.

Progress in Allergy. S.Karger, Basle.

Modern Trends in Immunology. Butterworth, London.

* *Immunological Reviews* (ed. G. Moller). Munksgaard, Copenhagen.

Contemporary Topics in Molecular Immunology. Plenum Press, New York.

Contemporary Topics in Immunobiology. Plenum Press, New York.

Protides of the Biological Fluids. Pergamon Press, Oxford.

* In depth treatment

Current information

Current Titles in Immunology, Transplantation & Allergy. MSK Books, London.

Immunology Today. Elsevier Science Publications, Amsterdam. (The immunologist's 'newspaper'.)

Major journals

Nature, Lancet, Science, J.Exp.Med., Immunology, J.Immunology, Clin.Exp.Immunology, Mol.Immunol., Immunopharmacology, Infect & Immunity, Int.Arch.Allergy, Cell.Immunology, European J.Immunology, Scand.J.Immunol., Clin.Immunol. & Immunopath., J.Clin.Immunol., J.Immunogenetics, J.Immunol.Methods, J.Reticuloendoth.Soc., Tissue Antigens, Immunogenetics, Human Immunol., Transplantation, Ann.d'Immunologie, Cancer Immunol.Immunotherapy, J.Allergy Clin.Immunol., Clin.Allergy, Ann.Allergy, J.Clin.Lab.Immunology, Parasitic Immunol.

2

The Immunoglobulins

The association of antibody activity with the classical γ-globulin fraction of serum was shown many years ago by Tiselius and Kabat. They hyperimmunized rabbits with pneumococcal polysaccharide to produce a high concentration of circulating antibody and then examined the effect of absorbing the serum with antigen on the electrophoretic profile. Only the γ-globulin fraction was significantly reduced after removal of antibody (figure 2.1). With the recognition of heterogeneity in the types of molecules which can function as antibodies, it has now become customary to use the general term 'immunoglobulin'. In each species, the immunoglobulin molecules can be subdivided into different classes on the basis of the structure of their 'backbone' (rather than on their specificity for given antigens). Thus, in the human for example, five major structural types or classes can be distinguished: immunoglobulin G (abbreviated to IgG), IgM, IgA, IgD and IgE.

The basic structure of the immunoglobulins

The antibody fraction of serum consists predominantly of one group of proteins with molecular weight around 150,000 (sedimentation coefficient 7S) of which the major component is IgG, and another of molecular weight 900,000 (19S IgM). The IgG antibodies can be split by papain into three fragments (R.R. Porter). Two of these are identical and are able to combine with antigen to form a soluble complex which will not precipitate; these are therefore univalent antibody fragments and are given the nomenclature Fab ('fragment

Figure 2.1. Association of antibody activity with γ-globulin serum fraction. Hyperimmune serum is separated into major fractions by electrophoresis before (a) and after (b) absorption with antigen. Only the γ-globulin fraction is reduced.

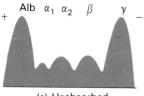

(a) Unabsorbed

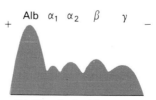

(b) Absorbed with antigen

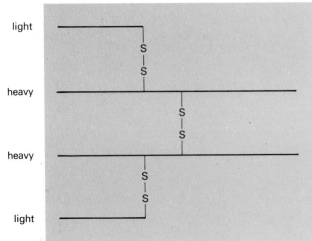

N–terminal   C–terminal

light

heavy

heavy

light

Figure 2.2. Antibody model proposed by R.R. Porter with two heavy and two light polypeptide chains held by interchain disulphide bonds. In the diagram the amino-terminal residue is on the left for each chain.

antigen binding'). The third fragment has no power to combine with antigen and is termed Fc ('fragment crystallizable' obtainable in crystalline form). Another proteolytic enzyme, pepsin, cleaves the Fc part from the remainder of the antibody molecule, leaving a large fragment (5S) which can still precipitate with antigen and is formulated as F(ab')$_2$ since it is clearly still divalent.

Antibodies can also be broken down into their constituent peptide chains. First the disulphide bonds linking different chains must be broken by reduction with *excess* of a sulphydryl reagent. The reduced molecule still has a sedimentation coefficient of 7S because the chains are held together by non-covalent forces but they can be separated by lowering the pH into two sizes of peptide chain termed *light* and *heavy chains* (G.M. Edelman).

On the basis of these findings Porter put forward a symmetrical four-peptide model for antibody consisting of two heavy and two light chains linked together by interchain disulphide bonds (figure 2.2). The formation of the various fragments by proteolysis and reduction is represented in figure 2.3.

Purified IgG antibodies when visualized in the electron microscope by negative staining can be seen to be Y-shaped molecules whose arms can swing out to an angle of 180° through the papain and pepsin sensitive region acting as a hinge (figure 2.4). Amino acid analysis of the hinge region has revealed an unusual feature—a large number of proline residues; because of its structure, proline prevents the peptide chain assuming α-helix conformation, and so this stretch of the chain is extended and accessible to proteolytic enzymes.

Elegant confirmation of the correctness of these general

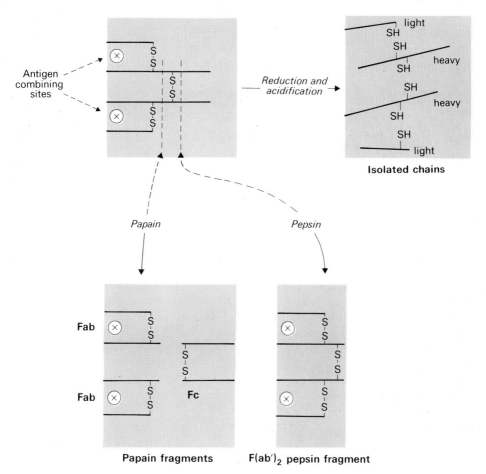

Reduction and acidification →

Isolated chains

Papain

Pepsin

Fab

Fab Fc

Papain fragments

F(ab')₂ pepsin fragment

Figure 2.3. Degradation of immuno-globulin to constituent peptide chains and to proteolytic fragments showing divalence of pepsin F(ab')₂ and univalence of the papain Fab. After pepsin digestion the pFc′

fragment representing the C-terminal half of the Fc region is formed. The portion of the heavy chain in the Fab fragment is given the symbol Fd.

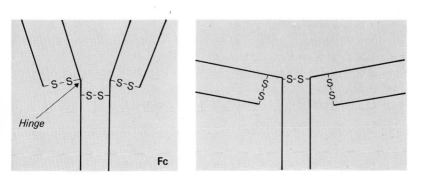

Hinge

Fc

Figure 2.4. Illustrating the flexibility of the immunoglobulin molecule at the hinge

region. Compare with conformation of immunoglobulin molecules in figure 2.5.

23

views on the structure of the antibody molecule has come from studies using a divalent hapten, bis-N-dinitrophenyl (DNP)-octamethylene-diamine:

$$NO_2-\langle\bigcirc\rangle-NH-CH_2CH_2CH_2CH_2CH_2CH_2CH_2CH_2-NH-\langle\bigcirc\rangle-NO_2$$
$$\qquad\quad NO_2 \qquad\qquad\qquad\qquad\qquad\qquad\qquad\qquad NO_2$$

where the two haptenic DNP groups are far enough apart not to interfere with each other's combination with antibody. When mixed with purified IgG antibody to DNP, the divalent hapten brings the antigen-combining sites on two different antibodies together end to end; when viewed by negative staining in the electron microscope a series of geometric forms are observed which represent the different structures to be expected if a Y-shaped hinged molecule with a combining site at the end of each of the two arms of the Y were to complex with this divalent hapten. Triangular trimers, square tetramers and pentagonal pentamers may be readily discerned (figure 2.5). The way in which these polymeric forms arise is indicated in figure 2.6. The position of the Fc fragment and its lack of involvement in the combination with antigen are apparent from the shape of the polymers formed using the pepsin $F(ab')_2$ fragment (figure 2.5e).

Variations in structure of the immunoglobulins

Any attempt to analyse the amino acid structure of the immunoglobulins in normal serum is bedevilled by the incredible number of different molecules present. This heterogeneity may be inferred from analysis by immuno-electrophoresis, the principle of which is explained in figure 2.7. It is evident that the immunoglobulins occur in different classes of molecules and also that they have a very wide range of electrophoretic mobilities within each class, ranging in the case of IgG, from slow γ- to α_2-globulin (figure 2.8). This range of mobilities is due to different net charges on the different immunoglobulin molecules and is indicative of variations in amino acid structure (e.g. replacement of a neutral residue such as valine with a basic amino acid like lysine will tend to increase the net charge by $+ 1$). Even 'purified' antibodies directed against a simple hapten may show a wide spectrum of electrophoretic mobilities since, as mentioned in the previous chapter, they represent a variety of antibodies of varying degrees of fit for various shapes on the hapten surface.

The answer to this seemingly insoluble problem of analysing amino acid structure has come from study of the *myeloma proteins*. In the human disease known as multiple myeloma, one cell making one particular individual immunoglobulin

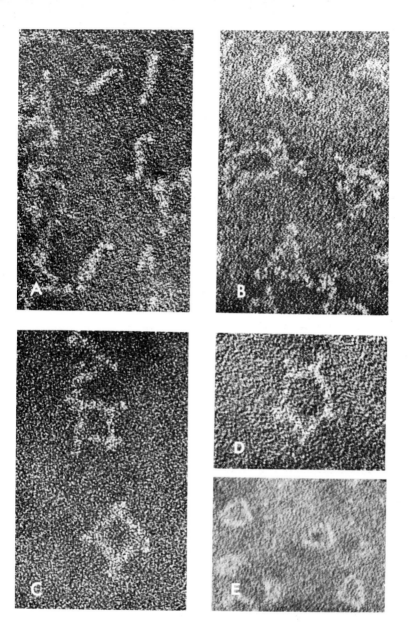

Figure 2.5. (a)–(d) Electron micrograph (× 1,000,000) of complexes formed on mixing the divalent DNP hapten with rabbit anti-DNP antibodies. The 'negative stain' phosphotungstic acid is an electron-dense solution which penetrates in the spaces between the protein molecules. Thus the protein stands out as a 'light' structure in the electron beam. The hapten links together the Y-shaped antibody molecules to form (a) dimers, (b) trimers, (c) tetramers and (d) pentamers (cf. figure 2.6). The flexibility of the molecule at the hinge region is evident from the variation in angle of the arms of the 'Y'.

(e) As in (b); trimers formed using the $F(ab')_2$ antibody fragment from which the Fc structures have been digested by pepsin (× 500,000). The trimers can be seen to lack the Fc projections at each corner evident in (b). (After Valentine R.C. & Green N.M. (1967) *J.mol.Biol.* **27**, 615; courtesy of Dr Green and with the permission of Academic Press, New York.)

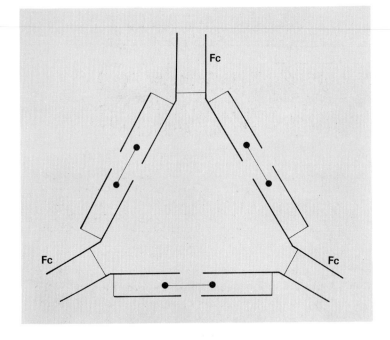

Figure 2.6. Three DNP antibody molecules held together as a trimer by the divalent hapten (●——●). Compare figure 2.5b. When the Fc fragments are first removed by pepsin, the corner pieces are no longer visible (figure 2.5e).

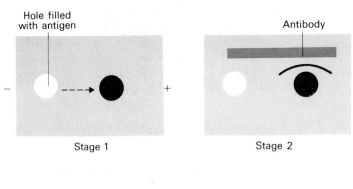

Hole filled with antigen

Antibody

Stage 1

Stage 2

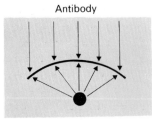

Antibody

Antigen

Figure 2.7. The principle of immuno-electrophoresis. *Stage 1 :* Electrophoresis of antigen in agar gel. Antigen migrates to hypothetical position shown. *Stage 2 :* Current stopped. Trough cut in agar and filled with antibody. Precipitin arc formed.

Because antigen theoretically at a point source diffuses radially and antibody from the trough diffuses with a plane front, they meet in optimal proportions for precipitation along an arc. The arc is closest to the trough at the point where antigen is in highest concentration.

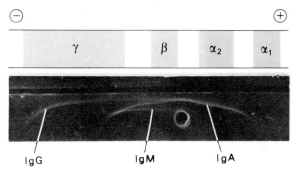

$\ominus$ $\oplus$

γ   β   α₂   α₁

IgG   IgM   IgA

Figure 2.8. Major human immunoglobulin classes demonstrated by immunoelectrophoretic analysis of human serum using a rabbit antiserum in the trough. The position of the main electrophoretic globulin fractions is indicated. Three of the five major immunoglobulin classes can be recognized: immunoglobulin G (IgG), immunoglobulin A (IgA) and immunoglobulin M (IgM). The IgG precipitin arc extends from the γ region well into the α_2-globulin mobility range.

divides over and over again in the uncontrolled way a cancer cell does, without regard for the overall requirement of the host. The patient then possesses enormous numbers of identical cells derived as a clone from the original cell and they all synthesize the same immunoglobulin—the myeloma or M-protein—which appears in the serum, sometimes in very high concentrations. By purification of the myeloma protein we can obtain a preparation of an immunoglobulin having a unique structure. These myeloma proteins have been studied in two ways: amino acid analysis and the recognition of major characteristic groups on the molecules using specific antibodies produced in experimental animals.

STRUCTURAL VARIATION IN RELATION TO
ANTIBODY SPECIFICITY

Amino acid analysis of a number of purified myeloma proteins has revealed that, within a given major immunoglobulin class such as IgG, the N-terminal portions of both heavy and light chains show quite considerable variations whereas the remaining parts of the chains are relatively constant in structure (figure 2.9). Each variable region has a basic overall amino acid structure which is common to a number of antibodies with differing specificities. They are said to belong to the same *subgroup* and to give an example, the heavy chain variable regions in a normal individual form three such subgroups (table 2.4, p. 42). This subgroup 'framework' structure cannot be related to antibody specificity since so many different antibodies belong to the same subgroup. What is striking, however, is the hypervariability in amino acid residues at certain positions in the peptide chain. For example, when 13 myeloma light chains were sequenced, 8 different amino acids were found at residue number 93, 6 at residue 94

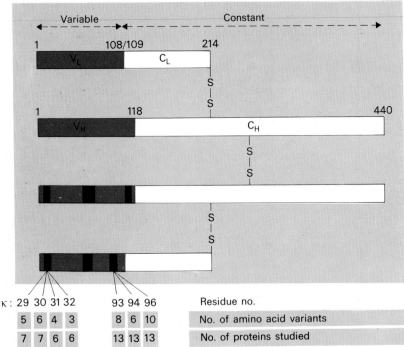

κ : 29 30 31 32	93 94 96	Residue no.		
5 6 4 3	8 6 10	No. of amino acid variants		
7 7 6 6	13 13 13	No. of proteins studied		

Figure 2.9. Showing the regions of IgG with relatively variable (▓) and constant (□) amino acid composition. The terms 'V region' and 'C region' are used to designate the variable and constant regions respectively, 'V$_L$' and 'C$_L$' are generic terms for these regions on the light chain and 'V$_H$' and 'C$_H$' specify variable and constant regions on the heavy chain. The amino acid residues are numbered starting from the N-terminal end. C$_L$ starts at residue 108 for κ-types and 109 for λ (see also figure 2.13). Examples are given of the degree of variation in amino acid residues seen in the κ light chain hypervariable regions (▓).

and 10 at residue 96 (figure 2.9). The most attractive view, supported by the latest X-ray analysis, is that these 'hot spots', three on the light and three on the heavy chain, lie relatively close to each other as peptide loops to form the antigen binding site (figures 2.10 and 2.15), their heterogeneity ensuring diversity in combining specificities through variation in the shape and nature of the surface they create (cf. p. 13). Thus each hypervariable region may be looked upon as an independent structure contributing to the complementarity of the binding site for antigen and perhaps one can speak of complementarity determinants.

That these variable regions of heavy and light chains both contribute to antibody specificity is suggested by experiments in which isolated chains were examined for their antigen combining power. In general, varying degrees of residual activity were associated with the heavy chains but relatively little with the light chains; on recombination, however, there was always a significant increase in antigen-binding capacity.

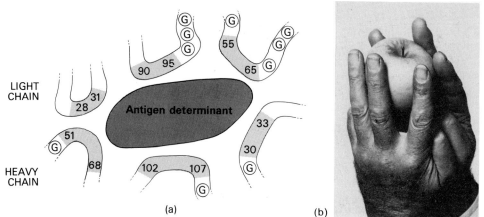

Figure 2.10. (a) Two-dimensional representation of an antigen binding site formed by spatial apposition of peptide loops containing the hypervariable regions (hot spots: 🔳) on light and heavy chains. Numbers refer to amino acid residues. Glycine residues (Ⓖ) are invariably present at the positions indicated whatever the specificity or animal species of the immunoglobulin. They are of importance in allowing peptide chains to fold back and form β-pleated sheet structures which enable the hypervariable regions to lie close to each other (figure 2.15). Wu and Kabat have suggested that the flexibility of bond angle in this amino acid is essential for the effective formation of a binding site. On this basis the greater frequency of invariant glycines on the light chain might indicate that coarse specificity for antigen binding was provided by the heavy chain and 'fine tuning' by the light chain. Through binding to different combinations of hypervariable regions and to different residues within each of these regions, each antibody molecule can form a complex with a variety of antigenic determinants (with a comparable variety of affinities). (b) A simulated combining site formed by apposing the three middle fingers of each hand, each finger representing a hypervariable loop. (Photograph by B.N.A. Rice; inspired by A. Munro!)

More direct attempts to identify the amino acid residues associated with the combining site have been made by Singer and others using a technique called 'affinity-labelling'. In this, a hapten is equipped with a chemically reactive side-chain which will form covalent links with adjacent amino acids after combination of the hapten with antibody, so labelling residues in the neighbourhood of the combining site. A modification introduced by Porter and his colleagues utilizes a 'flick-knife' principle. The hapten with an azide side-chain combines with its antibody and is then illuminated with ultraviolet light; this converts the azide to the reactive nitrene radical which will covalently link to almost any organic group with which it comes in contact (e.g. figure 2.11). The affinity label binds to both heavy and light chains *in the hypervariable regions*. There is no doubt that the electron microscopic studies with divalent hapten (cf. figures 2.5 and 2.6) show the antigen-combining sites to be associated with the N-terminal region of the molecule which at least bears out the overall view that the variable regions are implicated in antibody specificity.

VARIABILITY IN STRUCTURE UNRELATED TO ANTIBODY SPECIFICITY

Even the 'constant' portions of the immunoglobulin peptide chains which are not directly concerned in antigen binding

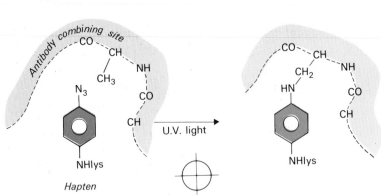

Hapten

Figure 2.11. Affinity labelling: The hapten binds to its antibody and the azide group activated by ultraviolet light loses N_2 forming a reactive radical which combines with an adjacent amino acid—in this hypothetical example an alanine residue. Analysis of the protein after digestion would show the alanine to be labelled with the hapten and implicate this residue in the combining site. Studies by Fleet G.W.J., Porter R.R. & Knowles J.R. (*Nature* 1969, **224**, 511) indicate that the affinity label combines with heavy and light chains in a ratio of approximately 3.5 : 1 in their system.

show considerable heterogeneity. This has largely been analysed through the recognition of characteristic groupings on the molecules by use of specific antisera raised usually in other species. Let us consider, for example, studies on human immunoglobulin light chains.

Light chains

A convenient source of human material is the urinary Bence-Jones' protein which is found in a proportion of patients with myeloma. The Bence-Jones' protein represents a dimer of light chains derived from the pool used in the synthesis of the myeloma protein. By raising antisera in rabbits to a number of Bence-Jones' proteins it was found that light chains could be divided into two groups (called *kappa* (κ) and *lambda* (λ)) depending upon their reactions with the antisera. The Bence-Jones' light chains of the κ-group all gave precipitin reactions with anti-κ sera but no reaction with anti-λ sera. Parallel reactions were always obtained with the parent myeloma protein as would be expected if they were derived from light chains produced by one clone of myeloma plasma cells (figure 2.12). The reactions with normal serum show that molecules with κ- and λ-chains are present. They occur on different molecules, i.e. no naturally occurring antibody has mixed κ and λ chains, and approximately 65% of the immunoglobulin molecules in normal serum are of κ-type, the remainder being λ-type. It is of interest that myeloma proteins of type κ occur with nearly twice the frequency of type λ, suggesting that cells synthesizing molecules with λ-chains carry the same risk of becoming malignant as those making κ-chains. The $\kappa : \lambda$ ratio varies in different species.

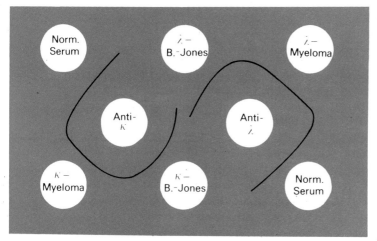

Figure 2.12. Precipitation reactions in agar-gel using antisera prepared against κ and λ Bence-Jones' proteins (urinary light chain dimers). The anti-κ reacted with κ but not λ light chains and gave reactions of 'identity' with the related myeloma protein and with normal serum. Parallel results were obtained with the anti-λ serum.

Heavy chains

Similar studies using antisera prepared against normal and myeloma proteins have established the existence of *five* major types of heavy chain in the human, each of which gives rise to a distinct immunoglobulin class. As mentioned earlier these are IgG, IgA, IgM, IgD and IgE. But whereas each immunoglobulin class is associated with a particular type of heavy chain, they all have κ- and λ-light chains; thus each myeloma protein so far studied, whatever its class, has possessed light chains of either κ- or λ-specificity (but never of both together).

We have already considered the view that the variable portion of the immunoglobulin molecule is bound up with antibody specificity and all classes have been shown to have binding affinity for antigen associated with the Fab regions. What of the constant region, particularly the Fc part of the heavy chain backbone which makes no contribution to specificity? Almost certainly the Fc structure directs the *biological activity* of the antibody molecule. As will be seen below, it determines to some extent the distribution of the immunoglobulin throughout the body, e.g. the selective passage of IgG across the placenta and the secretion of IgA into the external body fluids. But also, after combination with antigen, a new or enhanced activity such as the ability to fix complement or to bind effectively to macrophages may arise. It has been suggested that this occurs through an allosteric change in Fc conformation due to the opening of the 'hinge' Fc. However, the flexibility of the hinge makes this rather unlikely and physical measurements with nuclear magnetic resonance and electron spin probes only detect conformational changes in the Fab, not the Fc, region after complexing with antigen. The complement system (cf. p. 165) may be activated if the combination of antibody with antigen causes a shift in the relative spatial orientation of Fab and Fc fragments and permits access of the initiating complement component (C1) to the appropriate site in the Fc region; this contention is strengthened by the finding that IgG4 (a *sub-class* variant of IgG, see below) with a very short hinge can only activate complement when the Fc is cleaved from the Fab. Secondary biological properties of antibodies which are mediated through interaction with cell surface receptors for the immunoglobulin Fc may depend upon greatly increased binding to the cell due to the multivalent Fc sites present in an immune complex (cf. bonus effect of multivalency, p. 13) or the cross-linking of Fc receptors by the complex, or both mechanisms. Each of these biological functions may require a different type of Fc structure and hence amino acid sequence. Thus the multiplicity of Fc structures as expressed in the different immunoglobulin classes and subclasses may be looked upon as a system which has evolved to provide antibodies with different biological capabilities in relation to antigens.

In summary, the variable part provides specificity for binding antigen; the constant part is associated with different biological properties which vary from one immunoglobulin class to another, depending upon the primary structure, and which may require combination with antigen for their activation.

Immunoglobulin domains

In addition to the *interchain* disulphide bonds which bridge heavy and light chains, there are internal, *intrachain* disulphide links which form loops in the peptide chain (figure 2.13). As Edelman predicted, the loops are compactly folded to form globular domains (figure 2.15). These interact laterally through their hydrophobic regions (figure 2.14) forming V_H/V_L, C_{H1}/C_L and C_{H3}/C_{H3} diads; C_{H2} domains remain separate.

Different domains subserve separate functions. Thus the variable region domains (V_L and V_H) are responsible for the formation of a specific antigen-binding site. The C_{H1} region in IgG ($C\gamma1$) binds to the fourth component of the complement system (C4b), while the C_{H2} structure can attach C1q to initiate the classical complement sequence (cf. p. 165). Since the isolated C_{H2} domain has the same half-life as the parent IgG molecule, this region must be dominant in controlling the rate of metabolic degradation *in vivo*. Adherence to the monocyte surface is mediated largely through the terminal C_{H3} domain (figure 2.13) but synergism between C_{H2} and C_{H3} appears to be required for optimal binding to Fc

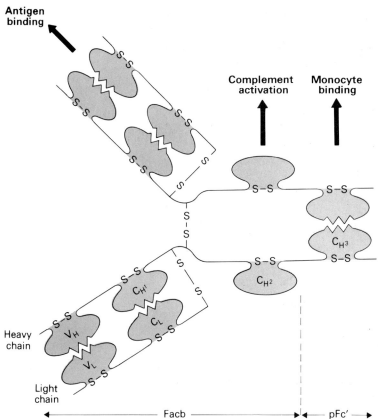

Figure 2.13. Immunoglobulin domains in IgG. Each loop in the peptide chain formed by an *intrachain* disulphide bond represents a single domain (shaded) and these are labelled V_H, C_{H1} etc. as indicated. They show considerable homology (i.e. similarities in amino acid structure) but each domain appears to be specialized for a specific function as shown. The involvement of the C_{H2} region in complement activation is indicated by the activity of the plasmin Facb fragment which contains the C_{H2} domain, and the inactivity of the $F(ab')_2$ fragment which lacks it. The active site is a hydrophobic region near the hinge. The pepsin pFc' fragment which bears the C_{H3} domain can bind directly to the monocyte surface and inhibit the formation of Fc rosettes with antibody-coated red cells. Staphylococcal protein-A reacts at the interface between C_{H2} and C_{H3}.

receptors on placental syncytiotrophoblast, polymorphonuclear leucocytes and K cells (p. 242).

Comparison of immunoglobulin classes

The physical and biological characteristics of the five major immunoglobulin classes in the human are summarized in tables 2.1 and 2.2. The following comments are intended to supplement this information.

Immunoglobulin G

During the secondary response IgG is probably the major immunoglobulin to be synthesized. Through its ability to

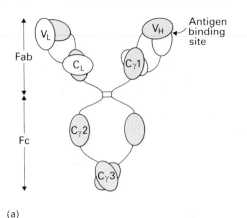

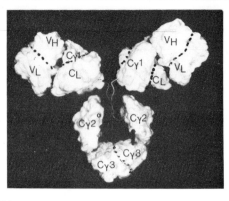

(a)

(b)

Figure 2.14. The disposition and inter-action of Ig domains in IgG. (a) Diagram showing apposing domains making contact through hydrophobic regions (after Dr A. Feinstein). The structures of these contact frameworks are highly conserved, an essential feature if different V_H and V_L domains are to associate in order to generate a wide variety of antibody specificities. These hydrophobic regions on the two complement fixing C_{H2} ($C\gamma2$) domains are partly masked by carbohydrate and remain independent so allowing the formation of a hinge region which is extremely flexible both with respect to variation in the angle of the Fab fragments and their rotation about the hinge peptide chain. Thus combining sites in IgG can be readily adapted to spatial variations in the presentation of the antigenic epitopes. (b) Space-filling model (courtesy of Dr A. Feinstein).

cross the placenta it provides a major line of defence against infection for the first few weeks of a baby's life which may be further reinforced by the transfer of colostral IgG across the gut mucosa in the neonate. IgG diffuses more readily than the other immunoglobulins into the extravascular body spaces where as the predominant species it carries the major burden of neutralizing bacterial toxins and of binding to micro-organisms to enhance their phagocytosis. The complexes of bacteria with IgG antibody activate complement thereby chemotactically attracting polymorphonuclear phagocytic cells (cf. p. 166) which adhere to the bacteria through surface receptors for complement and the Fc portion of IgG (Fcγ); binding to the Fc receptor then stimulates ingestion of micro-organisms through phagocytosis. In a similar way, the extracellular killing of target cells coated with IgG antibody is mediated through recognition of the surface Fcγ by K-cells bearing the appropriate receptors (cf. p. 242). The interaction of IgG complexes with platelet Fc receptors presumably leads to aggregation and vasoactive amine release but the physiological significance of Fcγ binding sites on other cell types, particularly lymphocytes, has not yet been clarified. Although unable to bind firmly to mast cells in human skin, IgG alone among the human immunoglobulins has the somewhat useless property of fixing to guinea pig skin. The thesis that the biological

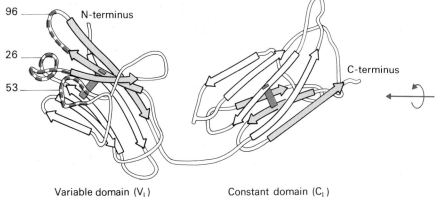

96 ——

N-terminus

26 ——

53 ——

C-terminus

Variable domain (V_L)   Constant domain (C_L)

Figure 2.15. Structure of the globular domains of a light chain (from X-ray crystallographic studies of a Bence-Jones' protein by Schiffler *et al.* (1973) *Biochemistry*, **12**, 4620). One surface of each domain is composed essentially of four chains (white arrows) arranged in an anti-parallel β-pleated structure stabilized by interchain H bonds between the amide CO. and NH. groups running along the peptide backbone, and the other surface of three such chains (grey arrows); the dark bar represents the intra-chain disulphide bond. This structure is characteristic of all immunoglobulin domains. Of particular interest is the location of the hypervariable regions (■▨■▨■) in three separate loops which are closely disposed relative to each other and form the light chain contribution to the antigen binding site (cf. figure 2.10). One numbered residue from each complementarity determinant is identified. To generate a Fab fragment (cf. figure 2.14), imagine a V_H–C_{H1} segment just like the V_L–C_L in the diagram, rotate it 180° around the axis of the arrow on the right of the figure and lay it on top of the V_L–C_L segment (Dr. A. Feinstein).

Table 2.1. Physical properties of major human immunoglobulin classes.

WHO designation	IgG	IgA	IgM	IgD	IgE
Sedimentation coefficient	$7S$	$7S, 9S, 11S$*	$19S$	$7S$	$8S$
Molecular weight	150,000	160,000 and dimer	900,000	185,000	200,000
Number of basic four-peptide units	1	1, 2*	5	1	1
Heavy chains	γ	α	μ	δ	ε
Light chains κ + λ	κ + λ	κ + λ	κ + λ	κ + λ	κ + λ
Molecular formula†	$\gamma_{2Z3\kappa_2}, \gamma_2\lambda_2$	$(\alpha_2\kappa_2)_{1-2}$ $(\alpha_2\lambda_2)_{1-2}$ $(\alpha_2\kappa_2)_2 S$* $(\alpha_2\lambda_2)_2 S$*	$(\mu_2\kappa_2)_5$ $(\mu_2\lambda_2)_5$	$\delta_2\kappa_2(\delta_2\lambda_2 ?)$	$\varepsilon_2\kappa_2, \varepsilon_2\lambda_2$
Valency for antigen binding	2	2, 4	5(10)	2	2
Concentration range in normal serum	8–16 mg/ml	1.4–4 mg/ml	0.5–2 mg/ml	0–0.4 mg/ml	17–450 ng/ml‡
% Total immunoglobulin	80	13	6	0–1	0.002
% Carbohydrate content	3	8	12	13	12

* Dimer in external secretions carries secretory component—S.
† IgA dimer and IgM contain J chain.
‡ ng = 10^{-9} g.

Table 2.2. Biological properties of major immunoglobulin classes in the human.

	IgG	IgA	IgM	IgD	IgE
Major characteristics	Most abundant Ig of internal body fluids particularly extravascular where it combats microorganisms and their toxins	Major Ig in sero-mucous secretions where it defends external body surfaces	Very effective agglutinator; produced early in immune response—effective first-line defence vs. bacteraemia	Most, if not all, present on lymphocyte surface	Protection of external body surfaces Recruits anti-microbial agents Raised in parasitic infections Responsible for symptoms of atopic allergy
Complement fixation					
Classical	++	−	+++	−	−
Alternative	−	±	−	−	
Cross placenta	+	−	−	−	−
Fix to homologous mast cells and basophils	−	−	−	−	+
Binding to macrophages and polymorphs	+	±	−	−	−

individuality of different immunoglobulin classes is dependent on the heavy chain constant regions, particularly the Fc, is amply borne out in relationship to the activities we have discussed such as transplacental passage, complement fixation and binding to various cell types, where function has been shown to be mediated by the Fc part of the molecule.

With respect to overall regulation of IgG levels in the body, the catabolic rate appears to depend directly upon the total IgG concentration whereas synthesis is largely governed by antigen stimulation so that in germ-free animals, for example, IgG levels are extremely low but rise rapidly on transfer to a normal environment.

Immunoglobulin A

IgA appears selectively in the sero-mucous secretions such as saliva, tears, nasal fluids, sweat, colostrum and secretions of the lung, genito-urinary and gastro-intestinal tracts where it clearly has the job of defending the exposed external surfaces of the body against attack by micro-organisms. It is present in these fluids as a dimer stabilized against proteolysis by combination with another protein—the secretory component which is synthesized by local epithelial cells and has a single peptide chain of molecular weight 60,000. The IgA is synthesized locally by plasma cells and dimerized intracellularly together with a cysteine-rich polypeptide called J-chain of molecular weight 15,000. If dimerization occurred randomly *after* secretion, dimers of mixed specificity would be formed which would not be as effective in combining with antigen as those of single specificity which would have a higher effective valency. The dimeric IgA binds strongly to secretory component present on the surface of the cell in which it was produced and the complex is then actively endocytosed, transported across the cytoplasm and secreted into the external body fluids (figure 2.16).

IgA antibodies function by inhibiting the adherence of coated micro-organisms to the surface of mucosal cells thereby preventing entry into the body tissues. Aggregated IgA binds to polymorphs and can also activate the alternative (p. 167) as distinct from the classical complement pathway which probably accounts for reports of a synergism between IgA, complement and lysozyme in the killing of certain coliform organisms. Human plasma contains relatively high concentrations of monomeric IgA and its role is still something of a mystery.

Immunoglobulin M

Often referred to as the macroglobulin antibodies because of their high molecular weight, IgM molecules are polymers of

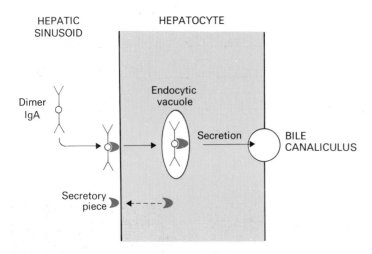

HEPATIC SINUSOID

HEPATOCYTE

Dimer IgA

Endocytic vacuole

Secretion

BILE CANALICULUS

Secretory piece

Figure 2.16. The mechanism of IgA secretion as exemplified by the transfer of circulating IgA into the bile. Dimeric IgA in the sinusoid binds to surface secretory piece thereby activating the uptake and secretion of the immunoglobulin. There is perhaps an analogy with the uptake of IgG into macrophages through stimulation of the surface IgG receptors.

five four-peptide subunits each bearing an extra C_H domain. As with IgA, polymerization of the subunits depends upon the presence of J-chain whose function may be to stabilize the Fc sulphydryl groups during Ig synthesis so that they remain available for cross-linking the subunits to give the structure shown in figure 2.17a. Under negative staining in the electron microscope, the free molecule in solution assumes a 'star' shape but when combined as an antibody with an antigenic surface membrane it can adopt a 'crab-like' configuration (figures 2.17b and c). The theoretical combining valency is of course 10 but this is only observed on interaction with small haptens; with larger antigens the effective valency falls to 5 and this must be attributed to some form of steric restriction due to lack of flexibility in the molecule. IgM antibodies tend to be of relatively low affinity as measured against single determinants (haptens) but, because of their high valency, they bind with quite respectable avidity to antigens with multiple epitopes (bonus effect of multivalency, p. 13).

For the same reason, these antibodies are extremely efficient agglutinating and cytolytic agents and since they appear early in the response to infection and are largely confined to the bloodstream, it is likely that they play a role of particular importance in cases of bacteraemia. The isohaemagglutinins (anti-A, anti-B) and many of the 'natural' antibodies to micro-organisms are usually IgM; antibodies to the typhoid

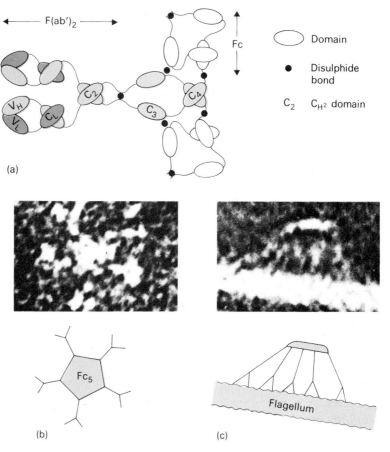

(a)

(b)

(c)

Figure 2.17. The structure of IgM: (a) The arrangement of domains in one of the five subunits showing how the pentamer is built up through the disulphide linkages between C_{H3} and C terminal regions (after Hilschman & Feinstein). Without too much aggravation, I hope the reader will appreciate that the hinge region in IgG (cf. figure 2.14) is replaced by a rigid pair of extra domains (C_{H2}), while the C_{H3} and C_{H4} domains in IgM are structurally equivalent to the C_{H2} and C_{H3} regions respectively in IgG. (b) As shown by electron microscopy of a human Waldenström's macroglobulin in free solution adopting a 'star'-shaped configuration. (c) As revealed in an E.M. preparation of specific sheep IgM antibody bound to *Salmonella paratyphi* flagellum where the immunoglobulin has assumed a 'crab-like' conformation in establishing its links with antigen. With the $F(ab')_2$ arms bent out of the plane of the central Fc_5 region, the C_{H3} complement binding domains are now readily accessible to the first component of complement (cf. p. 166). The Fc_5 constellation obtained by papain cleavage can activate complement directly. (Electron micrographs—kindly provided by Dr A. Feinstein and Dr E.A. Munn—are negatively stained preparations of magnification × 2,000,000, i.e. 1 mm represents 0.5 nm.)

'O' antigen (endotoxin) and the 'WR' antibodies in syphilis also tend to be found in this class. IgM would appear to precede IgG in the phylogeny of the immune response in vertebrates. We shall see later (p. 61) that monomeric IgM anchored into the surface membrane of certain lymphocytes has a receptor function.

Immunoglobulin D

This class was recognized through the discovery of a myeloma protein which did not have the antigenic specificity of IgG, A or M, although it reacted with antibodies to immunoglobulin light chains and had the basic four-peptide structure. The hinge region is particularly extended and although protected to some degree by carbohydrate, it may be this feature which makes IgD, among the different immunoglobulin classes, uniquely susceptible to proteolytic degradation, and account for its short half-life in plasma (2.8 days). An exciting development has been the demonstration that nearly all the IgD is present, together with IgM, on the surface of a proportion of blood lymphocytes where it seems likely that they may operate as mutually interacting antigen receptors for the control of lymphocyte activation and suppression. The even greater susceptibility of IgD to proteolysis on combination with antigen could well be implicated in such a function.

Immunoglobulin E

Only very low concentrations of IgE are present in serum and only a very small proportion of the plasma cells in the body are synthesizing this immunoglobulin. It is not surprising, therefore, that so far only six cases of IgE myeloma have been recognized compared with tens of thousands of IgC paraproteinaemias. IgE antibodies remain firmly fixed for an extended period when injected into human skin where they are probably bound to mast cells. Contact with antigen leads to degranulation of the mast cells with release of vasoactive amines. This process is responsible for the symptoms of hay fever and of extrinsic asthma when patients with atopic allergy come into contact with the allergen, e.g. grass pollen.

The main *physiological* role of IgE would appear to be protection of the external mucosal surfaces of the body by local recruitment of plasma factors and effector cells through triggering an acute inflammatory reaction. Infectious agents penetrating the IgA defences would combine with specific IgE on the mast cell surface and trigger the release of vasoactive agents and factors chemotactic for granulocytes, so leading to an influx of plasma IgG, complement, polymorphs and eosinophils (cf. p. 191). In such a context, the ability of eosinophils to damage IgG-coated helminths and the generous IgE response to such parasites would constitute an effective defence.

Antigenic analysis of IgG myelomas revealed further variation and showed that they could be grouped into four *subclasses* now termed IgG1, IgG2, IgG3 and IgG4. The differences all lie in the heavy chains which have been labelled $\gamma1$, $\gamma2$, $\gamma3$ and $\gamma4$ respectively. These heavy chains show considerable homology and have certain structures in common with each other—the ones which react with specific anti-IgG antisera—but each has one or more additional structures characteristic of its own subclass arising from differences in primary amino acid composition and in interchain disulphide bridging. These give rise to differences in biological behaviour which are summarized in table 2.3.

Two subclasses of IgA have also been found, of which IgA1, constitutes 80–90% of the total. The IgA2 subclass is unusual in that it lacks interchain disulphide bonds between heavy and light chains. Class and subclass variation is not restricted to human immunoglobulins but is a feature of all the higher mammals so far studied; monkey, sheep, rabbit, guinea-pig, rat and mouse.

OTHER IMMUNOGLOBULIN VARIANTS

Isotypes

The heavy chain constant region structures associated with the different classes and subclasses are termed isotypic variants, i.e. they are all present together in the serum of a normal subject. Other examples are provided by the types

Table 2.3. Comparison of human IgG subclasses.

	IgG1	IgG2	IgG3	IgG4
% Total IgG in normal serum	65	23	8	4
Electrophoretic mobility	slow	slow	slow	fast
Spontaneous aggregation	−	−	+++	−
Gm allotypes	a,z,f,x	n	bo,b1,b3, g,s,t, etc.	
Ga site reacting with rheumatoid factor*	+++	+++	−	+++
Combination with staphylococcal A protein	+++	+++	−	+++
Cross placenta	++	±	++	++
Complement fixation (C1 pathway)	+++	++	++++	±
Binding to monocytes	+++	+	+++	±
Binding to heterologous skin	++	−	++	++
Blocking IgE binding	−	−	−	+
Antibody dominance	Anti-Rh	Anti-dextran Anti-levan	Anti-Rh	Anti-Factor VIII

Other rheumatoid factors apparently react with Gm specific sites.

Table 2.4. Summary of immunoglobulin variants.

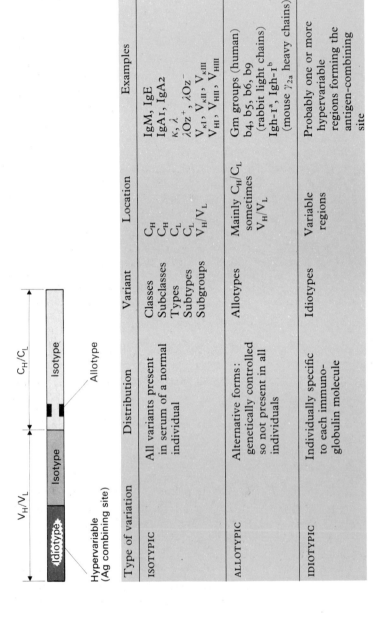

Type of variation	Distribution	Variant	Location	Examples
ISOTYPIC	All variants present in serum of a normal individual	Classes Subclasses Types Subtypes Subgroups	C_H C_H C_L C_L V_H/V_L	IgM, IgE IgA1, IgA2 κ, λ λOz^+, λOz^- $V_{\kappa I}$, $V_{\kappa II}$, $V_{\kappa III}$ V_{HI}, V_{HII}, V_{HIII}
ALLOTYPIC	Alternative forms: genetically controlled so not present in all individuals	Allotypes	Mainly C_H/C_L sometimes V_H/V_L	Gm groups (human) b4, b5, b6, b9 (rabbit light chains) Igh-1^a, Igh-1^b (mouse γ_{2a} heavy chains)
IDIOTYPIC	Individually specific to each immunoglobulin molecule	Idiotypes	Variable regions	Probably one or more hypervariable regions forming the antigen-combining site

V_H/V_L — C_H/C_L

Idiotype — Isotype — Isotype — Allotype

Hypervariable (Ag combining site)

and subtypes of the C_L domain and by the subgroups of the light and heavy chain variable regions (table 2.4).

Allotypes

These represent yet a further type of variation which depends upon the existence of allelic forms (encoded by alleles or alternative genes at a single locus). In somewhat the same way as the red cells in genetically different individuals can differ in terms of the blood group antigen system A, B, O, so the Ig heavy chains differ in the expression of their allotypic groups. Typical allotypes are the Gm specificities on IgG (Gm = *marker* on Ig*G*) which are recognizable by the ability of the individual's IgG to block agglutination of red cells coated with anti-rhesus D bearing the Gm allotype by sera from patients with rheumatoid arthritis containing the appropriate anti-Gm rheumatoid factors. Allotypic differences at a given Gm locus usually involve one or two amino acids in the peptide chain. Take, for example, the G1m(a) locus on IgG1 (table 2.3). An individual with this allotype would have the peptide sequence: Asp.Glu.Leu.Thr.Lys on each of his IgGI molecules. Another person whose IgG1 was a-negative would have the sequence Glu.Glu.Met.Thr.Lys., i.e. two amino acids different. To date, 25 Gm groups have been found on the γ-heavy chains and a further three (the Km—previously Inv groups) on the κ constant region.

Allotypic markers have also been found on the immunoglobulins of rabbits and of mice using reagents prepared by immunizing one animal with an immune complex obtained with antibodies from another animal of the same species. As in other allelic systems, individuals may be homozygous or heterozygous for the genes encoding the markers; these are expressed co-dominantly and are inherited in simple Mendelian fashion. Take, for example, the b4, b5 allotypes on rabbit light chains: an animal of b^4b^4 genotype would express the b4 allotype whereas a rabbit of b^4b^5 genotype derived from b^4b^4 and b^5b^5 parents would express the b4 marker on one fraction and b5 on another fraction of its immunoglobulin molecules.

Isoallotypes are horrendously small print: these are groups shared by 2 or more subclasses which are structurally antithetic to a Gm marker present in one class only, e.g. nG1m(a) is present on all IgG2 and IgG3 proteins but only on IgG1 molecules lacking G1m(a).

Idiotypes

We have seen that it is possible to obtain antibodies that recognize isotypic and allotypic variants; it is also possible to raise antisera which are specific for individual antibody molecules and discriminate between one monoclonal antibody and another or one myeloma protein and another independently of isotypic or allotypic structures. Such antisera define the individual determinants characteristic of each antibody, collectively termed the *idiotype* (Kunkel & Oudin). Not surprisingly, it turns out that the idiotypic determinants are located in the variable part of the antibody associated with the hypervariable regions which form the antigen-combining site (table 2.4; figure 2.18). Thus in many cases,

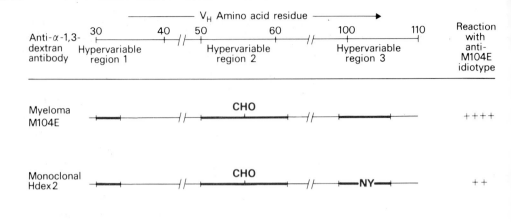

Anti-α-1,3-dextran antibody	Hypervariable region 1 (30—40)		Hypervariable region 2 (50—60)		Hypervariable region 3 (100—110)	Reaction with anti-M104E idiotype

V_H Amino acid residue →

Myeloma M104E			CHO			++++
Monoclonal Hdex2			CHO		NY	++
Monoclonal Hdex10			KK		VN	−

Figure 2.18. Association of idiotypic determinants with hypervariable regions. Three monoclonal immunoglobulins with anti-dextran activity were analysed. They were identical except for the amino acid substitutions shown (N = asparagine; Y = tyrosine; K = lysine; V = valine; CHO = carbohydrate). The idiotypic determinants (idiotopes) on the myeloma protein M104E were defined by an anti-idiotypic serum. Hdex2 which differed from M104E by just two amino acids in the 3rd hypervariable region shared some but not all the idiotypic determinants on M104E but Hdex10 with substitutions in the 2nd and 3rd hypervariable regions shared none. Reprinted by permission from *Nature*, **283**, 35. Copyright © 1980 MacMillan Journals Limited.

an anti-idiotypic serum directed against an anti-hapten antibody can block the binding of hapten. Anti-idiotypic sera which do not block are presumably directed to hypervariable regions not concerned in the binding of that hapten (figure 2.19). Anti-idiotypes which react with one antibody and no other are said to recognize *private* idiotypes and provide

Figure 2.19. Different possible relationships between the antigen or hapten-binding area (paratope) and the idiotypic determinant (idiotope) within the hypervariable regions. (a) Identical or overlapping paratope and idiotope; anti-idiotype blocks hapten binding. (b) Non-overlapping paratope and idiotype; anti-idiotype does not influence hapten binding.

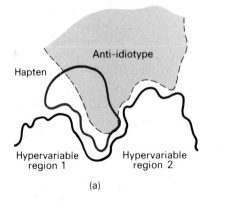

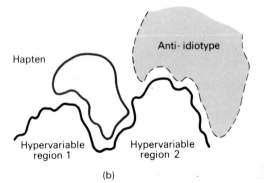

(a)   (b)

further support for the idea that each antibody has a unique structure. Frequently, antibody molecules of closely similar amino acid structure may, in addition, share idiotypes (e.g. MIO4E and Hdex2 in figure 2.18) and we then speak of *public* or *cross-reacting* idiotypes.

Anti-idiotypic sera provide useful reagents for demonstrating the same V region on different heavy chains and on different cells, for identification of specific immune complexes in patients' sera, for recognition of V_L type amyloid in subjects excreting Bence-Jones' proteins, for detection of residual monoclonal protein after therapy and perhaps for selecting lymphocytes with certain surface receptors. The reader will (or should be) startled to learn that it is possible to raise *auto*anti-idiotypic sera since this means that individuals can make antibodies to their own idiotypes. This has quite momentous consequences as will become apparent when we discuss the Jerne network theory in Chapter 4.

Summary

Immunoglobulins (Ig) have a basic four-peptide structure of two identical heavy and two identical light chains joined by interchain disulphide links. Papain splits the molecule at the exposed flexible hinge region to give two identical univalent antigen binding fragments (Fab) and a further fragment (Fc). Pepsin proteolysis gives a divalent Ag binding fragment $F(ab')_2$ lacking the Fc.

There are perhaps 10^8 or more different Ig molecules in normal serum. Analysis of myeloma proteins which are homogeneous Ig produced by single clones of malignant plasma cells has shown the N-terminal region of heavy and light chains to have a variable amino acid structure and the remainder to be relatively constant in structure. Each chain is folded into globular domains. The variable region domains bind Ag, and three *hypervariable* loops on the heavy and three on the light chain form the Ag binding site. The constant region domains of the heavy chain (particularly the Fc) carry out a secondary biological function after the binding of Ag, e.g. complement fixation and macrophage binding.

In the human there are five major types of heavy chain giving five *classes* of Ig. IgG is the most abundant Ig particularly in the extravascular fluids where it combats microorganisms and toxins; it fixes complement, binds to phagocytic cells and crosses the placenta. IgA exists mainly as a monomer (basic four-peptide unit) in plasma, but in the seromucous secretions where it is the major Ig concerned in the defence of the external body surfaces, it is present as dimer linked to a secretory component. IgM is a pentameric molecule, essentially intravascular, produced early in the immune response. Because of its high valency it is a very effective bacterial agglutinator and mediator of complement-dependent cytolysis and is therefore a powerful first-line defence against bacteraemia. IgD is largely present on the lymphocyte and probably functions as an Ag receptor. IgE binds firmly to mast cells and contact with antigen leads to local recruitment of anti-microbial agents through degranu-lation of the mast cells and release of inflammatory medi-ators. IgE is of importance in certain parasitic infections and is responsible for the symptoms of atopic allergy. Further diversity of function is possible through subdivision of classes into subclasses based on structural differences in heavy chains present in each normal individual.

Allotypic structural variations are controlled by allelic genes and provide genetic markers. Idiotypic determinants unique to a given immunoglobulin are recognizable by anti-idiotypic antibodies and are associated with the hyper-variable regions forming the Ag binding site.

Further reading

Benacerraf B. (ed.) (1975) *Immunogenetics and Immunodeficiency* (Articles by B. Frangione on Ig structure and by H.G. Kunkel & T. Kindt on allotypes and idiotypes). MTP Press, Lancaster, England.

Davies R.D., Padlan E.A. & Segal D.M. (1975) Immunoglobulin structure at high resolution. In *Contemporary Topics in Molecular Immunology*. Inman F.P. (ed.). Vol. 4, p. 127. Plenum Press, New York.

Edelman G.M. *et al.* (1969) Complete sequence of human IgGI. *Proc. Nat. Acad. Sci.* **63**, 78.

Givol D. (1979) The antibody combining site. *Int. Rev. Biochem.* **23**, 71.

Glynn L.E. & Steward M.W. (eds) (1977) *Immunochemistry : an Advanced Textbook*. John Wiley & Sons, Chichester.

Kabat E.A. (1976) *Structural Concepts in Immunology and Immuno-chemistry*, 2nd edn. Holt, Rinehart & Winston, New York.

Leslie R.G.Q. (1982) The characterization of cell receptors for IgG. *Immunology Today* **3**, 265.

Moller G. (ed.) (1978) Immunoglobulin E. *Immunol. Rev.* **41**.

Nisonoff A. (1982) *Introduction to Molecular Immunology*. Sinauer Associates, Massachusetts.

3

The Immune Response
I—Fundamentals

Two types of immune response

When antigen enters the body, two different types of adaptive immunological reaction may occur:

1 The synthesis and release of free antibody into the blood and other body fluids (*humoral immunity*). This antibody acts, for example, by coating bacteria to enhance their phagocytosis and by combination with and neutralization of bacterial toxins.

2 The production of 'sensitized' lymphocytes which are themselves the effectors of *cell-mediated immunity*. This confers protection against organisms such as the tubercle bacillus and viruses which are characterized by an ability to live and replicate *within* the cells of the host. In individuals immune to tubercle infection, the 'sensitized' lymphocytes interact with injected tuberculin antigen to produce the delayed type hypersensitivity skin response, well known as the Mantoux reaction. Cells of this type are also involved in the rejection of skin grafts.

Role of the small lymphocyte

The central importance of the lymphocyte for both types of immune response was established largely by the work of Gowans. By labelling the lymphocytes with radioisotope and following their fate in the body it could be shown that there is a pool of recirculating lymphocytes which pass from the blood into the lymph nodes, spleen and other tissues and back to the blood by the major lymphatic channels such as the thoracic duct (figure 3.1).

PRIMARY RESPONSE

When rats are depleted of their lymphocytes by chronic drainage of lymph from the thoracic duct by an indwelling cannula, they have a grossly impaired ability to mount a primary antibody response to antigens such as tetanus toxoid and sheep red blood cells, or to reject a skin graft. Immunological reactivity can be restored by injecting thoracic duct lymphocytes obtained from another rat. The same effect can be obtained if, before injection, the thoracic duct cells are

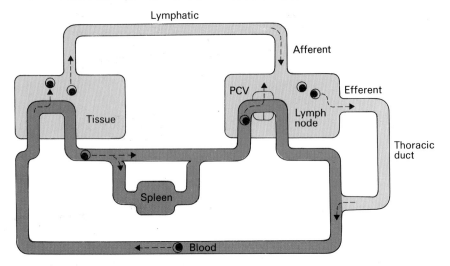

Figure 3.1. Traffic and recirculation of lymphocytes. Blood-borne lymphocytes enter the tissues and lymph nodes passing between the high cuboidal cells of the post-capillary venules (PCV) and leave via the draining lymphatics. The efferent lymphatics finally emerging from the last node in each chain join to form the thoracic duct which returns the lymphocytes to the bloodstream where it empties into the left subclavian vein (in the human). In the spleen, lymphocytes enter the lymphoid area (white pulp) from the arterioles, pass to the sinusoids of the erythroid area (red pulp) and leave by the splenic vein.

first incubated at 37°C for 24 hours under conditions which kill off large and medium-sized cells and leave only the small lymphocytes. Thus the small lymphocyte is necessary for the primary response of antigen.

Transfer experiments have also shown that small lymphocytes can become antibody synthesizing cells (plasma cells) and effector cells in cell-mediated immunity transplantation reactions.

SECONDARY RESPONSE—MEMORY

An immunologically 'virgin' rat, i.e. one which has had no previous contact with a specific antigen, may be inoculated with small lymphocytes from a rat which has already given a primary response to that antigen. Challenge of the recipient rat with antigen leads to a secondary type response with the rapid production of high-titre antibodies. If the recipient had not been injected with small lymphocytes from the 'primed' donor, a primary response with the relatively slow development of lower titre antibodies would have been seen (figure 3.2). Thus the small lymphocytes carry the *memory* of the first contact with antigen.

In the primary response, the relatively small number of virgin cells specific for the antigen are induced to *proliferate*;

48

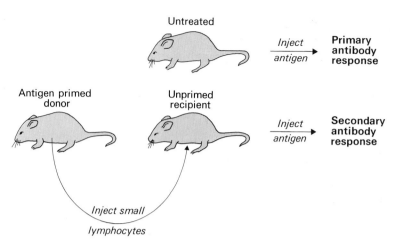

Untreated

Inject antigen → **Primary antibody response**

Antigen primed donor

Unprimed recipient

Inject antigen → **Secondary antibody response**

Inject small lymphocytes

Figure 3.2. Transfer of immunological memory by small lymphocytes from primed donor rat. In these transfer experiments, genetically identical animals of the same strain are used to prevent complications arising from transplantation reactions between the transferred lymphocytes and the host.

some go on to produce antibody- or cell-mediated immunity while others form an expanded population of antigen-sensitive memory cells which are capable of a faster response to antigen (figure 3.3). This combination of increase in cell number and more rapid maturation after antigen triggering is responsible for the characteristically brisk and heightened course of the secondary antibody response (cf. figure 1.2).

The thymus

This gland is organized into a series of lobules made up essentially of a meshwork of epithelial cells within which are packed aggregates of lymphocytes. The outer cortical area is densely populated with actively mitotic and some dying lymphoid cells and surrounds an inner medullary zone of prominent reticular dendritic and epithelioid cells with considerably fewer lymphocytes and isolated Hassall's corpuscles (figure 3.4). The occurrence of frequent thymic abnormalities in children with immunological deficiency disorders led to the suggestion that the thymus was related in some way to the development of immune responses (Good and colleagues). The relationship was clarified by Miller's demonstration that removal of the thymus gland in mice at birth led to:

1 decrease in circulating lymphocytes;
2 severe impairment of graft rejection;
3 reduced humoral antibody response to some but not all antigens (i.e. there are thymus-dependent and thymus-independent antigens);

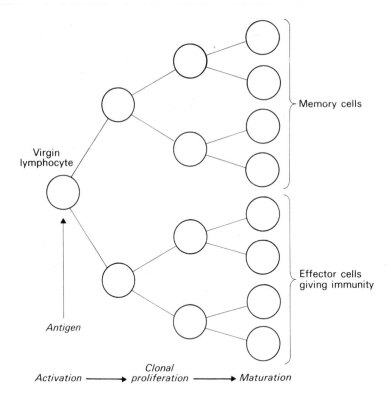

Virgin
lymphocyte

Antigen

Memory cells

Effector cells
giving immunity

Activation ⟶ *Clonal
proliferation* ⟶ *Maturation*

Figure 3.3. The cellular basis of the primary response. After stimulation by antigen the previously resting virgin lymphocyte proliferates and ultimately the daughter cells mature. Some become non-dividing memory cells and others the effector cells of humoral or cell-mediated immunity. Memory cells require fewer cycles before they develop into effectors and this shortens the reaction time for the secondary response. The expanded clone of cells with memory for the original antigen provides the basis for the greater secondary relative to the primary immune response. Priming with low doses of antigen can often stimulate effective memory without producing very adequate antibody synthesis.

4 wasting after 1–3 months—probably a result of inability to combat infection effectively since neonatally thymectomized mice reared under germ-free conditions did not waste.

X-irradiation of adult mice destroys the ability of their lymphocytes to divide and hence their immunological responsiveness. This can be restored by injection of bone marrow cells. However, bone marrow cells fail to restore cell-mediated immunity in X-irradiated adult mice which have been thymectomized; on the other hand, mature cells from adult spleen or lymph node were effective (figure 3.5). It is thus concluded that the thymus acts on primitive cells coming from the bone marrow to make them immunologically competent.

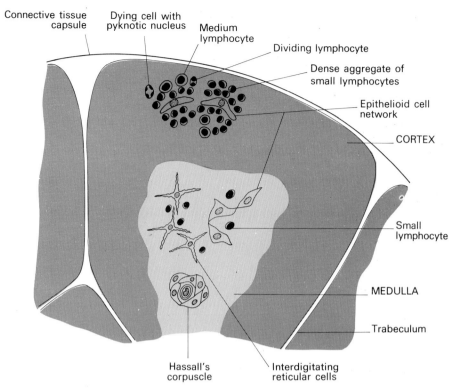

Connective tissue capsule
Dying cell with pyknotic nucleus
Medium lymphocyte
Dividing lymphocyte
Dense aggregate of small lymphocytes
Epithelioid cell network
CORTEX
Small lymphocyte
MEDULLA
Trabeculum
Hassall's corpuscle
Interdigitating reticular cells

Figure 3.4. Features of a thymus lobule. The medulla is continuous and sends finger-like processes into each lobule. The meshwork of epithelioid cells derived embryologically from the 3rd pharyngeal pouch and cleft forms an almost continuous cytoplasmic barrier around the blood vessels ('blood-thymus barrier'). Whorled, possibly degenerate aggregates of epithelial cells appear as the characteristic Hassall's corpuscles. Reticular dendritic cells of bone marrow origin are prominent in the medulla. The lymphocytes, particularly in the cortex, are densely packed and closely associated with the stromal cells. Single epithelial cells associated with very large numbers of thymocytes (? intracellular) have been termed 'nurse cells'. Rapidly dividing lymphocytes in the cortex are mostly immunologically immature and readily destroyed by cortisone; 90% are small, 1% large and the remainder are medium-sized. Lymphocytes in the medulla are more sparse and more cortisone resistant.

The Bursa of Fabricius

In chickens, another lymphoid organ termed the Bursa of Fabricius can be recognized. It is similar to the thymus and also embryologically derived from gut epithelium. Just as the thymus appears to act as a central lymphoid organ controlling the maturation of lymphocytes concerned largely with cell-mediated immunity, so the Bursa of Fabricius is responsible for the development of immunocompetence in cells destined to make humoral antibody. This differentiation of function may be readily seen from the results of the experiments documented in table 3.1: the thymus or bursa

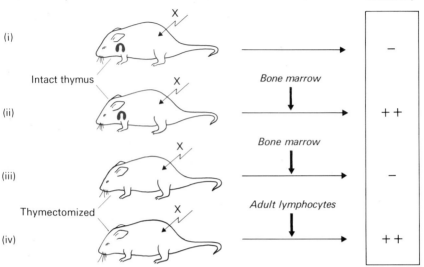

Cell-mediated immunity

(i) Intact thymus — X

(ii) Bone marrow — ++

(iii) Thymectomized — Bone marrow — −

(iv) Adult lymphocytes — ++

Figure 3.5. Maturation of bone marrow stem cells under the influence of the thymus to become immunocompetent lymphocytes capable of cell-mediated immune reactions. X-irradiation (X) destroys the ability of lymphocytes to mount a cellular immune response (i) but the stem cells in injected bone marrow can become immuno-competent and restore the response (ii) unless the thymus is removed (iii) in which case, only already immunocompetent lym-phocytes are effective (iv). Incidentally, the bone marrow stem cells also restore the levels of other formed elements of the blood (red cells, platelets, neutrophils, monocytes) which otherwise fall dramatically after X-irradiation and such therapy is crucial in cases where accidental or therapeutic expo-sure to X-rays or other anti-mitotic agents seriously damages the haemopoietic cells (cf. p. 117).

was removed from newborn chicks which were then irradi-ated to inactivate any competent lymphocytes which had already reached the peripheral tissues. After several weeks the chickens were tested and it was found that bursectomy had a profound effect on humoral antibody synthesis but did not unduly influence the cell-mediated reactions responsible

Table 3.1. Effect of neonatal bursectomy and thymectomy on the development of immunologi-cal competence in the chicken (From Cooper M.D., Peterson R.D.A., South M.A. & Good R.A. (1966) *J.exp.Med.* **123**, 75, with permission of the editors.)

All X-irradiated after birth	Peripheral blood lymphocyte count	Ig concn.	Antibody	Delayed skin reaction to tuberculin	Graft rejection
Intact	14,800	++	+++	++	++
Thymecto-mized	9,000	++	+	−	−
Bursectomized	13,200	−	−	+	+

for tuberculin skin reactivity and graft rejection. On the other hand, as in the mice, thymectomy grossly impaired cell-mediated reactions and had some effect on antibody production.

Two populations of lymphocytes: T- and B-cells

Thus primitive lymphoid cells from the bone marrow appear to differentiate into two small lymphocyte populations:

1 *T-lymphocytes,* processed by, or in some way dependent on, the thymus, and responsible for cell-mediated immunity;

2 *B-lymphocytes,* bursa-dependent, and concerned in the synthesis of circulating antibody.

Both populations on appropriate stimulation by antigen proliferate and undergo morphological changes (figure 3.6). The B-lymphocytes develop into the plasma cell series. The mature plasma cell (figure 3.7d and h) is actively synthesizing and secreting antibody and has a well-developed rough surfaced endoplasmic reticulum (figure 3.8c) characteristic of

Figure 3.6. Processing of bone marrow cells by thymus and gut-associated central lymphoid tissue to become immunocompetent T- and B-lymphocytes respectively. Proliferation and transformation to cells of the lymphoblast and plasma cell series occur on antigenic stimulation.

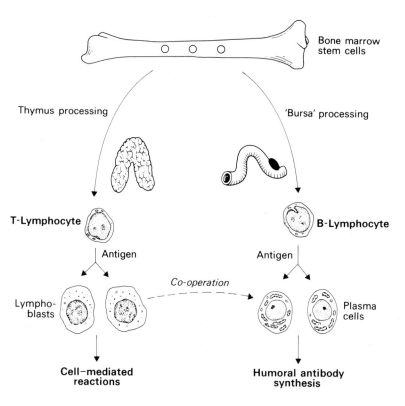

Figure 3.7. Light microscopy of cells involved in immune responses. (a) Small lymphocytes. Condensed chromatin gives rise to heavy staining of the nucleus. The cell on the left is a typical T-cell with receptors for IgM with a thin rim of cytoplasm. The other cell has more cytoplasm and azurophilic granules are evident; it bears receptors for IgG and sheep red cells and has therefore been defined as a T_G lymphocyte. Isolated platelets are visible. B-lymphocytes have a similar appearance. Giemsa stain × 2,500. (b) T_M lymphocytes. Acid esterase staining giving characteristic 'dot'-like appearance × 2,500. (c) Transformed lymphocyte (lymphoblast) following stimulation of lymphocytes in culture with a polyclonal activator. The large lymphoblasts with their relatively high ratio of cytoplasm to nucleus may be compared in size with the isolated small lymphocyte. One cell is in mitosis. May–Grünewald–Giemsa × 2,500. (d) Plasma cells. The nucleus is eccentric. The cytoplasm is strongly basophilic due to high RNA content. The juxta-nuclear lightly stained zone corresponds with the Golgi region. May–Grünewald–Giemsa × 2,500. (e) Monocyte, showing 'horseshoe-shaped' nucleus and moderately abundant pale cytoplasm with well-defined granules. A small lymphocyte with a more strongly stained nucleus is shown for comparison. Staining for peroxidase is frequently positive. Giemsa × 5,000. (f) Four polymorphonuclear leucocytes (neutrophils) and one eosinophil. The multi-lobed nuclei and the cytoplasmic granules are clearly shown, those of the eosinophil being heavily stained. Leishman stain × 2,000. (g) Macrophages in monolayer cultures after phagocytosis of mycobacteria (stained red). Carbol–Fuchsin counterstained with Malachite Green × 1,000. (h) Plasma cells stained to show intracellular immunoglobulin using a fluorescein-labelled anti-IgG (green) and a rhodamine-conjugated anti-IgM (red) × 2,500. (a), (b), (c) and (g) were photographed by Dr P.M. Lydyard. The material for (a) was supplied by Dr K. McLennan and (g) by Dr G. Rooke. (d) and (h) were given by Professor C. Grossi, (e) by Professor J. Stewart and (f) by Professor J.J. Owen.

Figure 3.8. (pp. 56–9). Electron microscopy of cells involved in immune responses (eosinophils may be seen in figure 7.21, mast cells in figure 9.6 and platelets in figure 10.12).

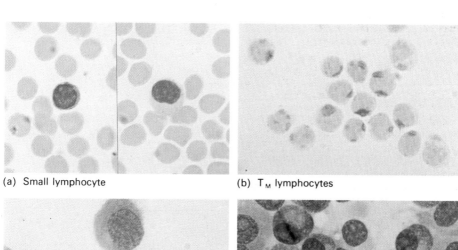

(a) Small lymphocyte

(b) T$_M$ lymphocytes

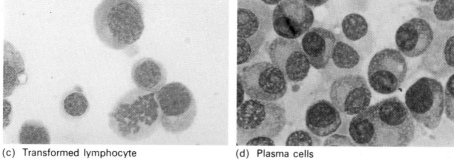

(c) Transformed lymphocyte

(d) Plasma cells

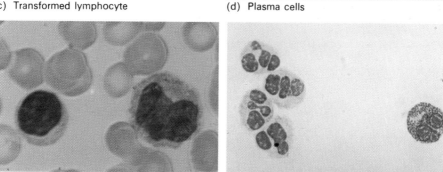

(e) Monocyte

(f) Neutrophils and eosinophil

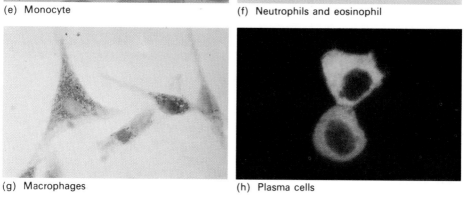

(g) Macrophages

(h) Plasma cells

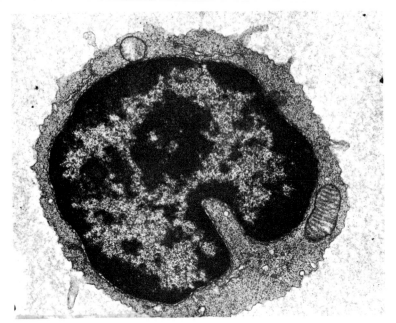

Figure 3.8. (a) Small T-lymphocyte with receptors for IgM. Indented nucleus with condensed chromatin, sparse cytoplasm: single mitochondrion shown and many free ribosomes but otherwise few organelles ($\times$ 13,000). B-lymphocytes are essentially similar with slightly more cytoplasm and occasional elements of rough-surfaced endoplasmic reticulum.

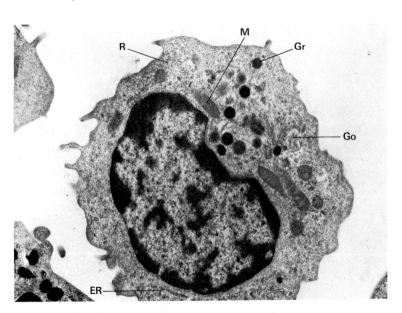

(b) T-lymphocyte with receptors for IgG ($\times$ 7,500). The more abundant cytoplasm contains several mitochondria (M), free ribosomes (R) with some elements of rough-surfaced endoplasmic reticulum (ER), prominent Golgi apparatus (Go) and characteristic membrane-bound electron-dense granules (Gr). The nuclear chromatin is less condensed than that of the T_M cell. (Courtesy of Drs A. Zicca and C.E. Grossi.)

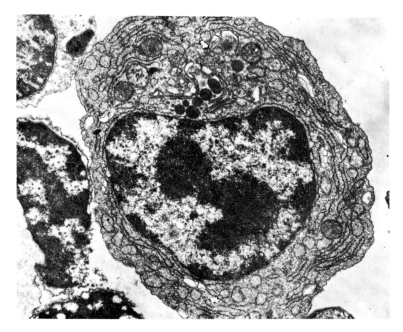

(c) Plasma cell (× 10,000). Prominent rough-surfaced endoplasmic reticulum associated with the synthesis and secretion of Ig.

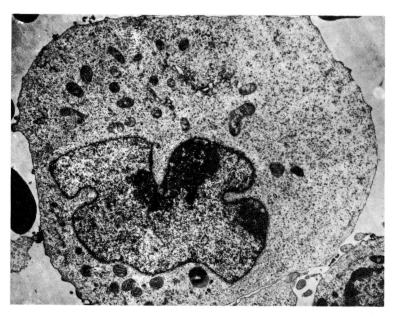

(d) Transformed lymphocyte (lymphoblast) (× 7,000). The nuclear chromatin is less condensed than in the small lymphocyte (a). The more extensive cytoplasm shows numerous mitochondria and free polyribosomes. (Courtesy Miss V. Petts.)

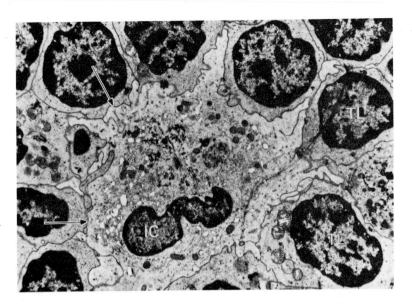

(e) Interdigitating cell (IC) in the thymus-dependent area of the rat lymph node. This is thought to be an antigen-presenting cell derived from the Langerhans' cell in the skin which travels to the node in the afferent lymph as a 'veiled' cell bearing antigen on its profuse surface processes. Intimate contacts are made with the surface membranes (arrows) of the surrounding T-lymphocytes (TL). The cytoplasm of the IC contains relatively few organelles and does not show Birbeck granules (racket-shaped cytoplasmic organelles, characteristic of the Langerhans' cell), but these granules appear after antigenic stimulation (× 2,000). (From Kamperdijk E.W.A., Hoefsmit E.Ch.H., Drexhage H.A. & Balfour B.H. (1980) In *Mononuclear Phagocytes*, 3rd edn. Van Furth R. (ed.). Rijhoff Publishers, The Hague. Courtesy of authors and publishers.)

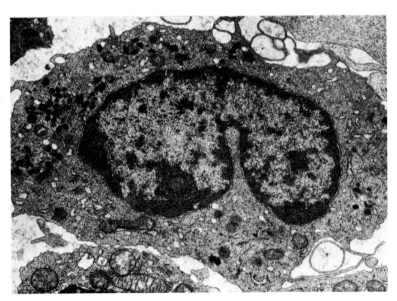

(f) Monocyte (× 10,000). 'Horseshoe' nucleus. Phagocytic and pinocytic vesicles, lysosomal granules, mitochondria and isolated profiles of rough-surfaced endoplasmic reticulum are evident.

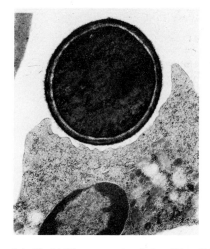
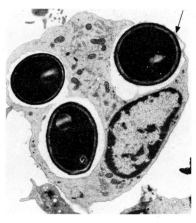

(g) (Left) Phagocytosis of *Candida albicans* by a polymorphonuclear leucocyte (neutrophil). Adherence to the surface initiates enclosure of the fungal particle within arms of cytoplasm. Lysosomal granules are abundant but mitochondria are rare

($\times$ 15,000). (h) (Right) Phagocytosis of *C. albicans* by a monocyte showing near completion of phagosome formation (arrowed) around one organism and complete ingestion of two others ($\times$ 5,000). (Figure 3.8 g–j courtesy of Dr H. Valdimarsson.)

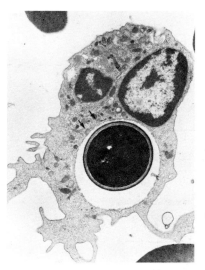
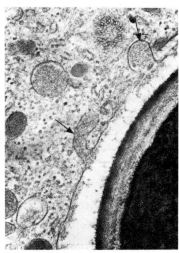

(i) (Left) Neutrophil 30 minutes after ingestion of *C. albicans*. The cytoplasm is already partly degranulated and two lysosomal granules (arrowed) are fusing with the phagocytic vacuole. Two lobes of the

nucleus are evident ($\times$ 5,000). (j) (Right) Higher magnification of (i) showing fusing granules discharging their contents into the phagocytic vacuole (arrowed). ($\times$ 33,000.)

a cell producing protein for 'export'. T-lymphocytes transform to lymphoblasts (figure 3.7c) which in the electron microscope are seen to have virtually no rough-surfaced endoplasmic reticulum although there are abundant free ribosomes, either single or as polysomes (figure 3.8d). This high ribosome content makes them basophilic so that they show superficial resemblance to plasmablasts in the light microscope but no antibody can be detected in their cytoplasm nor in their secretions. However, they do elaborate a series of soluble factors which act largely through the macrophage in establishing cell-mediated immunity, the other arm of this response being provided by a subpopulation of activated T-lymphocytes which are cytotoxic for virus-infected cells (cf. p. 75 and 76).

The anatomical equivalent of the bursa in man and other mammals does not seem to exist but experiments involving the culture of bone marrow or fetal liver *in vitro* make it seem likely that haemopoietic tissue itself provides the appropriate microenvironment for maturation of B-lymphocytes from precursor stem cells.

IDENTIFICATION OF B- AND T-LYMPHOCYTES

From the morphological standpoint it is difficult to differentiate T and B small lymphocytes at the light microscope level with conventional histological stains, although some differences are now becoming apparent in their enzyme content and their ultrastructure (figures 3.7a and b, 3.8a and b). Fortunately, the two populations differ strikingly in their surface markers (table 3.2) and these have been widely exploited.

Immunoglobulins are readily demonstrable on the surface of B- but not T-lymphocytes using an immunofluorescent technique with reagents such as fluorescein-labelled anti-immunoglobulin light chain (cf. figure 3.11b); this has also been shown in the electron microscope using peroxidase coupled (figure 6.13) or ^{125}I-labelled anti-Ig. Nearly all B-cells bear surface IgM, probably as monomer, but a proportion also stain with antisera directed against the Fc

Table 3.2. Tests for surface markers on human B- and T-cells.

Lymphocytes	Immunofluorescent staining for:		Rosette formation using sheep r.b.c. coated with:				Virus receptors	Approx. % of blood lymphocyte
	Ig	T3	Nothing	IgG	IgM	C3		
T	−	+ +	+ +	+	+ +	±	Measles	65–80
B	+ +	−	−	+ +	±	+ +	EB	8–15

portion of other Ig classes, particularly IgD. Antisera specific for the terminal heavy chain domain ($\not pFc'$; cf. p. 33) stain more weakly, suggesting attachment to the membrane through this region. The heavy chain of the surface IgM, which is present as a monomer, has an extra hydrophobic sequence relative to secreted pentameric IgM as revealed by its ability to bind detergent in the Fc region, to be labelled by lipophilic reagents and to insert itself into artificial membrane vesicles (liposomes). It must be supposed that the hydrophobic sequence anchors the molecule to the surface membrane and that removal of this sequence by mRNA splicing can be suitably arranged should the cell be turned on for Ig secretion as an antibody-forming cell (cf. figure 5.8, p. 138). I would now like to make an exceedingly important point. As we will see later, *each lymphocyte is programmed to make Ig of only one specificity and it is this Ig, placed on the B-lymphocyte surface, which is used as a specific receptor for antigen.*

In some circumstances, a proportion of T-cells do stain for surface immunoglobulin. This is not a product of the T-cell itself but is acquired by adsorption and probably represents immune complexes binding to receptors for the Ig Fc region which are displayed by some T-cells. These can be demonstrated by the formation of rosettes with red cells coated with IgG antibody, so-called 'Fcγ-rosettes'; clusters of red cells surround the lymphocyte to which they bind through the Fc of the coating IgG. Other T-cells have Fcμ receptors (i.e. binding sites for the Fc region of IgM heavy chains) and some features of these two subpopulations are contrasted in figures 3.7 and 3.8. Most, if not all, B-cells carry Fc receptors and form Fcγ-rosettes (figure 3.9a). In addition, approximately one half of the B-lymphocytes and perhaps some

Figure 3.9. B-cell rosettes—(a) diagrammatic representation of rosette formed with IgG (Y) coated erythrocytes binding to the receptor for Fcγ; (b) cluster of C3 coated red cells around B-lymphocyte (visualized in u.v. light after staining with acridine orange). (Courtesy of Dr A. Arnaiz-Villena.)

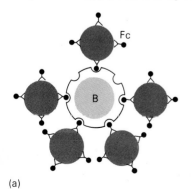

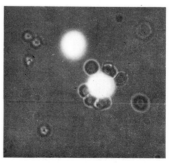

(a)   (b)

T-cells form clusters with red cells coated with the third component of complement (C3; cf. p. 166) (figure 3.9b).

Interestingly, human T-cells can be persuaded to form so-called 'spontaneous' rosettes with uncoated sheep erythrocytes, a useful if fortuitous reaction without any immunological foundation. The T-lymphocyte membrane also possesses a specific discriminating antigen, T3, which can be visualized by immunofluorescent staining with the appropriate monoclonal antibodies (cf. p. 91). In the mouse T-cells possess the Thy1 iso-antigenic system (watch for the old nomenclature—θ) which is acquired as the cells differentiate within the milieu of the thymus gland.

At the time of writing, the most popular means of enumerating lymphocyte populations in human blood is to use fluorescent anti-immunoglobulin for B-cells and anti-T3 or spontaneous rosette formation with neuraminidase-treated sheep erythrocytes for T-cells. Values given by these two tests usually add up to a few per cent short of 100%; without giving anything away, the remaining lymphocyte-like cells, negative on both counts, are termed 'null-cells' (figure 3.10).

For the unwearying seeker after truth, the plot diversifies. Aside from the implication above that B-cells may exist as subpopulations, only one of which bears a C3 receptor, different subsets of murine T-cells have been defined by the allelic forms of two genetic loci, Lyt1 and Lyt2. Cells destined to subserve 'helper' and 'lymphokine' activity (pp. 67 and 75 respectively) display the Lyt1 phenotype on their surface; the precursors of cytotoxic and suppressor T-cells (pp. 76 and 102) are Lyt1,2, but essentially express only the Lyt2 surface antigen as they become effector cells. In the human, monoclonal antibodies define the population bearing the T4 marker which includes the T-helper subset, and T8, which largely identifies cytotoxic/suppressor cells (cf. p. 294).

B- and T-cells can be separated by selective depletion of one or the other by rosette formation. For example, T-cells forming spontaneous sheep cell rosettes can be isolated by centrifugation over a 'density step' of Ficoll which holds back non-rosetting cells. T-lymphocytes can be recovered by mechanically disrupting the rosettes and recentrifuging over Ficoll to remove the sheep cells. Further fractionation may be effected by forming rosettes between the T-cells with Fcγ receptors and IgG-coated ox cells. Depletion of one population, say T-cells, by destruction with anti-T serum plus complement (cf. p. 163) has also been extensively employed. Another procedure involves affinity chromatography. B-lymphocytes can be selectively retained on solid phase columns to which anti-light chain is bound covalently, the effluent providing a T (+ null-cell) population virtually free of Ig-bearing B-cells; the column-bound cells can be released by elution with IgG. Passage down nylon wool columns depletes adherent T-cells and most B-

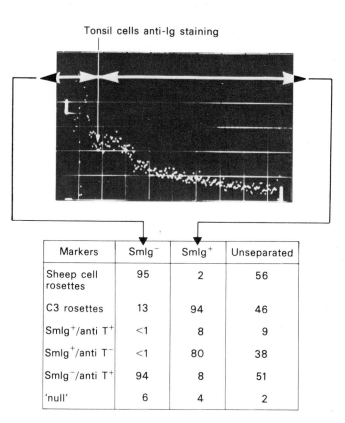

Tonsil cells anti-Ig staining

Markers	SmIg⁻	SmIg⁺	Unseparated
Sheep cell rosettes	95	2	56
C3 rosettes	13	94	46
SmIg⁺/anti T⁺	<1	8	9
SmIg⁺/anti T⁻	<1	80	38
SmIg⁻/anti T⁺	94	8	51
'null'	6	4	2

Figure 3.10. Separation of B- and T-cells from human tonsil lymphocytes by the fluorescence activated cell sorter. After staining with fluorescein-conjugated anti-Ig, the viable cells were analysed by flow cytofluorimetry to give the histogram shown (vertical axis = number of cells; horizontal axis, increasing relative fluorescence intensity). The lymphocytes were separated into a surface membrane Ig positive (SmIg⁺) and a negative (SmIg⁻) population depending upon the fluorescence intensity being either above or below the arbitrary cut-off point. Analysis of the % of cells positive for each marker (cf. p. 60) is shown. The anti-T serum was a fluorescent rabbit anti-monkey thymus made specific by absorption with B lymphoblastoid cell lines. 'Null' cells were negative with both anti-Ig and anti-T reagents. (Data kindly provided by Dr M.F. Greaves.)

lymphocytes. The prize for elegance (and expense) must go to the fluorescence activated cell sorter (FACS) designed by Herzenberg and colleagues (figure 3.10). Lymphocytes coated with fluorescently labelled antibodies directed against the surface antigens of one sub-population of cells, flow obediently in a single stream past a laser beam. Each fluorescent cell is charged and then separated from non-fluorescent and therefore uncharged cells in an electric field. The flow-through rate is approximately 10^4 cells/sec. The machine can also be used to measure the quantitative distribution of fluorescence within the lymphocyte population (flow cytofluorography).

LYMPHOCYTE SURFACE PHENOMENA

When viable B-lymphocytes are stained in the cold with a fluorescein-conjugated anti-Ig, the fluorescence is seen as

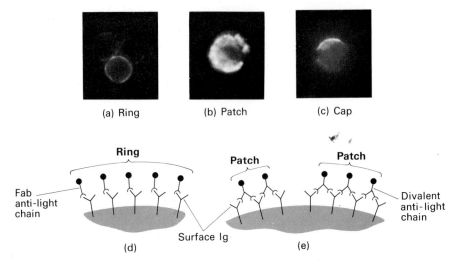

(a) Ring   (b) Patch   (c) Cap

Figure 3.11. Patterns of immunofluorescent staining of B-lymphocyte surface immunoglobulin using fluorescein-conjugated (●) anti-Ig (cf. p. 155 for discussion of technique). Provided the reaction is carried out in the cold to prevent pinocytosis, the labelled antibody cannot penetrate to the interior of the viable lymphocytes and reacts only with surface components. (a) Ring staining with monovalent (Fab) anti-Ig; (b) patch formation with whole anti-Ig; (c) cap formation on warming the cells in (b); (d) diagram of ring staining by monovalent anti-Ig; (e) diagram of patch formation by divalent anti-Ig. During cap formation, submembranous myosin becomes redistributed in association with the surface Ig and induces locomotion of the previously sessile cell in a direction away from the cap. (Photographs kindly provided by Drs A. Arnaiz-Villena & L. Hudson.)

patches on the cell surface (figure 3.11b). However, if the experiment is repeated using monovalent (Fab) anti-Ig, a smooth ring of surface fluorescence is observed (figure 3.11a). The interpretation of these findings is that the lymphocyte surface immunoglobulins are floating freely in the plasma membrane (like icebergs in a sea of lipid) and are agglutinated into little patches by the divalent anti-Ig (figure 3.11d and e). If the lymphocytes are now allowed to warm up, the patches coalesce to form a cap over one pole of the cell (figure 3.11c) and the complexes are taken into the cytoplasm by endocytosis leaving the surface free of immunoglobulin. The cell will resynthesize its surface immunoglobulin within a few hours if washed and incubated at 37° in fresh medium.

When rabbit lymphocytes are cultured in the presence of anti-Ig for a minimum of 16–20 hours, they go on to transform into blast-like cells (cf. figure 3.7c) and divide. Activation also occurs with the divalent F(ab')$_2$ pepsin fragment derived from the anti-Ig but not the monovalent Fab, with the strong implication that cross-linking and aggregation of surface Ig is an important step in B-lymphocyte stimulation, which would normally be brought about by antigen combining with complementary surface Ig receptors on those lymphocytes capable of synthesizing the appropriate antibody. However, the blast cells induced by such activation do not make antibody and current thinking is that in most circumstances additional non-specific signals are required, particularly for the triggering of antibody production by thymus-dependent antigens (i.e. those antigens which provoke a grossly depressed response in animals deprived of T-lymphocytes by neonatal thymectomy or other means: cf. p. 49).

Cellular co-operation in the antibody response

THE ROLE OF ANTIGEN-PROCESSING CELLS

The mononuclear cells of the monocyte-macrophage series have long been thought to play a central role in the induction of the immune response with respect to the presentation of antigen to lymphocytes. Studies on antibody formation in tissue culture reveal clusters of macrophages and lymphocytes with intimate cytoplasmic contacts between them; the antibody response to most antigens is largely abrogated when glass-adherent cells, predominantly macrophages, are first removed from the responding lymphoid population, and the defect can be overcome by the addition of macrophages. Furthermore, antigens such as bovine serum albumin provoke a vastly superior antibody response when injected together with adherent cells rather than as a free solution; interestingly the more thymus-dependent the response to a given antigen, the greater the enhancing effect due to these accessory cells.

Antigen trapping and concentration of antigen at the cell surface for effective presentation to the lymphocyte seems to be important. In general, when antigen is taken up by macrophages, a proportion is degraded by phagocytic digestion while part is fixed to the cell surface where it is thought to be in a strongly immunogenic state in some form of association with the Ia molecules encoded by the I region of the major histocompatibility complex (figure 3.12). Cells of the macrophage series adopt many morphological forms which vary greatly in their expression of these two mechanisms for handling antigens. Some, like the Kupffer cells of the liver, the alveolar macrophages or the lining cells of splenic cords, have well-developed lysosomal granules and are actively phagocytic. We may look upon them as 'professional phagocytes' largely destined for a life of microbe-crunching. In contrast with these men of violence, the dendritic macrophages of the lymph node cortex and skin (Langerhans' cells) are far more genteel; largely eschewing the degrading process

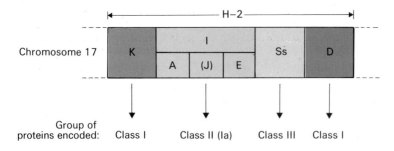

Figure 3.12. The genes encoding the major histocompatibility complex (MHC) in the mouse (designated H-2). The MHC is present in all higher vertebrates and was originally identified by Gorer through its predominant influence on the survival of grafts between mice by controlling the synthesis of 'histocompatibility' or 'transplantation' antigens which provoked violent immunological rejection (cf. p. 273). Different types of protein are encoded by the MHC genes and have been designated class I, II (the Ia antigens now being discussed) and III molecules, each class subserving different biological roles (cf. p. 295).

of phagocytosis, they prefer to incorporate antigen into their surface membranes for the more aristocratic purpose of presentation to, and activation of, lymphocytes. The large surface area of their elongated processes and high stable concentration of their membrane Ia make these cells ideal for this role. Antigen-antibody complexes formed in antigen-excess and containing the 3rd component of complement (C3b, p. 166) localize efficiently on the dendritic cells associated with lymphoid follicles where they persist for many weeks and can trap antigen-specific B-lymphocytes to generate B-cell memory. T-cells seem to communicate with a different species of dendritic macrophage, the interdigitating cell of the lymph node paracortical area; this is illustrated in figure 3.8e which shows the large area of close contact with the membranes of the surrounding T-lymphocytes rather well. Some of these, at least, derive from the dendritic Langerhans' cells of the skin which are thus able to transport antigen from the periphery for effective presentation to the lymph node T-cells. Although like conventional macrophages, the dendritic cells are derived from the bone marrow stem cells, they differ from them with respect to a number of surface markers and, of course, in their lack of phagocytic function. Indeed, one wonders whether the label 'macrophage' (literally 'big eater') should be applied at all; perhaps the term 'dendritic antigen-presenting cell' (APC) is safer and certainly more informative. Macrophages in the marginal zone of the spleen provide a further example of specialization of APC in their ability to handle certain thymus-independent antigens such as pneumococcus polysaccharide.

66

Attention has already been drawn to the fact that the antibody response to certain antigens is considerably depressed following neonatal thymectomy. However, we know from the work of Davies with chromosome (T6) marked thymus cells, that the T-lymphocytes do not themselves secrete antibody even though they actively divide after contact with antigen. This involvement of the T-lymphocyte in antibody synthesis without itself producing antibody is now seen to be due to a form of *co-operation* by the T-cell which helps the antigenic stimulation of B-lymphocytes to be more effective (figure 3.6). Using an irradiated mouse (which cannot itself make an immune response) as a 'living test-tube', Claman and his colleagues showed that thymocytes or bone marrow cells (containing B-cell precursors) injected together with sheep red cells brought about only poor or modest antibody production. When T- and B-cells were injected together, there was a very marked increase in the number of cells engaged in antibody synthesis (table 3.3).

The cellular origin of the antibody-forming cells was elegantly demonstrated by Miller and his colleagues in co-operation experiments involving transfer of T-cells and bone marrow from genetically different mouse strains. The antibody-forming cells in the recipient spleen were studied *in vitro* by the Jerne plaque technique (p. 87) and could be inhibited only by an antiserum to the transplantation antigens of the strain providing the bone marrow, *not* the thymus cells (figure 3.13).

At the molecular level, further light on the nature of co-operation has been shed by the experiments with carrier-hapten conjugates. The reader may recall that haptens are small groups which can combine with preformed antibody but fail to stimulate antibody synthesis unless coupled with an antigenic carrier (usually a protein; cf. p. 7). Both Mitchison and Rajewsky have shown that primed B-cells make a secondary antibody response to a hapten bound to protein carrier only when T-cells primed to the carrier ('helper cells') are also present (figure 3.14). In other words, when T-cells recognize and respond to carrier determinants, they help B-lymphocytes specific for the hapten to develop into

Table 3.3. Co-operation of bone marrow and thymus cells in production of antibody to sheep red cells in irradiated recipient.

Irradiated recipient given antigen plus:	Antibody response
Spleen cells	+ + +
Thymocytes (T-cells)	±
Bone marrow (B-cells)	+
Thymocytes and bone marrow	+ + +

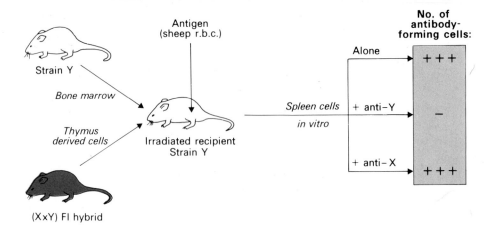

	No. of antibody-forming cells:
Alone	+++
+ anti–Y	−
+ anti–X	+++

Figure 3.13. Bone marrow origin of antibody-forming cells. Antibody-forming cells were studied in the antigen-stimulated recipient of a bone marrow/thymus mixture. Antibodies to the transplantation antigens of the strain providing bone marrow inhibited the plaque-forming cells whereas antibodies specific for the thymocyte donor were ineffective (based on Miller J.F.A.P. & Mitchell G.F. (1968) *J.exp.Med.* **128**, 821: in these studies thymus-derived cells from the thoracic duct were used).

antibody-forming cells, presumably by providing an accessory signal (figure 3.15).

SOLUBLE FACTORS IN CO-OPERATION

The mechanisms underlying co-operation are becoming clearer. They involve complex interactions between antigen-presenting macrophages, T-cells and B-cells in which association of the carrier determinants with Ia molecules of the major histocompatibility complex is crucial (figure 3.12, p. 66) and in which various soluble factors are implicated. The first stage is antigen-driven; T-helper cells activated by their interaction with antigen-presenting macrophages stimulate resting B-cells to divide in a relatively limited fashion, the daughter cells becoming blast-like (cf. figure 3.7c) and exhibiting surface receptors for B-cell growth factor (figure 3.16). Subsequent stages are independent of antigen and are driven by soluble factors derived from the helper T-cells. Thus, B-cell growth factor greatly expands the numbers of activated B-cells through reaction with their surface receptors and finally, a B-cell maturation factor brings the proliferation to a halt and instructs the progeny to become plasma cells secreting antibody.

RELEVANCE TO ANTIGENICITY

When discussing the question of antigenicity in Chapter 1 (p. 16) we were largely preoccupied with the factors governing

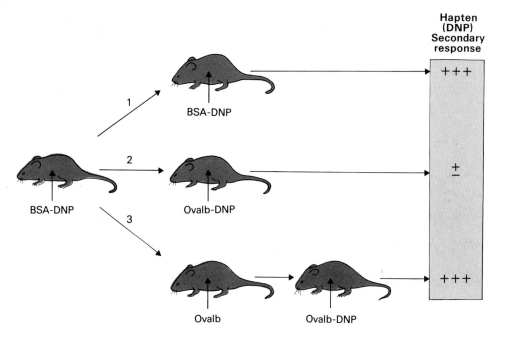

Figure 3.14. Carrier-hapten co-operation showing that a secondary response to the hapten (dinitrophenyl group—DNP) is only obtained when cells are primed to both carrier and hapten.

1 After priming with an injection of DNP linked to bovine serum albumin (BSA) as a carrier, later inoculation with the same BSA–DNP combination gives a secondary response to DNP.

2 If the primed animals are challenged instead with DNP on a different carrier, ovalbumin, there is no secondary response.

3 However, if animals primed with BSA–DNP are further primed with ovalbumin, challenge with Ovalb–DNP will now give a secondary response. Similar results can be obtained using lymphoid cell transfers from primed animals into irradiated recipients. The 'helper-cells' with specificity for the carrier can be shown to be T-cells by the use of anti-Thy1 serum or thymectomized donors.

Figure 3.15. T-B *co-operation*. The T-cells on recognizing carrier determinants on the antigen provide a co-operative signal which activates B-cells that recognize hapten and enables them to mature into antibody-secreting plasma cells. Co-operation only occurs when the carrier and hapten determinants are covalently linked, strongly suggesting that the antigen acts as a 'bridge' between the T-helper and the B-cell.

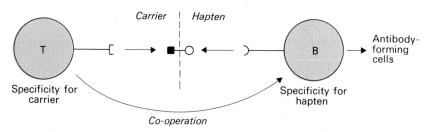

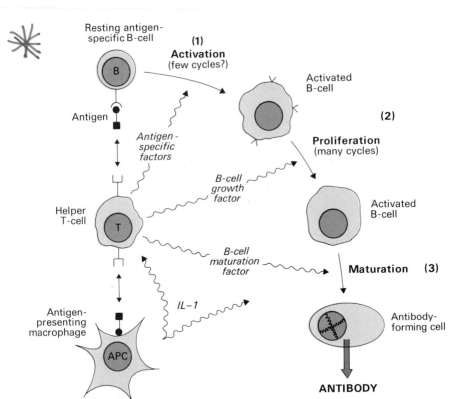

Figure 3.16. T-B co-operation in the response to a carrier-hapten (■—●). Stage 1—*Activation*: helper T-cells activated by the soluble factor interleukin-1 (IL-1) produced by their interaction with the antigen-presenting macrophage, stimulate the resting antigen-specific B-cell through an antigen 'bridge' and drive it into a few cycles of division with the help of antigen-specific soluble factors, giving rise to daughter blast cells with surface receptors for B-cell growth factor (<). Stage 2—*Proliferation*: these cells now undergo extensive division under the influence of B-cell growth factor produced by activated T-helpers. Stage 3—*Maturation*: finally these cells are switched from division into antibody production by B-cell maturation factor, a further soluble mediator produced by the helper T-cell. Stage 1 is antigen-specific and involves restriction by the major histocompatibility Ia molecules (cf. figure 4.6); stages 2 and 3 are not antigen-specific or Ia restricted.

the shape of the antigenic determinant and its fit with the antibody site without considering the initiation of an antibody response. If a single determinant binds to a B-lymphocyte surface receptor, no cross-linking will result (figure 3.17a) and the cell will not be activated (remember the definition of a hapten—combines with antibody but will not stimulate antibody synthesis). Certain linear antigens which are not readily degraded in the body and which have an appropriately spaced, highly repeating determinant— pneumococcus polysaccharide, D-amino acid polymers and polyvinylpyrrolidine for example—are thymus independent in that they can stimulate B-cells directly without the need

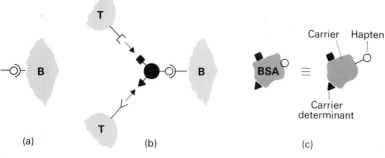

(a)   (b)   (c)

Carrier   Hapten

Carrier
determinant

Figure 3.17. Response to a simple protein antigen looked at from the carrier-hapten standpoint. A small protein such as bovine serum albumin has several determinants but all are different, so that the molecule itself cannot cross-link B-cell receptors and therefore behaves as a monovalent hapten with respect to each determinant (cf. (a)). Only if other determinants can be recognized by T-cells can appropriate co-operation be provided for B-cell stimulation (b). Thus the determinants on the protein act in a 'carrier' function for each other (c).

for T-cell help. They persist on the surface of the antigen-specific B-cell to which they bind with great avidity through their multivalent attachment (cf. p. 14) to the specific Ig receptors, thereby causing cross-linking and the stimulation of IgM but not IgG antibody synthesis (figure 3.18a; critical matrix model). Other antigens such as bacterial lipopolysaccharide with inherent mitogenic activity may also trigger IgM-producing cells independently of T-cells by binding passively to the surface immunoglobulin and providing an activation signal through a mitogen receptor on the B-cell (figure 3.18b; non-specific activation model).

Antigens which cannot fulfil the molecular requirements for direct stimulation must use their other determinants as carriers (figure 3.17b) to evoke an accessory signal through T-cell co-operation (figure 3.18c). Such help from the T-cell must be even more essential for those cases where a determinant appears only once on each molecule, thereby acting in effect as a monovalent hapten. This will usually be the case with proteins which have little or no symmetry such as bovine serum albumin where it will be appreciated that each determinant can only activate its specific B-cell by calling upon the carrier function of the others (figure 3.17c). To a first approximation larger molecules tend to be better antigens because they have more determinants capable of acting as carriers. Where an animal lacks T-cells capable of recognizing potential carrier determinants there will be a correspondingly poor response to the hapten even if hapten-specific B-cells are present. T-cell participation, possibly involving isotype-specific T-helpers, appears to be mandatory for the switch from the synthesis of IgM to antibodies of IgG and other classes, while activated B-cells

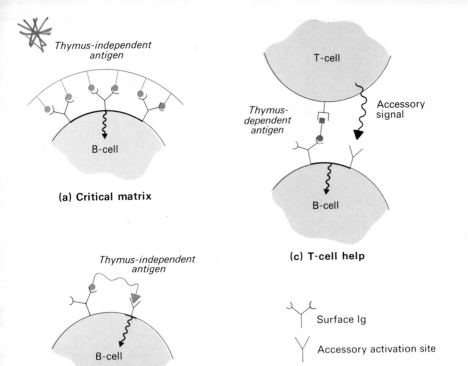

(a) Critical matrix

(c) T-cell help

(b) Non-specific activation

Surface Ig

Accessory activation site

Figure 3.18. Models of B-cell triggering. (a) Thymus independent antigen (TI-Ag) with repeating determinants trigger the cell by forming a critically spaced matrix of cross-linked immunoglobulin receptors; an Lyb 3^+5^+ B-cell subset responds to these antigens and was recognized through its absence in CBA/N mice which have a sex-linked immunodeficient (xid) response to polysaccharide antigens. (b) Thymus-independent antigen with inherent poly-clonal activating ability is focused on the B-cell through the immunoglobulin recep-tors. (c) Thymus-dependent antigen binds to surface immunoglobulin receptors and the carrier determinants are recognized together with the major histocompatibility Ia molecules (p. 66), by T-cells which provide an accessory stimulating signal. The importance of Ig receptors as active participants in the triggering process is seen by the proliferation induced by anti-Ig (cf. p. 64) and by the fact that *resting* B-cells from male animals cannot be stimulated by the accessory signal provided by T-helpers specific for the male antigen on the B-cell surface, anti-Ig again being required. Bret-scher & Cohn have suggested that the signal through Ig receptors alone without T-cell help tolerizes the cell (cf. p. 115).

bearing a regulatory idiotype can be expanded by anti-idiotype helpers (cf. figure 4.15, p. 109).

The cell-mediated immune response

Immunity to those infectious organisms which have devel-oped the capacity for living and multiplying *within* the cells of the host is masterminded by the T-lymphocytes indepen-dently of the B-cells. Thus infections with intracellular facul-tative parasites such as tubercle and leprosy bacilli, budding viruses like smallpox and parasites such as *Toxoplasma*, pose serious problems for children with thymic insufficiency in contrast to infants with primary immunoglobulin deficiency who cope relatively well with these organisms. Support for this view is also afforded by studies on thymectomized and bursectomized chicks and by the demonstration that T-cells from mice which had recovered from infection with TB could passively confer immunity on previously uninfected animals into which they had been injected (cf. figure 7.12).

THE ACTIVATION OF T-CELLS

The T-cells are antigen-sensitive in that they show specificity for antigen in their response to carriers, in delayed hypersensitivity reactions and in their cytotoxicity for virally infected cells or allogeneic (cf. p. 76) targets. The fact that such cytotoxic cells can be specifically adsorbed on to fibroblasts bearing the transplantation antigens to which the animal was initially sensitized clearly indicates that T-cells do have surface receptors which recognize antigen, although it must be said that the nature of these receptors is still hotly debated. The presence of binding sites on different T-lymphocytes for $Fc\gamma$ and $Fc\mu$ led to the inevitable suggestion that the antigen receptors were nothing more than exogenously acquired cytophilic antibody, but the ability of neonatally bursectomized chickens and of a-γ-globulinaemic children to mount specific cell-mediated hypersensitivity responses is powerful evidence that T-cells possess their own endogenous receptors independently of B-cells and their products. This view is reinforced by the phenomenon of selective T-cell tolerance (p. 113) and clinched by the experimental isolation of numerous antigen-specific T-cell clones and hybridomas (p. 94) in each of which a population of identical T-cells derived from a single parent (just as myeloma cells are progeny of a single B-cell) can be propagated in tissue culture and shown to be stimulated selectively by the antigen which triggered the original parent cell; in other words, T-cells maintain their antigen-specific responses even after prolonged cell division *in vitro* in the absence of B-cells.

The nature of the T-cell receptor will be discussed more extensively in Chapters 5 and 9. Suffice it to say now that it is not a conventional Ig molecule and that a curious feature is its ability to recognize antigen in association with Ia molecules of the major histocompatibility complex (p. 66) on the surface of the antigen-presenting macrophage. This contact between the cells leads to release of the soluble mediator interleukin-1 (IL-1) from the macrophage which synergizes with the signal received through the T-cell receptor to activate the lymphocytes. The early stages of T-cell activation

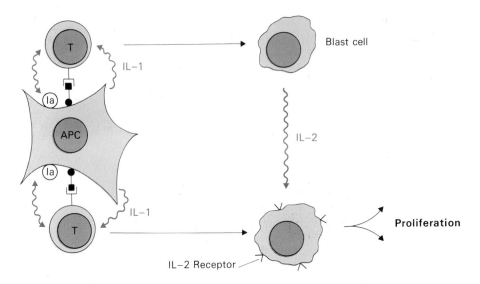

Figure 3.19. Initiation of the cell-mediated immune response. Recognition of the antigen (●—■)-Ia complex on the antigen-presenting macrophage (APC) by the T-cell receptor, leads to mutual interaction of macrophage and resting T-cell which becomes activated through the synergistic action of interleukin-1. The expression of interleukin-2 receptors on activated blasts allows them to undergo proliferative expansion under the influence of IL-2 produced by another activated T-subpopulation.

involve a calcium-mediated increase in the intracellular cGMP concentration although the details are not yet ready to be engraved on tablets of stone. The influx of extracellular calcium ions is thought to bring about the release of arachidonic acid from phosphatidyl inositol by stimulation of a membrane phospholipase; arachidonic acid in turn can be metabolically converted via the lipoxygenase pathway to the hydroperoxyeicosatetranoic acids (HPETEs), their hydroxy-forms (HETEs) and leukotriene B$_4$ which can stimulate guanylate cyclase. The increased cGMP together with calcium ions derepresses the appropriate genes in the resting lymphocyte nucleus and new synthesis of RNA and protein occurs, producing blast-like cells with nuclear and cytoplasmic enlargement (figure 3.7c) and surface receptors for a soluble T-cell growth factor known as interleukin-2 (IL-2). Similar events, in what is probably a separate T-subset, spark off the production of IL-2 itself which will, of course, act to expand the blasts bearing IL-2 receptors (figure 3.19). We know there to be several different T-cell subpopulations specialized to deal with various immune effector functions. Consequent upon activation, one or more of these subpopulations releases a number of soluble factors, another develops cytotoxic powers while a proportion become memory cells which can give an enhanced secondary response just like primed

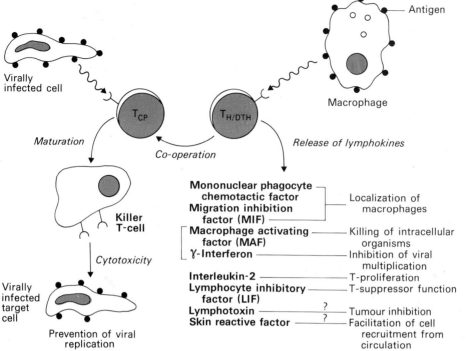

Figure 3.20. The cell-mediated immune response. This operates through the generation of cytotoxic T-cells and the release of lymphokines through the stimulation of two distinct T-subpopulations, the cytotoxic cell precursor (T_{CP}) and the T-helper/inducer/delayed type hypersensitivity cells ($T_{H/DTH}$) which themselves can probably be divided into functional subsets. Different lymphokines may be produced by different lymphocyte subsets. The intense proliferation induced by antigenic stimulation has not been shown but is an essential factor in the amplification of the response.

B-cells; together, these phenomena form the basis of cell-mediated immunity.

THE TWO ARMS OF THE CELL-MEDIATED RESPONSE

Proliferation and differentiation of the stimulated T-cells provides the mechanism for amplification of the cell-mediated immune response which depends upon these two major effector mechanisms—the generation of cytotoxic cells and the release of biologically active soluble factors (termed 'lymphokines' by Dumonde) which modulate the behaviour of other cells, particularly the mononuclear phagocytes (monocytes and macrophages) (figure 3.20).

Lymphokines

The supernatant fluid recovered after stimulating sensitized lymphocytes with antigen possesses several biological activities, some of which have been ascribed to different molecular species. These lymphokines have molecular weights of the order of 20,000–80,000. Among them is a group which directly influences the movement and activity of macrophages. *Macrophage chemotactic factor* causes an accumulation of mononuclear phagocytes at the site of antigen-mediated lymphokine release; this can be demonstrated in Boyden chambers where monocytes or macrophages move across Millipore membranes into the chamber containing higher concentrations of factor. Once attracted, the cells are discouraged from leaving by macrophage *migration inhibition factor* (MIF); interaction with the cells appears to involve a fucose residue on MIF and a useful control for its assay is abrogation of a positive test by added fucose. Stimulation by *macrophage activating factor* (MAF) produces significant morphological changes with a ruffling of the surface membrane which gives the cell an 'angry' appearance, and leads to an increase in lysosomal enzyme content and a heightened ability to kill off ingested intracellular organisms. The movement of monocytes from blood vessels into the extravascular spaces is facilitated by another lymphokine, the *skin reactive factor* which also increases capillary permeability. *Immune* or *γ-interferon*, which inhibits intracellular viral replication, is identical with MAF.

The role of IL-2 in expanding T-cell populations has already been alluded to but another lymphokine *lymphocyte inhibitory factor* (LIF), which inhibits the proliferation of lymphocytes could well be related to T-suppressor function. *Lymphotoxin*, although only mildly cytolytic for certain cultured cell lines, showed quite marked cytostatic activity and one is tempted to postulate a role in the constraint of tumour growth. Other biological activities which have been ascribed to lymphokines include effects on the migration and adhesiveness of polymorphs and eosinophils and on the aggregation of platelets.

Cytotoxic T-cells

Viral infection can generate a population of killer T-cells which are specifically cytotoxic for host cells infected with that virus. Similarly, a graft from a genetically dissimilar member of the same species (allogeneic graft) provokes the formation of cytotoxic T-cells directed against target cells bearing the major histocompatibility antigens of the donor. Just as B-cells require growth and maturation factors from helper T-cells, so precursors of cytotoxic T-cells are clonally expanded by IL-2 after activation by antigen and develop into killer cells under the influence of a distinct maturation factor.

The first stage in the killing sequence, which may be followed *in vitro*, involves intimate binding of effector to target through recognition of the target antigens by surface receptors on the T-cell; this stage is Ca^{2+} independent and cytochalasin B sensitive. Within a matter of minutes, a change occurs in the target cell, a 'kiss of death' so to speak, which leads irrevocably to cytolysis; this phase is Ca^{2+} dependent and cytochalasin insensitive. Thus by carrying out the binding step in the absence of Ca^{2+} and then allowing cytolysis to proceed by adding Ca^{2+} and cytochalasin (which inhibits cell movement and prevents binding to further target cells), each cytotoxic cell should theoretically lyse only one target. Enumeration of cytotoxic T-cells, by counting the number of killed allogeneic targets in this way, gives an estimate of approximately 1% of the spleen lymphocytes. This high proportion of cells committed to each major histocompatibility specificity is striking and implies a special relationship between T-cells and such antigens. In this context it should be noted that effective killing is only seen when the T-cells are sensitized to molecules (usually class I; figure 3.12) of the major histocompatibility complex or a determinant (e.g. viral) recognized in association with these molecules (cf. p. 293).

The anatomical basis of the immune response

The complex cellular interactions which form the basis of the immune response take place within the organized architecture of peripheral, or secondary, lymphoid tissue which includes the lymph glands, spleen and unencapsulated tissue lining the respiratory, alimentary and genito-urinary tracts.

LYMPH NODE

The encapsulated tissue of the lymph node contains a meshwork of reticular cells and their fibres organized into sinuses. These act as a filter for lymph draining the body tissues and possibly bearing foreign antigens which enters the subcapsular sinus by the afferent vessels and diffuses past the lymphocytes in the cortex to reach the macrophages of the medullary sinuses (figure 3.21d) and thence the efferent lymphatics (figures 3.1 and 3.21a). What is so striking about the organization of the lymph node is that the T- and B-lymphocytes are very largely separated into different anatomical compartments.

B-cell areas

The follicular aggregations of B-lymphocytes are a prominent feature of the outer cortex. In the unstimulated node

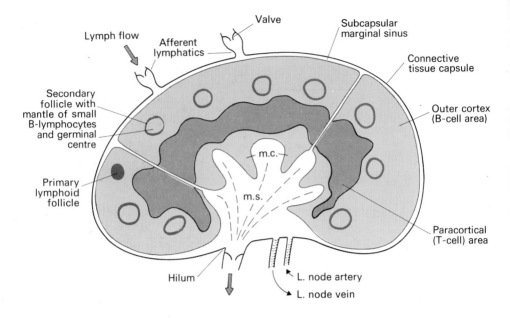

Valve
Lymph flow
Afferent lymphatics
Subcapsular marginal sinus
Connective tissue capsule
Secondary follicle with mantle of small B-lymphocytes and germinal centre
Outer cortex (B-cell area)
m.c.
m.s.
Primary lymphoid follicle
Paracortical (T-cell) area
Hilum
L. node artery
L. node vein

m.c. Medullary cords
m.s. Medullary sinuses

(a)

Figure 3.21. Lymph node. (a) Diagrammatic representation. (b) Human lymph node, low power view. (c) Medulla stained with methyl green pyronin to show the basophilic (pink) cytoplasm of the plasma cells with their abundant ribosomes. (d) Medullary sinus of lymph node draining site of lithium carmine injection showing macrophages which have phagocytosed the colloidal dye. (e) Node from mouse immunized with the thymus-independent antigen, pneumococcus polysaccharide SIII, revealing prominent stimulation of secondary follicles with germinal centres. (f) Methyl green pyronin stain of lymph node draining site of skin painted with the contact sensitizer oxazolone, highlighting the generalized expansion and activation of the paracortical (T-cell) area, the T-blasts being strongly basophilic. (g) The same study in a neonatally thymectomized mouse shows a lonely primary nodule (follicle) with complete lack of cellular response in the paracortical area.
SS, subcapsular sinus; PN, primary nodule; SF, secondary follicle; LM, lymphocyte mantle of SF; GC, germinal centre; PA, paracortical area; MC, medullary cords; MS, medullary sinus; PC, plasma cell; SM, sinusoidal macrophage. ((b) photographed by Dr P.M. Lydyard, (c) photographed by Dr K.A. MacLennan, (d) courtesy of Anatomy Dept., Middlesex Hospital Medical School, (e), (f) and (g) courtesy of Dr M. de Sousa and Prof. D.M.V. Parrott.)

they are present as spherical collections of cells termed *primary nodules* but after antigenic challenge they form *secondary follicles* (figure 8.6, p. 224) which consist of a corona or mantle of concentrically packed resting small B-lymphocytes surrounding a pale-staining *germinal centre* which contains large, often proliferating, B-blasts, scattered conventional reticular macrophages and the specialized dendritic macrophages with elongated cytoplasmic processes and few, if any, lysosomes. Germinal centres are greatly enlarged

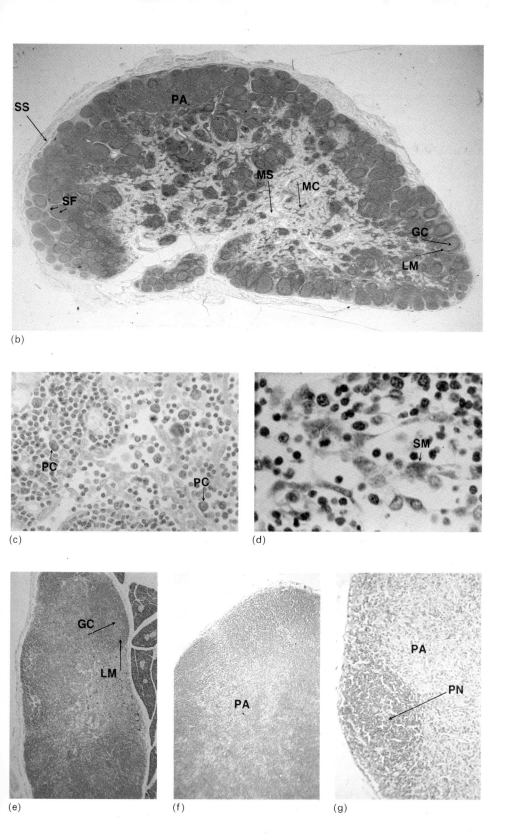

(b)

(c)

(d)

(e)

(f)

(g)

in secondary antibody responses and it is reasonable to regard them as important sites of B-cell memory. Following antigenic stimulation, differentiating plasmablasts appear and become plasma cells in the medullary cords of lymphoid cells which project between the medullary sinuses (figure 3.21c). The remainder of the outer cortex is also essentially a B-cell area with scattered T-cells.

T-cell areas

T-cells are largely confined to a region of the node referred to as the paracortical (or thymus-dependent) area (figure 3.21a); if one looks at nodes taken from children with selective T-cell deficiency (figure 8.6) or neonatally thymectomized mice (figure 3.21g), the paracortical region is seen to be virtually devoid of lymphocytes. Furthermore, when a T-cell-mediated response is elicited in a normal animal, say by a skin graft or by painting chemicals such as picryl chloride on the skin to induce contact hypersensitivity, there is a marked proliferation of cells in the thymus-dependent area and typical lymphoblasts are evident (figure 3.21f). In contrast, stimulation of antibody formation by the thymus-independent antigen, pneumococcus polysaccharide SIII, leads to proliferation in the cortical lymphoid follicles with development of germinal centres while the paracortical region remains inactive reflecting the inability to develop cellular hypersensitivity to the polysaccharide (figure 3.21e). As would be expected, nodes taken from children with congenital hypogammaglobulinaemia associated with failure of B-cell development are conspicuously lacking in primary and secondary follicular structures. This segregation of B- and T-lymphocyte areas tends to favour models of co-operation which involve soluble factors rather than antigen-bridging of T- and B-cells but the separation of cell types is not absolute.

Lymphocyte traffic

Lymphocytes enter the node through the afferent lymphatics and by passage across the specialized cuboidal epithelium of the postcapillary venules (cf. figure 3.1). This traffic of lymphocytes between the tissues, the bloodstream and the lymph glands enables antigen-sensitive cells to seek the antigen and to be recruited to sites at which a response is occurring, while the dissemination of memory cells and their progeny enables a more widespread response to be organized throughout the lymphoid system. Thus, antigen-reactive cells are depleted from the circulating pool of lymphocytes within 24 hours of antigen first localizing in the lymph nodes or spleen; several days later, after proliferation at the site of antigen localization, a peak of activated cells appears in the thoracic duct. When antigen reaches a node in a primed animal, there is a dramatic fall in the output of cells in the efferent lymphatics, a phenomenon described variously as 'cell shutdown' or 'lymphocyte trapping' and which probably results from the antigen-induced release of a T-cell soluble factor (cf. the lymphokines, p. 75); this is followed by an output of activated blast cells which peaks at around 80 hours.

SPLEEN

On a fresh section of spleen, the lymphoid tissue forming the white pulp is seen as circular or elongated grey areas within the erythrocyte-filled red pulp consisting of splenic cords lined with macrophages and venous sinusoids. As in the lymph node, T- and B-cell areas are segregated (figure 3.22). The spleen is a very effective blood filter removing effete red and white cells and responding actively to blood-borne antigens, the more so if particulate. Plasmablasts and mature plasma cells are present in the marginal zone extending into the red pulp.

UNENCAPSULATED LYMPHOID TISSUE

The respiratory, alimentary and genito-urinary tracts are guarded immunologically by subepithelial accumulations of lymphoid tissue which are not constrained by a connective tissue capsule. These may occur as diffuse collections of lymphocytes, plasma cells and phagocytes throughout the lamina propria of the intestinal wall with only isolated solitary follicles (figure 3.23a) or as more clearly organized tissue with well-formed follicles (figure 3.23b). In man, the latter includes the lingual, palatine and pharyngeal tonsils, the small intestinal Peyer's patches and the appendix. It has been suggested that the unencapsulated lymphoid tissue forms a separate interconnected system, the mucosal-associated lymphoid tissue (MALT), within which cells committed to IgA or IgE synthesis may circulate.

In the gut, cells leave the Peyer's patches, presumably after antigenic stimulation, and ultimately drain into the blood from the thoracic duct and pass into the lamina propria where many become IgA-forming cells. This maturation of antibody-forming cells at a site distant from that at which antigen triggering has occurred is seen in the lymph node where plasma cells develop in the medullary cords and the spleen where they are found predominantly in the marginal zone. My guess is that this movement of cells acts to prevent the generation of high local concentrations of antibody in the

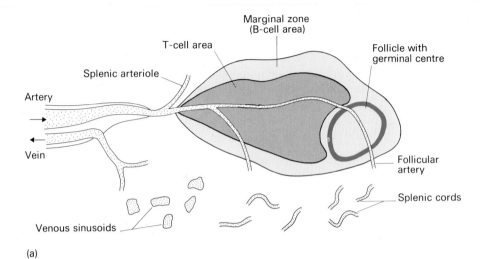

(a)

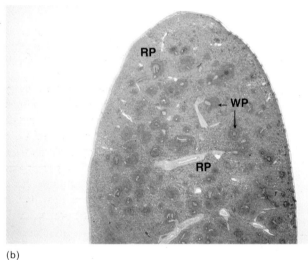

(b)

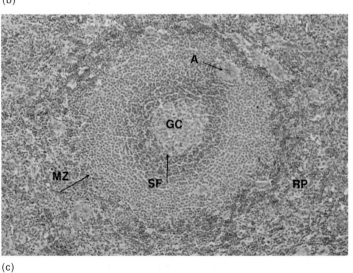

(c)

Figure 3.22.
Spleen. (a) Dia-
grammatic rep-
resentation. (b)
Low power view
showing lymphoid
white pulp (WP)
and red pulp (RP).
(c) High power
view of secondary
follicle (SF) with
germinal centre
(GC) surrounded
by periarteriolar
(T-cell) lymphoid
tissue, showing
arteriole (A), mar-
ginal zone (MZ)
and red pulp (RP).
((b) Photographed
by Dr P.M.
Lydyard and (c) by
Dr K.A. MacLen-
nan.)

82

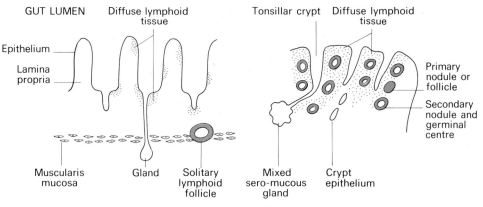

GUT LUMEN   Diffuse lymphoid tissue   Tonsillar crypt   Diffuse lymphoid tissue

Epithelium

Lamina propria

Muscularis mucosa   Gland   Solitary lymphoid follicle

Primary nodule or follicle

Secondary nodule and germinal centre

Mixed sero-mucous gland   Crypt epithelium

(a) Diffuse lymphoid tissue in lamina propria   (b) Well-formed lymphoid tissue of a tonsil

Figure 3.23. Unencapsulated lymphoid tissue.

region of the macrophage-processed antigen to avoiding neutralization of the antigen and premature shutting off of the immune response.

A few days after a secondary response, activated memory B-cells can be shown to migrate to the bone marrow where they mature into plasma cells. Bone marrow is a much neglected site of antibody synthesis which proves to be a major source of serum Ig contributing up to 80% of the total Ig secreting cells in the 100 week-old mouse. The peripheral lymphoid tissue responds rapidly to antigen, but only for a relatively short time, whereas bone marrow starts slowly and gives a long-lasting massive production of antibody to antigens which repeatedly challenge the host.

Summary

Lymphocytes mediate adaptive immune responses which involve a first phase of induction or activation, a second phase of clonal proliferation and a final phase in which a proportion of the lymphocytes become effector cells and the remainder an expanded population of memory cells able to provide secondary responses. T-lymphocytes, which mature under the influence of the thymus, mediate cellular immunity and B-lymphocytes, which mature in the bone marrow in mammals (bursa of Fabricius in birds), become antibody-forming cells responsible for humoral immunity. T- and B-cells are recognized by different surface markers: human T-cells form rosettes with sheep erythrocytes and have the T3 marker, while B-cells have surface Ig which functions as a receptor for antigen.

Macrophages, particularly the dendritic form, present

antigen together with class II(Ia) molecules of the major histocompatibility complex on their surface for reacting with and triggering antigen-sensitive lymphocytes. In the thymus-dependent response to a hapten linked to an immunogenic carrier, T-cells reacting to the carrier help B-cells to be triggered by the hapten to form anti-hapten antibody. In the response to a typical protein, one determinant is like a hapten combining with the B-cell surface Ig receptor, and the remaining determinants act as carrier to which the T-cell binds. The B-cell is activated by synergistic signals from its Ig receptor and the T-cell and then, under the influence of B-cell growth factor and B-cell maturation factor provided by the T-cell, sequentially undergoes proliferation and maturation to produce a clone of antibody-forming cells. Poorly digested, linear, highly polymeric antigens such as pneumococcus polysaccharide, and antigens with inherent polyclonal activating ability like bacterial lipopolysaccharide, can stimulate IgM-producing B-cells directly without T-cell help and are termed thymus-independent antigens. Normally, T-cells are needed for the switch to production of antibodies of IgG and other classes.

Cell-mediated immunity, which provides the main defence against intracellular organisms, depends upon the interaction of specific receptors (not conventional Ig) on the surface of T-lymphocytes with antigen in association with Ia molecules of the major histocompatibility complex on the surface of antigen-presenting macrophages. The T-cells are activated by the combination of antigen and macrophage-derived interleukin-1, and are expanded by a T-cell growth factor, interleukin-2, produced by a subpopulation of the activated T-cells. One set of effector T-cells elaborate soluble factors (lymphokines) which are concerned with the provision of 'help' for T- and B-lymphocytes, the recruitment and activation of cells of the mononuclear-phagocytic system and the inhibition of viral replication; another population becomes cytotoxic for target cells bearing the antigen.

The immune response occurs most effectively in structured secondary lymphoid tissue. The lymph nodes filter and screen lymph flowing from the body tissues while spleen filters the blood. B- and T-cell areas are separated. B-cell structures appear in the lymph node cortex as primary follicles or secondary follicles with germinal centres after antigen stimulation; T-cells occupy the paracortical area; plasma cells synthesizing antibody appear in medullary cords which penetrate the macrophage-lined medullary sinuses. Lymphoid tissue guarding the G.I. tract is unencapsulated and somewhat structured (tonsils, Peyer's patches, appendix) or present as diffuse cellular collections in the lamina propria. Together with the subepithelial accumulations of cells lining the respiratory and genito-urinary tracts, they form the so-called mucosal-associated lymphoid tissue system. Bone marrow is a major site of antibody production.

Further reading

See references at the end of Chapter 4.

4

The Immune Response
II—Further Aspects

Synthesis of humoral antibody

DETECTION OF ANTIBODY-FORMING CELLS

Immunofluorescence

Cells containing antibody within their cytoplasm can be identified by the 'sandwich' technique (see figure 6.11c). For example, a cell making antibodies to tetanus toxoid if treated first with the antigen will subsequently bind a fluorescein labelled anti-tetanus antibody and can then be visualized in the fluorescence microscope (cf. figure 3.7h).

Plaque techniques

Antibody-secreting cells can be counted by diluting them in an environment in which the antibody formed by each individual cell produces a readily observable effect. In one of the most widely used techniques, developed from the original method of Jerne and Nordin, the cells from an animal immunized with sheep erythrocytes are suspended together with an excess of sheep red cells and complement within a shallow chamber formed between two microscope slides. On incubation the antibody-forming cells release their immunoglobulin which coats the surrounding erythrocytes. The complement (cf. p. 163) will then cause lysis of the coated cells and a plaque clear of red cells will be seen around each antibody-forming cell (figure 4.1). Direct plaques obtained in this way largely reveal IgM producers since this antibody has a high haemolytic efficiency. To demonstrate IgG synthesizing cells it is necessary to increase the complement binding of the erythrocyte-IgG antibody complex by adding a rabbit anti-IgG serum; this develops the 'indirect plaques' and can be used to enumerate cells making antibodies in different immunoglobulin subclasses, provided the appropriate rabbit antisera are available. The method can be extended by coating an antigen such as pneumococcus polysaccharide on to the red cell, or by coupling hapten groups to the erythrocyte surface.

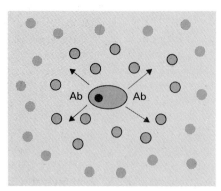

Secreted antibody coats surrounding red cells

(a)

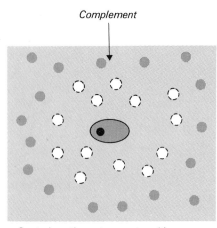

Complement

Coated erythrocytes are lysed by complement to form plaque with antibody-forming cell at centre

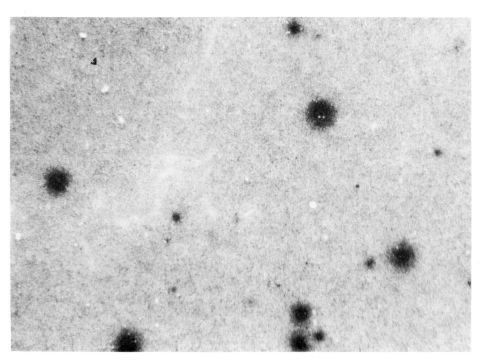

(b)

Figure 4.1. Jerne plaque technique for enumerating antibody-forming cells (Cunningham modification). (a) The direct technique for cells synthesizing IgM haemolysin is shown. The indirect technique for visualizing cells producing IgG haemolysins requires the addition of anti-IgG to the system. The difference between the plaques obtained by direct and indirect methods gives the number of 'IgG' plaques. (b) Photograph of plaques which show as circular dark areas under dark-ground illumination (courtesy of Mr C. Shapland, Ms P. Hutchings & Dr D. Male).

In the normal antibody-forming cell there is a rapid turnover of light chains which are present in slight excess. Defective control occurs in many myeloma cells and one may see excessive production of light chains or complete suppression of heavy chain synthesis. Interchain disulphide bridges may form while the heavy chains are still attached to the ribosomes (figure 4.2) but the sequence in which the intermediates arise varies with the nature of the immunoglobulin. Using 'pulse and chase' techniques with radioactive amino acids it was found that the build-up of both light and heavy chains proceeds continuously starting from the N-terminal end. Furthermore, isolation of the mRNA for each type of chain has shown them to be of appropriate size to allow synthesis of the complete peptides. The evidence is, therefore, against the view that either chain can be formed by joining together two preformed lengths of peptide and it is now thought that the messenger regions for variable and constant regions are spliced together before leaving the nucleus.

ABNORMAL IMMUNOGLOBULIN SYNTHESIS

In Chapter 2 we discussed the production of unique monoclonal immunoglobulins in multiple myeloma where there is an uncontrolled proliferation of a single clone of Ig-

Figure 4.2. Synthesis of mouse IgG2a immunoglobulin. As the H-chains near completion, adjacent peptide chains can spontaneously cross-link through their constant regions. It is thought that the light chains may aid release of the terminal chains from the ribosome by forming the L–H–H molecule. Combination with a further light chain would yield the full immunoglobulin L–H–H–L (based on Askonas B.A. & Williamson A.R. (1968) *Biochem. J.* **109**, 637). The order in which the interchain disulphide bridges are formed varies in different immunoglobulins depending on the relative strengths of the bonds as assessed by susceptibility to reduction.

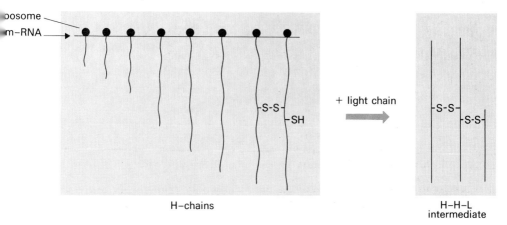

ribosome
m–RNA

–S–S–
–SH

+ light chain

–S–S–
–S–S–

H–chains

H–H–L
intermediate

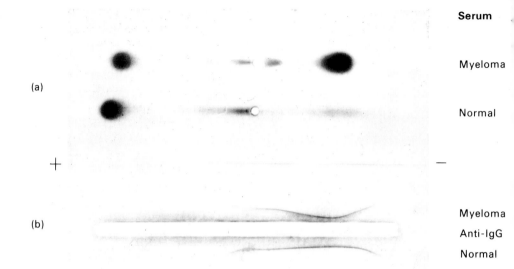

Myeloma

(a)

Normal

+   −

Myeloma

(b)   Anti-IgG

Normal

Figure 4.3. Myeloma serum with an 'M' component. (a) Agar gel electrophoresis showing strong band in γ-globulin region. (b) Immunoelectrophoresis against anti- IgG serum revealing the 'bump' or 'bow' in the precipitin arc. (Courtesy Dr F.C. Hay.)

producing plasma cells. IgG, IgA, IgD and IgE myeloma has been reported in frequencies which parallel their serum concentration; Waldenström's macroglobulinaemia represents a closely comparable situation involving monoclonal IgM production. The myeloma or 'M' component in serum is recognized as a tight band on paper electrophoresis (all molecules in the clone are of course identical and have the same mobility) and as an abnormal arc on immunoelectrophoresis with a 'bump' caused by the monoclonal protein (figure 4.3a and b). 'M' bands have been found in the sera of a number of individuals who have no clinical signs of myeloma; the comparative rarity with which invasive multiple myeloma develops in these people and the constant level of the monoclonal protein over a period of years suggests the presence of benign tumours of the lymphocyte-plasma cell series.

Amyloid Between 10 and 20% of patients with myeloma develop widespread amyloid deposits which contain the variable region of the myeloma light chain. Being identical, the variable region fragments polymerize and form the characteristic amyloid fibrils which are recognizable by their green birefringence on staining with Congo Red. Other components in amyloid have not yet been characterized. The fibrils are relatively resistant to digestion and accumulate in the ground substance of connective tissue where they can lead to pathological changes in the kidneys, heart and brain. Amyloid can also be formed secondarily to chronic inflammatory conditions such as rheumatoid arthritis and familial Mediterranean fever but in this case involves the polymerization of a unique substance, Amyloid A (AA) protein derived from the N-terminal part of a serum precursor (SAA) of molecular weight 90,000. SAA behaves as an acute phase protein in that its concentration increases rapidly in response to tissue injury or inflammation. Levels rise with age and the minority of individuals with high values are those most likely to develop amyloid.

Heavy chain disease is a rare condition in which quantities of abnormal heavy chains are excreted in the urine—γ-chains in association with malignant lymphoma and α-chains in cases of abdominal lymphoma with diffuse lympho-plasmacytic infiltration of the small intestine. The amino acid sequences of the N-terminal regions of these heavy chains are normal but they have a deletion extending from part of the variable domain through most of the C_{H1} region so that they lack the structure required to form cross-links to the light chains. One idea is that the defect arises through faulty coupling of V and C region genes (cf. p. 135).

MONOCLONAL ANTIBODIES

A fantastic technological revolution has been achieved by Milstein and Köhler who devised a technique for the production of 'immortal' clones of cells making single antibody specificities by fusing normal antibody-forming cells with an appropriate B-cell tumour line. These so-called 'hybridomas' are selected out in a tissue culture medium which fails to support growth of the parental cell types, and by successive dilutions or by plating out, single clones can be established (figure 4.4). These clones can be propagated in spinner culture or grown up in the ascitic form in mice when quite prodigious titres of monoclonal antibody can be attained. Remember that even in a good antiserum, over 90% of the Ig molecules have little or no avidity for the antigen, and the 'specific antibodies' themselves represent a whole spectrum of molecules with different avidities directed against different determinants on the antigen. What a contrast is provided by the monoclonal antibodies where all the molecules produced by a given hybridoma are identical (figure 4.5): they have the same Ig class and allotype, the same variable region, structure, idiotype, affinity and specificity for a given epitope.

Whereas the large amount of non-specific relative to antigen-specific Ig in an antiserum means that background binding to antigen in any given immunological test may be uncomfortably high, the problem is greatly reduced with a monoclonal antibody preparation since all the Ig is antibody, thus giving a much superior 'signal : noise' ratio. By being directed towards single epitopes on the antigen, monoclonal antibodies frequently show high specificity in terms of their low cross-reactivity with other antigens. Occasionally,

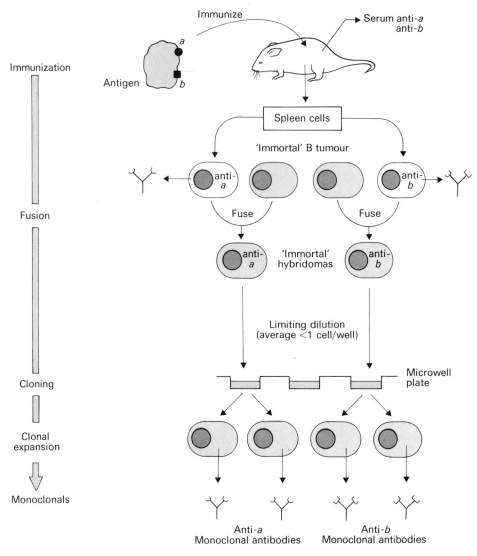

Figure 4.4. Production of monoclonal antibodies. Mice immunized with an antigen bearing (shall we say) two epitopes, *a* and *b*, develop spleen cells making anti-*a* and anti-*b* which appear as antibodies in the serum. The spleen is removed and the individual cells fused in polyethylene glycol with constantly dividing (i.e. 'immortal') B-tumour cells selected for a purine enzyme deficiency and often for their inability to secrete Ig. The resulting cells are distributed into micro-well plates in HAT (hypoxanthine, aminopterin, thymidine) medium which kills off the perfusion partners, at such a high dilution that *on average* each well will contain less than one hybridoma cell. Each hybridoma being the fusion product of a single antibody-forming cell and a tumour cell will have the ability of the former to secrete a single species of antibody and the immortality of the latter enabling it to proliferate continuously, clonal progeny providing an unending supply of antibody with a single specificity—the monoclonal antibody. In this example, we considered the production of hybridomas with specificity for just two epitopes, but the same technique enables monoclonal antibodies to be raised against complex mixtures of multiepitopic antigens. Fusions using rat cells instead of mouse may have certain advantages in giving a higher proportion of stable hybridomas, and monoclonals which are better at fixing human complement, a useful attribute in the context of therapeutic application to humans involving cell depletion.

Figure 4.5. Heterogeneity of IgG anti-hapten (dinitrophenyl : DNP) antibodies purified from the serum of an immunized animal contrasting with the homogeneity of a monoclonal IgG anti-DNP as shown by Scatchard plot of hapten binding. If r represents the average number of DNP molecules bound to each antibody molecule, of affinity constant k and number of binding sites n, in the presence of a free antigen concentration $[Ag]$, then from the mass-action equation of equilibrium relationships (p. 12) it can be shown that:

$$r/[Ag] = nk - rk$$

Thus, a Scatchard plot of $r/[Ag]$ against r for a single antibody species will be a straight line of slope k as seen for the monoclonal antibody; the deviation from a straight line given by anti-DNP from the antiserum clearly indicates the existence of antibodies with different affinities as may be confirmed by the binding of labelled

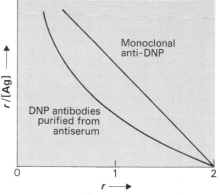

(Average No. hapten mol. bound/mol. Ab)

DNP to many different bands after separation of the individual antibodies by isoelectric focusing of the serum. Extrapolating to $r/[Ag] = 0$ (at infinitely high concentration of antigen) gives the number of binding sites on each IgG molecule as 2 (cf. p. 5 and figure 2.5).

however, one sees quite unexpected binding to antigens which react poorly, if at all, with a specific antiserum because this usually contains a group of different antibodies reacting with a given 'patch' on the antigen surface; the antiserum defines the overall shape of the patch by the 'average' shape of this group of antibodies, whereas a monoclonal antibody reacts with an epitope which may only be a part of the 'patch', and this smaller region may bear enough similarity to the surface of another antigen to allow the monoclonal antibody to bind. Inappropriate binding with a monoclonal antibody may also occur because only some of the hypervariable complementarity regions may be involved in the reaction with the original antigen, leaving the possibility of adventitious affinity for an unrelated antigen through the other parts of the binding site. In the antiserum, the several antibodies directed to a given patch will all differ in their ability to bind in this way to unrelated antigens so that this effect will be diluted out and not become apparent. The problem can be circumvented by using a group of monoclonals directed to the same 'patch' on the antigen.

A tremendous advantage of the monoclonal antibody as a reagent is that it provides a single standard material for all laboratories throughout the world to use in an unending supply if the immortality and purity of the cell line is nurtured; antisera raised in different animals, on the other hand, may be as different from each other as chalk and cheese. The monoclonal approach again shows a clean pair of heels relative to conventional strategies in the production of antibodies specific for individual components in a complex mixture of antigens, which, for example, one may wish to do in trying to identify which of a set of antigens on a given parasite can generate antibodies which are protective for the host. Whereas in the prehybridoma era we would have tried to purify individual antigens from the complex mixture and then raised antibodies to each component, now we would make a large number of hybridomas from the spleen of an animal immunized with the complete antigen mixture and separate the individual hybridomas by simple cloning. It must be clear that we now have in our hands a really powerful technique whose applications are truly legion. Some of these are touched upon in table 4.1 to give the reader an inkling of what is possible but the potential defies the imagination; the separation of individual cell types with specific surface markers (lymphocyte subpopulations, neural cells, etc.), diagnosis of lymphoid and myeloid malignancies, tissue typing, radioimmunoassay, serotyping of micro-organisms, elucidation of the fine structure of the antibody combining site and the basis for variability, immunological intervention with passive antibody, anti-idiotype inhibition or 'magic bullet' therapy with cytotoxic agents coupled to antitumour specific antibody—these and many other areas will all be transformed by hybridoma technology.

Hybridomas producing human antibodies would be particularly valuable for therapeutic purposes. It is possible to fuse human antibody-forming cells with mouse tumour lines but the mixed hybrids tend to be unstable and shed chromosomes. Progress in finding an effective human tumour line as a partner is slow. An alternative is to transform antigen-enriched lymphocytes to cell lines by polyclonal stimulation with EB virus and the successful isolation of a clone making anti-rhesus D (p. 244) has recently been reported.

The principle of immortalizing and cloning out individual cell types by fusion to a tumour cell is widely applicable but for the immunologist there is a special interest in the ability to generate helper and suppressor hybridomas by fusion of activated T-cells with T-lymphoma lines which produce a variety of antigen-specific and non-specific helper and suppressor factors.

IMMUNOGLOBULIN CLASSES

The synthesis of antibodies belonging to the various immunoglobulin classes proceeds at different rates. Usually there is an early IgM response which tends to fall off rapidly. IgG antibody synthesis builds up to its maximum over a longer time period. On secondary challenge with antigen, the time

Table 4.1. Some applications of monoclonal antibodies.

1	Enumeration of human lymphocyte subpopulations	Anti-T3 identifies all mature T-cells Anti-T4 identifies subset containing T-helpers Anti-T8 identifies cytotoxic/suppressor T-cells
2	Cell depletion	Cocktail of anti-T3 monoclonals + complement kills T-cells in human bone marrow to prevent graft vs host reaction (p. 277)
3	Cell isolation	Separation of murine Lyt1 +ve T-cells by monoclonal anti-Lyt1 in the FACS (p. 63)
4	Probing function of cell surface molecules	Anti-T8 inhibits killing by cytotoxic T-cells Anti-Ia monoclonal inhibits T-cell response to macrophage-processed Ag
5	Blood grouping	Anti-A monoclonal provides more reliable standard reagent than conventional antisera
6	Diagnosis in cancer	Monoclonal anti-T-ALL allows differentiation from non-T-ALL (cf. p. 122) Follicle centre cell lymphoma identified by peroxidase-labelled anti-common ALL in tissue sections
7	Imaging	Radioactive anti-carcinoembryonic antigen (p. 303) used to localize colonic tumours or secondaries by scanning
8	Analysis of complex antigen mixtures	Identification of the 'protective' antigen in parasite suitable for vaccine production Identification of antigenic 'patch' on acetyl choline receptor involved in experimental myasthenia gravis (p. 345)
9	Analysis of embryological relationships	Separate monoclonals to neurons of neural tube and neural crest origin help to define embryological derivation of cells in nervous system Monoclonals to Ag on chick prosencephalon reveal a concentration gradient on the dorso-ventral axis of the retina; ? positional information for forming specific synapses
10	Monoclonal mutants	Mutants lacking Fc structures used for *in vivo* neutralization of toxic drugs, e.g. digoxin overdose, or for defining biological roles of Fc domains

Comment: The cell surface differentiation molecules characteristic for a given cell type govern the relationship with other cells and the response to soluble factors. It is gratifying that the detailed identification of these molecules by monoclonal antibodies is proving to be such a successful strategy.

course of the IgM response resembles that seen in the primary. By contrast, the synthesis of IgG antibodies rapidly accelerates to a much higher titre and there is a relatively slow fall-off in serum antibody levels (figure 4.6). The same probably holds for IgA and in a sense both these immuno-

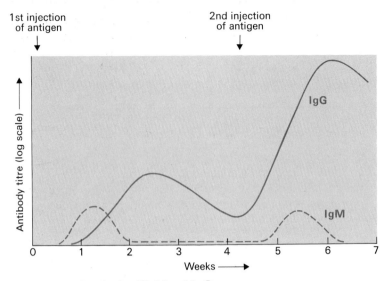

Figure 4.6. Synthesis of IgM and IgG
antibody classes in the primary and secondary responses to antigen.

globulin classes provide the main *immediate* defence against
future penetration by foreign antigens.

There is evidence that individual cells can switch over
from IgM to IgG production. Several days after immunization with salmonella flagella, isolated cells taken into micro-
drop cultures were shown to produce both IgM and IgG
immobilizing antibodies. In another study it was shown that
antigen challenge of irradiated recipients receiving relatively
small numbers of lymphoid cells, produced splenic foci of
cells, each synthesizing antibodies of different heavy chain
class bearing a single idiotype; the common idiotype suggests
that each focus is derived from a single precursor cell whose
progeny can form antibodies of different class.

Antibody synthesis in certain classes shows considerable
dependence upon T-co-operation in that the responses in
T-deprived animals are strikingly deficient; such is true of
mouse IgG1, IgE and part of the IgM antibody responses.
Immunopotentiation by complete Freund's adjuvant, a
water-in-oil emulsion containing antigen in the aqueous
phase and a suspension of killed tubercle bacilli in the oily
phase (p. 219), seems to occur, at least in part, through the
activation of helper T-cells which stimulate antibody production in T-dependent classes. The prediction from this
that the response to T-independent antigens (e.g. pneumococcus polysaccharide, p. 70) should not be potentiated by
Freund's adjuvant is borne out in practice; furthermore, as
would be expected, these antigens evoke primarily IgM antibodies and poorly defined immunological memory as do T-
dependent antigens injected into thymectomized hosts.

Thus, in rodents at least, the switch from IgM to IgG appears to be under T-cell control (cf. p. 71). Another class-specific effect which must be mentioned is the tremendous enhancement of IgE responses by helminths and even by soluble extracts derived from them.

Genetic control of the antibody response

GENES AFFECTING GENERAL RESPONSIVENESS

Mice can be selectively bred for high or low antibody responses through several generations to yield two lines, one of which consistently produces high titre antibodies to a variety of antigens and the other, antibodies of relatively low titre (Biozzi & colleagues). Out of the 10 or so different genetic loci involved, one or more affect macrophage behaviour. The two lines are comparable in their ability to clear carbon particles or sheep erythrocytes from the blood by phagocytosis, but macrophages from the high responders retain a far higher proportion of added antigen in an undegraded (and presumably) immunogenic form on their surface (cf. p. 65). On the other hand, the low responders survive infection by *Salmonella typhimurium* better and their macrophages support much slower replication of listeria (cf. p. 194) suggesting a dichotomy in the ability of macrophages to subserve humoral as compared with cell-mediated immunity.

IMMUNE RESPONSE LINKED TO IMMUNOGLOBULIN GENES

A large proportion of the antibodies made by the A/J strain of mice in response to the hapten p-azo-phenylarsonate, bear a common or cross-reacting idiotype (p. 45) somewhat coarsely referred to by the immunological fraternity as the ARS idiotype. Breeding experiments have shown that the capacity to produce this idiotype is inherited and is linked to the genetic markers for the immunoglobulin constant region, i.e. there is a gene coding for the variable region of the antibody and it occurs on the chromosome carrying the genes for the constant region. These findings would lead one to suppose that we inherit genes which enable us to make particular antibodies and that the capacity to produce an antibody response would be limited by the repertoire of specificities encoded by the genes on this chromosome. However, as we shall see in the next chapter, the mechanisms for generating antibody diversity from the available genes are so powerful that immunodeficiency is unlikely to occur as a consequence of a poor Ig variable region gene repertoire.

It will be recalled that the major histocompatibility complex (MHC) was first recognized by its predominant influence on the survival of grafts within each species through control of the synthesis of antigens which provoke intense immunological rejection (figure 3.12; p. 66). The MHC antigens are highly polymorphic (literally 'many shapes') due to the existence of several *alternative* genes (alleles) at each locus, each coding for a different antigen. It has been found that the antibody responses to a number of thymus-dependent antigenically simple substances are determined by genes—the so-called immune response or Ir genes—which are linked chromosomally to the MHC. Thus in mice, where the MHC is referred to as the H-2 region, all strains belonging to the H-2^b group respond well to the synthetic branched polypeptide antigen (T,G)-A--L (a polylysine backbone with sidechains of polyalanine randomly tipped with mixed tyrosine and glutamyl residues), whereas mice of H-2^k specificity which bear a different set of allelic genes in the H-2 region, respond poorly. We say that mice of the H-2^b haplotype (i.e. a particular set of H-2 genes) are high responders to (T,G)-A--L because they possess the appropriate Ir gene. With another synthetic antigen, (H,G)-A--L, having histidine in place of tyrosine, the position is reversed, the 'poor (T,G)-A--L responders' now giving a good antibody response and the 'good (T,G)-A--L responders' a weak one, showing that the capacity of a particular strain to give a high or low response varies with the individual antigen (table 4.2). These relationships are only apparent when antigens of highly restricted structure are studied because the response to each single determinant is controlled by an Ir gene and it is highly unlikely that the different determinants on a complex antigen will all be associated with consistently high or consistently low responder Ir genes; rather would one expect an average of randomly high and low responder genes since the various determinants on most thymus-dependent complex antigens are structurally unrelated. Thus H-2 linked immune responses have been observed not only with relatively simple polypeptides, but also with transplantation antigens from another strain and autoantigens where merely one or two determinants are recognized as foreign by the host. With complex antigens, H-2 linkage is only seen when the dose administered is so low that just one immunodominant determinant is recognized by the immune system. In this way, reactions controlled by Ir genes are distinct from the overall responsiveness to a variety of complex antigens which is a feature of the Biozzi mice (above).

Table 4.2. H-2
linked immune
responses to syn-
thetic polypeptide
antigens.

Antigen	Antibody response	
	H-2^b	H-2^k
(T,G)-A--L	High	Low
(H,G)-A--L	Low	High

See text for definition of terms
used. (After McDevitt H.O. &
Sela M. (1965) *J. Exp. Med.* **122**,
517.)

H-2I gene control of T-B co-operation

The Ir genes do not appear to affect B-cell triggering by
T-independent antigens but rather control the co-operative
response to T-dependent antigens, particularly the initial
triggering of T helpers by macrophage-processed (often
called 'nominal') antigen. Studies with recombinant strains
of mice have localized these genes within the I region of the
H-2 histocompatibility complex. Antisera raised between
strains have identified different Ia antigens (i.e. antigens
encoded by I region genes) as products of three genetic subregions, I-A, I-J and I-E (figure 3.12); each subregion is
multi-allelic and gives rise to a number of polymorphic gene
products certain of which may endow their host with high
responder and others with low responder status to restricted
determinants. The Ia molecules controlled by the I-A and
I-E subregion almost certainly represent the immune
response gene product since (i) anti-Ia monoclonals reacting
with I-A or I-E molecules (depending on the antigen) block
the stimulation of primed T-cells by antigen presented on
syngeneic macrophages, and (ii) a point mutation in the I-A
subregion in one strain led to a change in the Ia molecule at a
site affecting its polymorphic specificity, greatly reduced the
antigen-induced T-cell proliferation *in vitro* and changed the
mice from high to low responder status with respect to their
thymus-dependent antibody response to antigen *in vivo*.

It should be realized that these studies on genetic control
have not only drawn our attention to the connexion between
Ia molecules and high or low response, but also to the way in
which they contribute to the intercellular reactions in T-B
co-operation. Ia molecules are largely expressed on the
surface of B-cells and macrophages, particularly the dendritic
variety and we have seen that antigens 'processed' by
macrophages are presented to T-cells in some form of association with the surface Ia. Helper T-lymphocytes recognize
this antigen-Ia complex in much the same way that cytotoxic
T-cells have to recognize antigen on the target cell associated

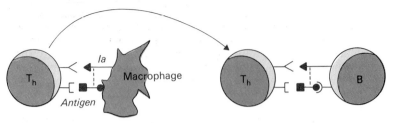

(a) Induction of helper T-cells   (b) Effector phase of T co-operation

Figure 4.7. H-2 linked immune response gene product (Ia) and T-B co-operation. Experimentally it can be shown that T-helper cells are most effective when the B-cells bear the same Ia specificity as the macrophages used for priming the T-cells. (a) The T-helpers are stimulated by antigen presented by the macrophage in some form of association (- - - - -) with Ia; (b) they can then co-operate with B-cells displaying the same Ia-antigen complex (although in this case the antigen is bound by surface Ig receptors). Other studies indicating the presence of Ia specificities on soluble 'helper' factors suggest the existence of further mechanisms of Ir gene involvement. Remember that subsequent stages in B-cell activation are non-antigen specific (cf. figure 3.16).

with other MHC products, H-2D and H-2K (cf. figure 10.17, p. 293). The activated helper cells could then trigger an Ia-bearing B-cell which had bound the antigen to its surface Ig receptors since it would recognize the same antigen-Ia combination it first saw on the macrophage (figure 4.7).

The mechanism by which Ia molecules influence responder status is still a controversial issue with powerful protagonists for the major hypotheses concerning poor response: defective macrophage presentation and defective T-cell recognition.

(a) *Defective presentation.* On this view the Ia on the macrophage of the poor responder phenotype is unable to form the correct association of the nominal antigen to present a given determinant effectively to the specific T-cell (so-called 'determinant selection'). The isolation of T-cell clones from high responders immunized with the antigen on low responder macrophages, which can be stimulated by antigen presented on poor responder macrophages, suggests that these macrophages can present antigen if the right T-cells are there to see it. Supporters of determinant selection say that under these circumstances the macrophages might have been presenting a different determinant on the antigen. Another problem with this hypothesis is the difficulty in understanding how the polymorphic region on the Ia molecule can carry out the dual function of associating specifically with antigen (a kind of primitive antigen recognition) and being recognized by the responding T-cell.

(b) *Defective T-cell recognition.* This holds that poor response is due to an Ia-induced 'hole' in the T-cell repertoire so that the antigen-Ia duo cannot be perceived. Jerne postulated that T-cells start out with a set of receptors which recognize major histocompatibility polymorphic determinants and that diversity is generated in the thymus, through T-cells with self-reacting receptors being forced to mutate until they no longer recognize self. On this basis, poor responder Ia phenotypes would produce mutant receptors which were unable to recognize structures for the particular antigen. The 'cross-tolerance' hypothesis of Ebringer provides an alternative mechanism by which MHC products could drive holes in the T-cell repertoire; originally, it was postulated that low response resulted from similarity in shape between the antigen and the individual's own MHC to which tolerance had, of course, already been established. This would predict that the F1 cross between high and low responder strains would be a low responder whereas the opposite is usually the case. A modification of this hypothesis states that tolerance occurs to self-molecules in association with an MHC component and that in the low responder, the antigen resembles some self-component in the context of the low responder MHC which tolerizes the relevant T-cells, whereas this is not true for the high responder MHC; on this basis, the T-cells which recognize antigen plus high responder Ia are not tolerized in the F1 which is therefore a responder (got it?!).

These hypotheses are not mutually exclusive. Poor presentation of antigen by macrophage would lead to low response, while good presentation could lead to a high response if the antigen did not resemble self in the context of the MHC and a low responder if it did. Other circumstances may also lead to poor antibody responses associated with the MHC. In some instances, low responders carry an I-J gene concerned in the synthesis of dominant amounts of a T-suppressor factor (see below) which acts to limit T-cell co-operation by overwhelming the helper cells.

Factors influencing the genetic control of the antibody response are summarized diagrammatically in figure 4.8.

Regulation of the immune response

In addition to the genetic factors influencing the immune response discussed above, feedback mechanisms must operate to limit antibody production; otherwise, after antigenic stimulation we would become overwhelmed by the responding clones of antibody forming cells and their products, a clearly unwelcome state of affairs as may be clearly seen in multiple myeloma where control over lymphocyte proliferation is lost. Since antigen is needed to drive the division and differentiation of lymphocytes, the concentration of antigen must be a major regulating factor. As antigen is catabolized by body enzymes and neutralized or blocked by antibody so will its concentration fall and its ability to sustain the immune response be progressively weakened. The role of antibody in diverting antigen to immunogenically inoffensive sites in the body to prevent primary sensitization is clearly evident from the protection against rhesus immunization afforded by administration of anti-D to mothers at risk (p. 246) and the inhibitory effect of maternal antibody on the peak titres obtained on vaccinating infants. Removal of circulating antibody by plasmapheresis during an on-going response leads to an increase in synthesis, whereas injection of preformed IgG antibody markedly hastens the fall in the number of antibody-forming cells, suggesting that such antibodies must exert an important feedback control on overall

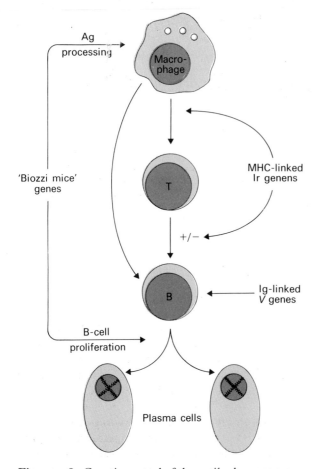

Figure 4.8. Genetic control of the antibody response.

synthesis. It is unlikely that this is achieved by simple neutralization of antigen since whole IgG is so much more effective than its $F(ab')_2$ fragment in switching off the reaction;
there is some evidence that cross-linking the antigen and Fc
receptors on the B-cell through surface-bound antigen
enables the IgG to block the productive phase of the T-
dependent B-cell response.

SUPPRESSOR T-CELLS

T-cells provide a distinct regulatory system. Not only can
they amplify the B-cell response through their helper activity, but there is now a body of evidence showing there to be a
separate T-cell population with a *suppressor* function. If mice
are made unresponsive by injection of a high dose of sheep
red cells, their T-cells will suppress specific antibody formation in normal recipients to which they have been transferred
(Gershon's 'infectious tolerance'; figure 4.9). Adult thymec-

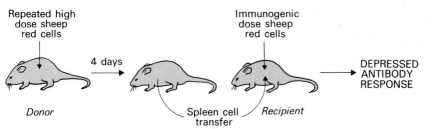

Repeated high
dose sheep
red cells

Immunogenic
dose sheep
red cells

4 days

Donor

Spleen cell
transfer

Recipient

DEPRESSED
ANTIBODY
RESPONSE

Figure 4.9. Demonstration of T-suppressor cells. Spleen cells from a donor injected with a high dose of antigen, depress the antibody response of a syngeneic animal to which they have been transferred. The effect is lost if the spleen cells are first treated with anti-Thy1 serum plus complement showing that the suppressors are T-cells (after Gershon R.K. & Kondo K. (1971) *Immunology* **21**, 903: in these studies mice were thymectomized, irradiated and reconstituted with bone marrow and thymocytes).

tomy in the mouse leads to a fall in the suppressor T-cell population, thereby increasing the response to T-independent antigens and preventing the fall-off in IgE antibody to haptens coupled with Ascaris extracts which occurs in intact animals. Furthermore, thymocytes from a young New Zealand Black (NZB) mouse can suppress autoantibody formation when injected into older diseased mice.

Helper and suppressor T-cells in the mouse have been distinguished in several ways. Suppressors are more vulnerable to adult thymectomy, x-irradiation and cyclophosphamide, and bind to sepharose-linked histamine-albumin conjugates, supposedly through surface histamine receptors. Unlike T-helpers, they can be depleted by passage down immunosorbent columns containing the specific antigen and whereas helpers are of phenotype Lyt 1 (cf. p. 62), suppressors are Lyt 2 and bear I-J determinants. In general terms the helper cells may be looked upon as inducers of the effector cells for humoral and cell-mediated immunity and it now appears that they are also responsible for the generation of T-suppressors which exert negative feedback control on the helper cells (figure 4.10). There is evidence that this suppression can be mediated by antigen. In the first place, soluble antigen-specific I-J positive suppressor factors have been well characterized. Secondly, experiments with lysozyme suggest that one determinant on the molecule can suppress the response to all the other determinants and it is not easy to see how a T-helper reacting with one epitope can be influenced by a T-suppressor directed against another structurally different epitope on the same molecule unless the two types of T-cell communicate in some way through an antigen bridge. However, interaction can also occur through recognition of an idiotype on the T-helper receptors by an

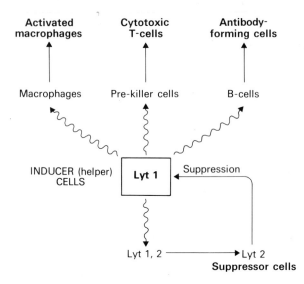

Activated macrophages **Cytotoxic T-cells** **Antibody-forming cells**

Macrophages   Pre-killer cells   B-cells

INDUCER (helper) CELLS   **Lyt 1**   Suppression

Lyt 1, 2 ──────→ Lyt 2

Suppressor cells

Figure 4.10. Immunoregulatory feedback circuit showing the central position of Lyt 1 cells in the induction (⤳) of T-dependent responses and in the generation of T-suppressors which in turn inhibit the Lyt 1 cells. The Lyt 1 population is heterogeneous but a proportion expresses the Qa-1 antigen encoded by genes which map between the H-2D and Tla loci (cf. figure 10.5). Both Lyt 1:Qa-1$^+$ and Lyt 1:Qa-1$^-$ are involved in optimal collaboration with B-cells but only the former are able to generate suppressors; thus the balance between Qa-1$^+$ and Qa-1$^-$ subsets may strongly influence the outcome of a given immune response (after Cantor H. & Gershon R.K.). Yet more complexity: an Lyt 1 cell with binding sites for the lectin *Vicia villosa* can act as a 'contrasuppressor' which protects the helper against suppression. The equivalent of Lyt 1:Qa-1$^+$ cells in the human are the suppressor-inducers bearing the T4 and TQ1 markers identified by monoclonal antibodies; the T4$^+$:TQ1$^-$ set is the counterpart of Lyt 1:Qa-1$^-$.

anti-idiotype on the suppressors and this will be discussed further in the next section.

Non-antigen specific T-suppression also occurs. Mouse T-lymphocytes when stimulated by the polyclonal activator concanavalin A (cf. p. 260) in culture are able to inhibit a variety of antibody responses. In the human, T-cells with receptors for Fcγ (IgG Fc) suppress the help given by T-cells with Fcμ receptors for the polyclonal stimulation of B-cells by pokeweed mitogen (cf. p. 260) and these findings may have relevance for the immunosuppressive action of IgG antibody described above and the stimulatory effect of IgM reported by Henry & Jerne. It has also been shown that immunoglobulin synthesis by normal B-lymphocytes following pokeweed stimulation in culture can be blocked by T-cells from a small proportion of patients with acquired hypo-γ-globulinaemia, with the clear implication that immunoglobulin production in the patient was restricted by active suppressor T-cells. This polyclonal B-cell inhibition contrasts with the antigen-specific suppression seen, for example, in the high dose sheep cell experiment mentioned

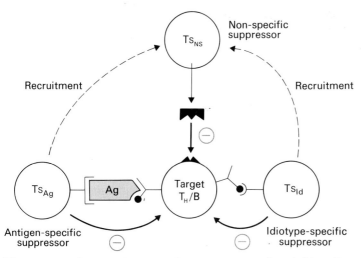

Figure 4.11. Suppression (⊖) of target T-helper or B-cells by different types of T-suppressors. Note the similarity between the antigen-specific suppressor and the helper in figure 3.15 (p. 69) where the antigen bridge allows either negative or positive signals respectively to be delivered to the target cell. ▰▰ = non-specific suppressor factor.

above, and it seems that both non-specific and antigen-specific soluble suppressor factors can be demonstrated, mirroring the situation with T-helper factors. It has been postulated that a crowding out of acceptor sites on the macrophage by such molecules could be responsible for *antigenic competition*, the situation in which one T-dependent antigen can block the response to another. Awareness of this phenomenon in vaccination programmes involving more than one antigen is of self-evident importance.

In summary, helper and suppressor T-cells act respectively as accelerator and braking systems to regulate the immune response. The suppressor system is proving to be complex, involving antigen and idiotype specific cells which finally recruit suppressors able to release non-specific effector factors (figure 4.11).

IDIOTYPIC NETWORKS

Jerne's network hypothesis

The hypervariable loops on the immunoglobulin molecule which go to form the antigen combining site have individual characteristic shapes which can be recognized by the appropriate antibodies as idiotypic determinants (cf. p. 43). There are hundreds of thousands, if not more, different idiotypes in one individual, virtually all of them present in very low concentrations at birth and therefore unlikely to produce self-tolerance.

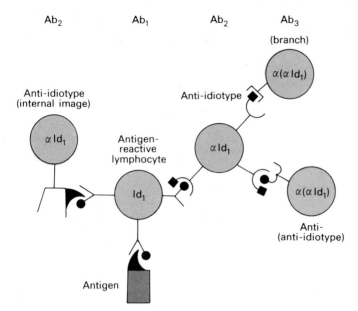

Ab₂   Ab₁   Ab₂   Ab₃

Figure 4.12. Elements in an idiotypic network in which the antigen receptors on one lymphocyte recognize an idiotype on the receptors of another. T-helper, T-suppressor and B-lymphocytes interact through idiotype–anti-idiotype reactions; either stimulation or suppression may result. One of the anti-idiotype sets may bear an idiotype of similar shape to (i.e. provides an *internal image* of) the antigen. The same idiotype (●) may be shared by two receptors of different specificity (since the several hypervariable regions provide a number of potential idiotypic determinants and a given idiotype does not always form part of the epitope binding site), so that the anti-(anti-Id_1) does not necessarily bind the original antigen. (The following abbreviations are often employed: α = anti; Id = idiotype; Ab_1 = Id; Ab_2 = αId; Ab_3 = $\alpha(\alpha Id)$).

Jerne reasoned brilliantly that the great diversity of idiotypes would to a considerable extent mirror the diversity of antigenic shapes in the external world. Thus, he said, if lymphocytes can recognize a whole range of foreign antigenic determinants, they should be able to recognize the idiotypes on other lymphocytes. They would therefore form a large network or series of networks depending upon idiotype–anti-idiotype recognition between lymphocytes of the various T- and B-subsets (figure 4.12) and the response to an external antigen perturbing this network would be conditioned by the state of the idiotypic interactions.

Evidence for idiotypic networks

There is no doubt that the elements to form an idiotypic network are present in the body. Individuals can be immunized against idiotypes on their own antibodies, and such auto-anti-idiotypes have been identified during the course of responses induced by antigens. Anti-idiotypic specificities

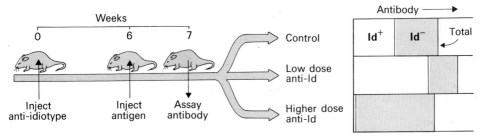

Figure 4.13. Modulation of a major idiotype in the antibody response to antigen by anti-idiotype. In the example chosen, the idiotype is present in a substantial proportion of the antibodies produced in controls injected with antigen alone (i.e. this is a public or cross-reacting Id; p. 45).

Pretreatment with 10 ng of a monoclonal anti-Id greatly expands the Id^+ antibody population whereas prior injection of 10 μg of anti-Id completely (or almost completely) suppresses expression of the idiotype without having any substantial effect on total antibody production.

can be demonstrated on both T-helpers and T-suppressors. For example, during the induction of suppression to the p-azo-phenylarsonate group by intravenous injection of hapten-conjugated lymphocytes, antigen-specific T-suppressors bearing the major ARS idiotype (p. 97) appear first, but these give rise to second-order anti-idiotype suppressor cells. Antigen and idiotype specific T-helpers have been demonstrated in the response to various antigens, the former MHC-restricted and the latter not, and both are required for optimal antibody synthesis (cf. Lyt 1^+Qa-1^- and Lyt 1^+Qa-1^+ helpers in legend to figure 4.10).

Furthermore, idiotypic interactions can modulate the immune response. Quite low doses of anti-idiotype, of the order of nanograms, can greatly enhance the expression of that idiotype in the response to a given antigen, whereas doses in the microgram range lead to suppression (figure 4.13).

Regulation by idiotype interactions

There has been a series of investigations based on the following protocol. Antigen is injected into $animal_1$ and the antibody produced, Ab_1 (idiotype), is purified and injected into $animal_2$. Ab_2 (anti-idiotype) so formed is purified and used to immunize $animal_3$ and so on (figure 4.14). Consistently, it is found that Ab_2 (anti-Id_1) recognizes an idiotype (Id_1) on Ab_1 which is also strongly present in Ab_3. Ab_4 behaves like Ab_2 in seeing the common idiotype on Ab_1 and Ab_3. Nonetheless, although Ab_1 and Ab_3 share idiotypes, only a small fraction of Ab_3 reacts with the original antigen. This is the result one would expect if the idiotype was a cross-reacting Id (public Id) present on a variety of antibodies (and by

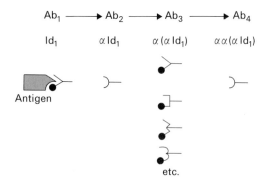

$$Ab_1 \longrightarrow Ab_2 \longrightarrow Ab_3 \longrightarrow Ab_4$$

$$Id_1 \qquad \alpha\,Id_1 \qquad \alpha\,(\alpha\,Id_1) \qquad \alpha\alpha\,(\alpha\,Id_1)$$

Antigen

etc.

Figure 4.14. Ab_1 produced by the antigen is injected into a second animal to produce Ab_2; this in turn is purified and injected into animal$_3$ and so on. Ab_2 and Ab_4 both react with an idiotype (●) on Ab_1 and Ab_3 but only a fraction of Ab_3 reacts with the original antigen. Bona & Paul (*Immunol. Today* 1982, **3**, 230) interpret the results in terms of a common regulatory idiotype Id_1 shared by many antibodies other than those reacting with the original antigen but recruited by the injection of anti-Id_1 (Ab_2) which stimulates the range of lymphocytes whose receptors bear this common or cross- reacting idiotype. On this basis, one can understand the paradoxical finding of Oudin & Cazenave that not all the Ig mole- cules bearing a given Id in response to an antigen can function as specific antibody. The presence of large amounts of Id_1 in Ab_3 also suggests that the linear relation- ship through the cross-reacting Id_1 is dominant, with relatively insignificant branching through the variety of 'private' idiotypes on Ab_2 molecules (cf. figure 4.12) because of the low frequency of such idiotypes and their anti-idiotypes.

implication B-cell receptors) of different specificities. As may be seen in figure 4.14, the anti-Id_1 (Ab_2), when injected into animal$_3$, would react with all B-cells bearing Id_1 and pre- sumably trigger them to produce Id_1 antibodies, only a frac- tion of which have specificity for the original antiserum.

Such frequently occurring idiotypes seem to be provoked fairly readily with anti-Id and are therefore candidates for regulatory Id which can be under some degree of control by a limited idiotypic network. Germane to this idea are the observations that antibodies with utterly distinct specificities, directed against totally different epitopes on the same antigen, often bear a common or cross-reacting idiotype. Pre- sumably, the first clone of antibodies to be formed which bears a dominant cross-reacting Id generates a population of regulatory T-helper cells which recognize this Id; from the complex mixture of B-lymphocytes activated by the other epitopes on the antigen, these T-helpers in turn selectively recruit those with Id positive receptors (figure 4.15). We can now see how the antigen and idiotype specific T-helpers syn- ergize in the antibody response, the latter expanding Id posi- tive clones induced by the former.

Given that regulation can occur through interaction with public or cross-reactive idiotypes, what is its importance relative to antigen-mediated control? Although the answer will vary with different antigens, my prejudice is that in

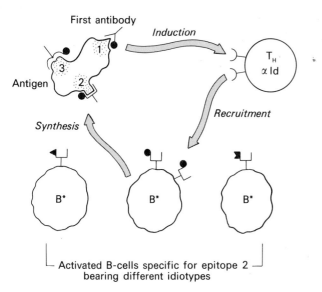

First antibody

Induction

T_H
α Id

Antigen

Recruitment

Synthesis

B*

B*

B*

Activated B-cells specific for epitope 2 bearing different idiotypes

Figure 4.15. Role of anti-idiotypic T-helper in recruiting antibodies with specificities for the different epitopes on an antigen but bearing the same public or cross-reacting idiotype. The first antibody bearing a cross-reacting Id induces αId T-helpers which are assumed to recruit Id$^+$ B-cells already activated by antigen; if resting Id$^+$ cells were recruited the amount of non-specific Ig synthesized might be wastefully high. It is worth considering whether memory αId T-helpers could be responsible for the phenomenon of 'original antigenic sin' in which a second infection with influenza virus involving an antigenically related but not identical strain generates antibodies with a higher titre for the strain which produced the first infection.

general the antigen-directed systems will dominate, with idiotypic networks providing accessory amplification and suppressive loops since (a) it seems most likely that antigen recognition and elimination were the driving forces behind selection for an adaptive immune response and therefore one wants the system to be sensitive to the presence and concentration of antigen, and (b) there would seem to be little point in Id and anti-Id squabbling about control of the response after antigen had been eliminated. The Id network could allow the response to 'tick over' for extended periods and maintain the memory-cell population, while the presence of primed T-helpers directed against a common Id on the various memory B-cells specific for a given antigen would increase their rate of mobilization during a secondary response.

Manipulation of the immune response through idiotypes

The idiotypic network provides interesting opportunities to manipulate the immune response, particularly in hypersensitivity states such as autoimmune disease, allergy and graft rejection. However, normally the B-cell response is so diverse that suppression by anti-Id is likely to prove difficult; even when the response is dominated by a public Id and that Id is suppressed, compensatory expansion of Id negative clones ensures that the fall in the total antibody titre is relatively undramatic (cf. figure 4.13). Perhaps ways can be developed to restrict this Id negative compensation, particularly if the total number of idiotypes is small as might conceivably be the case with IgE antibody synthesis in patients with atopic allergy. It is possible that T-helper cells may express a narrow spectrum of idiotypes thereby being more susceptible to suppression by Id autoimmunization. Reports that 'vaccination' with irradiated lines of helper T-cells specific for brain or thyroid antigens prevents the induction of experimental autoimmunity against the relevant organ, are encouraging. Sporadic success has been obtained with the strategy of autoimmunizing rats of strain A with antibodies (AαB) raised in A against the transplantation antigens of strain B so that the T-cell mediated rejection of a subsequent strain B graft is suppressed, presumably because the anti-idiotypic response (anti-[AαB]) inactivates lymphocytes capable of recognizing the graft by virtue of the AαB receptors on their surface. A totally different approach would be to use monoclonal anti-Id of the 'antigen internal image' set (figure 4.12) to stimulate antigen-specific T-suppressors capable of turning off B-cells directed to other epitopes on the antigen through bridging by the antigen itself (cf. figure 4.11).

Since we know that anti-Id can also stimulate antibody production by changing the conditions, it might be possible to use 'internal image' monoclonal anti-Ids as 'surrogate' antigens for immunization in cases where the antigen is difficult to obtain in bulk—for example, antigens from parasites such as filaria or the weak embryonic antigens associated with some cancers. Another example is where protein antigens obtained by chemical synthesis or gene cloning fail to fold into the configuration of the native molecule; this is not a problem with the anti-Id which by definition has been selected to have the shape of the antigenic epitope.

At this stage, if the reader is feeling a little groggy, try a glance at figure 4.16 which attempts a summary of the main factors currently thought to modulate the immune response.

Immunological tolerance

AT BIRTH

Over 20 years ago Owen made the intriguing observation that non-identical (dizygotic) twin cattle, which shared the same placental circulation and whose circulations were

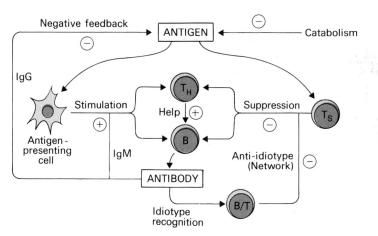

Figure 4.16. Regulation of the immune response. T_H = T-helper cell; T_S = T-suppressor cell. T-help for cell-mediated immunity will be subject to similar regulation. Some of these mechanisms may be interdependent; for example, one could envisage anti-idiotypic antibody acting in concert with a suppressor T-cell by binding to its Fc receptor, or suppressor T-cells with specificity for the idiotype on T_H or B-cells. To avoid too many confusing arrows, I have omitted the recruitment of B-cells by anti-idiotypic T-helpers and direct activation of anti-idiotype T-suppressors by idiotype-positive T-helpers.

thereby linked, grew up with appreciable numbers of red cells from the other twin in their blood; if they had not shared the same circulation at birth, red cells from the twin injected in adult life would be rapidly eliminated by an immunological response. From this finding Burnet & Fenner conceived the notion that potential antigens which reach the lymphoid cells during their developing immunologically immature phase in the perinatal period can in some way specifically suppress any future response to that antigen when the animal reaches immunological maturity. This, they considered, would provide a means whereby unresponsiveness to the body's own constituents ('self') could be established and thereby enable the lymphoid cells to make the important distinction between 'self' and 'non-self'. On this basis, any foreign cells introduced into the body around the perinatal period should trick the animal into treating them as 'self' components in later life and the studies of Medawar and his colleagues have shown that *immunological tolerance* or unresponsiveness can be artificially induced in this way. Thus neonatal injection of CBA mouse cells into newborn A strain animals suppresses their ability to immunologically reject a CBA graft in adult life (figures 4.17 and 4.18). Tolerance can also be induced with soluble antigens; for example, rabbits injected with bovine serum albumin at birth fail to make antibodies on later challenge with this protein.

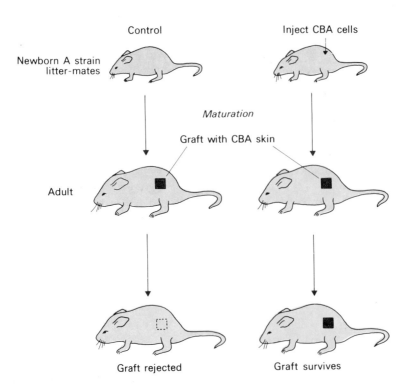

Control　　　　　　　　Inject CBA cells

Newborn A strain
litter-mates

Maturation

Graft with CBA skin

Adult

Graft rejected　　　　　Graft survives

Figure 4.17. Induction of tolerance to foreign CBA skin graft in A strain mice by neonatal injection of antigen (after Bill- ingham R., Brent L. & Medawar P.B. (1953) *Nature* **172**, 603).

Figure 4.18. CBA skin graft on fully toler- ant A strain mouse showing healthy hair growth eight weeks after grafting (courtesy of Prof. L. Brent).

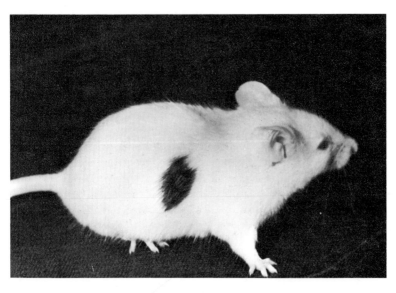

It is now recognized that tolerance can be induced in the adult as well as the neonate, although in general much higher doses of antigen are required. Surprisingly, repeated injection of *low* doses of certain antigens such as bovine serum albumin (BSA) which are weakly immunogenic, established a state of tolerance as revealed by a poor antibody response on challenge with BSA in a strongly antigenic form (in complete Freund's adjuvant—see p. 219). It was shown subsequently that this 'low zone tolerance' could also be achieved with more powerful antigens provided an immunosuppressive drug such as cyclophosphamide was given to inhibit antibody synthesis during the low dose treatment.

Thus, there is a 'low zone' and a 'high zone' in terms of antigen predosage for tolerance induction. Elegant studies by Weigle and co-workers have pinpointed the T-cell as the target for tolerance at low antigen levels while both B- and T-lymphocytes are made unresponsive at high antigen dose (table 4.3). Thus, for 'thymus-dependent' antigens at dose levels where the T-cells play a major co-operative role in antibody formation, the overall immunological performance of the animal will reflect the degree of reactivity of the T-cell population. In other words, the T-cells guide the reaction and when they are tolerant the B-cells will not respond.

Protein antigens are more tolerogenic (able to induce tolerance) when in a soluble rather than an aggregated or particulate form which can be readily taken up by macrophages, and it seems that molecules are more likely to be tolerogenic if they escape processing by macrophages before presentation to the lymphocyte. Persistence of antigen is

Table 4.3. Effect of antigen dose on tolerance induction in T- and B-cells.

Tolerogen administered (mg)	% Tolerance induced		
	T-cells	B-cells	Donor spleen
0.1	96	9	62
0.5	99	56	97
2.5	99	70	99

After induction of tolerance to aggregate-free human IgG in mice, the reactivity of thymocytes and bone marrow cells (containing B-cells) was assessed by transfer to irradiated recipients with either bone marrow or thymus respectively from normal donors. The degree of tolerance induced in the donor is shown in the final column. Low antigen doses tolerize the T-cells. B-cells become unresponsive at higher doses. The T-cell activity largely dictates the response of the spleen as a whole (from Chiller J.M., Habicht G.S. & Weigle W.O. (1971) *Science* **171**, 813).

required to maintain tolerance. In Medawar's experiments the tolerant state was long-lived because the injected CBA cells survived and the animals continued to be chimaeric (i.e. they possessed both A and CBA cells). With non-living antigens such as BSA, tolerance is gradually lost, the most likely explanation being that in the absence of antigen, newly recruited immunocompetent cells which are being generated throughout life, are not being rendered tolerant. Since recruitment of newly competent T-lymphocytes is drastically curtailed by removal of the thymus, it is of interest to note that the tolerant state persists for much longer in thymectomized animals.

MECHANISMS

Immunological 'silence' It is self-evident that the immune system will be tolerant of its own body components if it cannot communicate with them—we might then speak of a state of immunological 'silence'. Since virtually all body components are likely to be T-dependent because they lack the molecular qualities of T-independence (p. 70), they will not become immunogenic unless they associate with Ia. Thus, many surface molecules which are restricted to cells lacking Ia, e.g. TSH receptors on the thyroid, would not normally be capable of activating self-reactive lymphocytes (unless they were shed from the surface in large amounts and then presented by an Ia positive macrophage). It is conceivable, although there is no evidence for this to date, that unresponsiveness might arise from an innate inability to present certain self-antigens in association with Ia. Immunological silence would also result if an individual has no genes coding for lymphocyte receptors directed against particular self determinants; analysis of the experimentally induced auto-antibody response to cytochrome c suggests that only those parts of the molecule which show species variation are auto-antigenic whereas the highly conserved regions do appear to be silent.

Clonal deletion The exceptional vulnerability of the neonate to tolerance induction has led to the suggestion that during lymphocyte development, the cell goes through a phase in which contact with antigen leads to death or permanent inactivation. In support of this view, the surface Ig of very early B-cells can be capped at much lower concentrations of anti-IgM than are required by adult cells and remarkably, after endocytosis of the caps, the surface receptors are resynthesized by the adult cells but not by the early B-lymphocytes which are now effectively aborted through their inability to 'see' antigen. In Medawar's experiments it has been argued that tolerance is a result of T-suppressor activity rather than clonal deletion. However, animals made fully tolerant by neonatal injection of donor cells are devoid of mixed lymphocyte (p. 276) and cytotoxic T-cell reactivities against donor antigens and do not possess cells which suppress these reactivities in lymphocytes from a normal mouse of the same strain. Also, tolerance can be abrogated by the transfer of normal syngeneic (same strain) lymphocytes, which should not be possible if T-suppressor cells were dominant.

T-suppression Low zone tolerance to protein antigens has been shown in at least one case to be mediated by T-suppressors directed against T-helpers and a suppressor mechanism will probably prove to be the most common basis for this phenomenon. The inferior immunogenicity of soluble, as distinct from aggregated or particulate, antigen may be ascribed to weak stimulation of T-helpers through poor macrophage processing in contrast to effective activation of suppressor cells which do not require macrophage presentation. T-suppression has been recognized to be a major factor in transplantation tolerance in *adults* induced by a cocktail of donor antigen, pertussis vaccine and anti-lymphocyte serum.

Helplessness T-cells are more readily tolerized than B-cells and, as a result, a number of self-reacting B-cells are present in the body which cannot be triggered by T-dependent self-components since the T-cells required to provide the necessary T-B help are already tolerant—you might describe the B-cells as helpless. If we think of the determinant on a self-component which combines with the receptors on a self-reacting B-cell as a hapten and another determinant which has to be recognized by a T-cell as a carrier (cf. figure 3.16), then tolerance in the T-cell to the carrier will prevent the provision of T-cell help and the B-cell will be unresponsive. There are further consequences of helplessness, because if the self-reactive determinants cross-link B-cell receptors in the absence of T-cell signals, the B-cell should become tolerized as predicted by the 1 and 2 signal hypothesis of Bretscher & Cohn (p. 72); in fact, B-cell tolerance to haptenic determinants is readily produced when the hapten is presented to the B-cell on a thymus-independent carrier or on a carrier such as autologous IgG, to which the individual is already tolerant.

It is likely that self-tolerance involves all these mechanisms to varying degrees and that while clonal deletion is of prime importance early in life, T-suppression becomes a dominant factor later (figure 4.19). It should be stressed that these terms, early and late, apply to the life of the lymphocyte, not

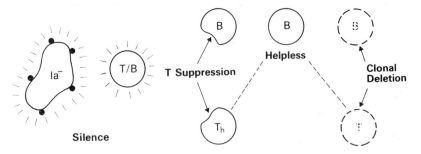

Figure 4.19. Mechanisms of self-tolerance. Unresponsiveness will result if self-components and lymphocytes will not speak to each other (self determinant (●) on Ia negative cell or lymphocyte lacks receptors), if T- or B-cells are T-suppressed or clonally deleted, or if T-dependent B-cells are deprived of T-help.

of the host. If an adult is irradiated and reconstituted with immature lymphocytes in the form of bone marrow cells, the animal behaves as a neonate with respect to the ease of tolerance induction with low doses of antigen.

Ontogeny of the immune response

Haemopoiesis originates in the early yolk sac but as embryogenesis proceeds, this function is taken over by the fetal liver and finally by the bone marrow where it continues throughout life. The haemopoietic stem cell which gives rise to the formed elements of the blood and the cells of the lymphoreticular system (figure 4.20) can be shown to be multipotent, to seed other organs and to renew itself through the creation of further stem cells.

T-CELLS AND THE THYMUS

Stem cells attracted to the thymus by a chemotactic factor differentiate within the microenvironment of the epithelioid cells where they proliferate extensively and acquire characteristic early T-cell markers (figure 4.21). Under the influence of the epithelioid cells, and in some cases also the dendritic reticular cells of the medulla, the thymocytes differentiate further to form distinct functional subpopulations with the competence to respond in the mixed lymphocyte reaction (p. 276), mediate allograft cytotoxicity (p. 76), generate carrier-specific help for B-cells and produce lymphokines for cell-mediated immunity ('delayed-type hypersensitivity' cells); cortisone-sensitive cells with potential suppressor function appear in the cortex. Presumably self-tolerance and the ability to recognize self-MHC specificities which provide the basis for haplotype restricted T-cell responses to antigen (p. 292) are also acquired at this stage.

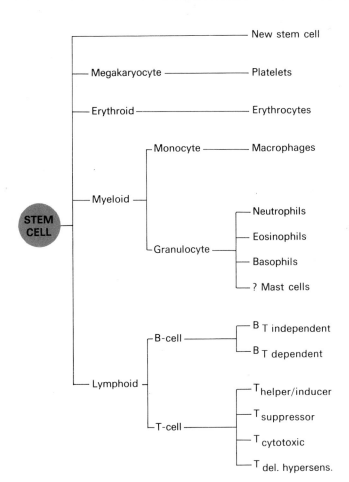

Figure 4.20. The multipotent haemopoietic stem cell. The classification of B- and T-cell subsets is still tentative as is the relationship between basophils and mast cells.

Some cells move directly from the cortex into the periphery and others (future helper and delayed-type hypersensitivity cells which must learn to react with macrophages?) migrate to the medulla, a proportion staying there for a curiously long time.

Earlier experiments on the partial restitution of immunocompetence in thymectomized females through pregnancy were taken to imply that a soluble thymic product (derived from the fetal thymuses) was responsible, at least in part, for the influence of the gland on T-cell maturation. Several different soluble thymic extracts have been prepared and active preparations isolated, usually on the basis of their ability to promote the appearance of T-cell differentiation markers (Thy1 in the mouse, T3 or sheep cell receptors in the human) and a variety of T-cell functions on culture with bone marrow cells *in vitro*. Of the many peptide hormones which have been isolated from these crude thymic 'soups', four have been characterized and chemically synthesized: thymulin (formerly FTS; 9 amino acids), thymosin α_1 (28

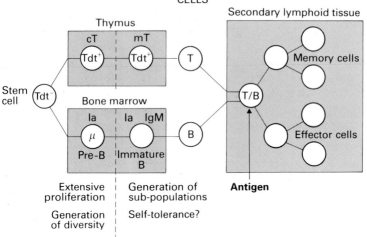

ANTIGEN-
INDEPENDENT
DIFFERENTIATION

CIRCULATING
IMMUNO-
COMPETENT
CELLS

ANTIGEN-DEPENDENT
MATURATION

Secondary lymphoid tissue

Thymus

cT | mT

Tdt^+ — Tdt^+ — T

Stem cell Tdt^-

Bone marrow

Ia | Ia | IgM

μ — ◯

Pre-B | Immature B

B

T/B

Memory cells

Effector cells

Extensive proliferation | Generation of sub-populations

Generation of diversity | Self-tolerance?

Antigen

Figure 4.21. Differentiation and maturation of human B- and T-cells.
Tdt = Terminal deoxynucleotidyl transferase; cT = cortical T-cell surface antigen; mT = mature T-cell surface antigen. The early replicating cells in the thymus and bone marrow are in the majority. Thymocytes are educated to recognize self-MHC haplotype (cf. p. 295). Tolerance to self-antigens is induced in the immature B- and T-cells within the primary lymphoid organs. Ia$^+$, μ^- pre-B cell precursors are Tdt$^+$; the Tdt enzyme may be involved as one of the mechanisms controlling the generation of diversity. In the mouse, the earliest thymocytes acquire surface Thy1; this then increases in surface density and is accompanied by the Tla antigen (p. 274); cells ready to leave the thymus have lost Tla and have a reduced Thy1.

amino acids), thymosin β_4 (43 amino acids) and thymopoietin (49 amino acids; a pentapeptide TP-5 has the activity of the full molecule). Preliminary studies with fluorescent antibodies make one suspect that the various hormones will prove to be synthesized by different thymic epithelial cells. Thymulin blood levels fall steadily with age as the thymus involutes, and precipitously in certain autoimmune disorders (SLE and NZB mice—Chapter 11) at a time corresponding roughly with the onset of disease. Thymosin α_1, aside from its influence on T-cell differentiation, has a neuroendocrine function and provides an immunoregulatory signal acting through the central nervous system to influence corticosterone levels. Each of the hormones is being subjected to intense and widespread clinical trials in attempts to correct immunodeficiencies, to prevent relapse in treated cancer patients and to restore the balance of regulatory cells in autoimmune diseases. This is a dynamic field of study with great potential and undoubtedly these peptides will be shown to influence many facets of T-cell biology; the present position may best be described as being in a state of flux.

THE DIFFERENTIATION OF B-CELLS

The microenvironment for the differentiation of B-cells is provided by the bursa of Fabricius in the chicken and the bone marrow itself in mammalian species (a nameless immunologist regularly slays his students by recalling that 'the bursa is strictly for the birds'). The early, rapidly dividing pre-B cells display cytoplasmic μ chains but no light chains (figure 4.21). It is likely that the genetic mechanisms responsible for the generation of receptor diversity (in T-cells as well) operate at this stage. In the immature B-cell, the receptor for which the cell is finally programmed is inserted into the plasma membrane as a specific IgM molecule. As immune competence emerges, the ability to mount an antibody response to each of a defined series of antigens appears sequentially and in the same order in different members of the same species, suggesting that the individual genes in the antibody V gene repertoire are recruited for receptor synthesis in a predetermined fashion. Immature B-cells have a lower density of surface immunoglobulins than primed lymphocytes and, unlike their mature counterparts, have difficulty in resynthesizing them after they have been stripped from the cell by treatment with anti-Ig which leads to 'shedding' or endocytosis. As discussed previously, this phenomenon could be related to the finding that bone marrow cells are easier to tolerize by exposure to thymus-dependent antigens than mature lymphocytes and that tolerance can be more readily induced in the newborn as compared with the adult. The relevance to the establishment of 'self-tolerance' to circulating body components at this stage hardly needs stressing; almost certainly, comparable events occur in the thymus.

At the next stage of differentiation, the cell develops a commitment to producing a particular antibody class and either bears surface IgM alone or in combination with IgA or IgG. The further addition of surface IgD now marks the readiness of the virgin B-cell for priming by antigen. Some cells, therefore, bear surface Ig of three different classes; M, G and D or M, A and D, but all Ig molecules on a single cell have the same idiotype and therefore are derived from the same V_H and V_L genes. IgD is lost on antigenic stimulation so that memory cells lack this Ig. At the terminal stages in the life of a fully mature plasma cell, virtually all surface Ig is shed. Injection of anti-μ (anti-IgM heavy chain) into chick embryos prevents the subsequent maturation of IgM and IgG antibody-producing cells, whereas anti-γ inhibits only

119

IgG development. Whether the switch from IgM production to other classes is partly antigen-driven (cf. p. 97) or occurs entirely as a result of microenvironmental factors is still unresolved. In the embryonic chicken bursa, a regular switch from IgM to IgG is observed and it seems possible that local influences in the gut will prove to be responsible for the predominant development of IgA bearing cells. These cells are generated in Peyer's patches, pass into the blood via the thoracic duct and return to populate the diffuse lymphoid tissue in the lamina propria of the gut.

THE NEONATAL PERIOD

Lymph node and spleen remain relatively underdeveloped in the human even at birth except where there has been intra-uterine exposure to antigens as in congenital infections with rubella or other organisms. The ability to reject grafts and to mount an antibody response is reasonably well developed by birth but the immunoglobulin levels with one exception are low particularly in the absence of intra-uterine infection. The exception is IgG which is acquired by placental transfer from the mother, a process dependent upon Fc structures specific to this Ig class. This material is catabolized with a half-life of approximately 30 days and there is a fall in IgG concentration over the first three months accentuated by the increase in blood volume of the growing infant. Thereafter the rate of synthesis overtakes the rate of breakdown of maternal IgG and the overall concentration increases steadily. The other immunoglobulins do not cross the placenta and the low but significant levels of IgM in cord blood are synthesized by the baby (figure 4.22). IgM reaches adult levels by nine months of age. Only trace levels of IgA, IgD and IgE are present in the circulation of the newborn.

LYMPHOID MALIGNANCIES

Lymphoid cells at almost any stage in their differentiation or maturation may become malignant and proliferate to form a clone of cells which are virtually 'frozen' at a particular developmental stage because of defects in maturation. At one time it was thought that maturation arrest occurred at the stage when the cell first became malignant but we now know that the tumour cells can be forced into differentiation by agents such as phorbol myristate acetate and the current view is that cells may undergo a few differentiation steps after malignant transformation before coming to a halt. The demonstration of a myeloma protein idiotype on the cytoplasmic μ chains of pre-B cells in the same patient certainly favours the idea that the malignant event had occurred in a

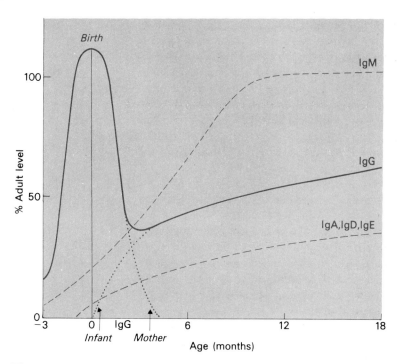

Figure 4.22. Development of serum immunoglobulin levels in the human (after Hobbs J.R. (1969) in *Immunology and Development.* Adinolfi M. (ed.). p. 118. Heinemann, London).

pre-B cell whose progeny formed the plasma cell tumour. However, an alternative explanation could be transfection of normal pre-B cells by an oncogene complex from the myeloma cells possibly through a viral vector. With the exciting discovery of a C-type retrovirus associated with certain human T-cell leukaemias (HTLV), this is an interesting possibility. The virus is likely to have the same relationship to the T-cell as Epstein–Barr virus (EBV) does to the B-cell, introducing an oncogene which drives the cell to unrestrained division.

Immunodeficiency is a common feature in patients with lymphoid malignancies. Take multiple myeloma for example: the levels of non-myeloma immunoglobulin may be grossly depressed and the patients susceptible to infection with pyogenic bacteria. It is worth mentioning Hodgkin's disease at this point because defects in cell-mediated immunity are so striking, even in early stage I or stage II patients. In fact, half the deaths in this malignant lymphoma are accounted for by infections with intracellular organisms such as *Pneumocystis* or cytomegalovirus. The origin of the characteristic Reed–Sternberg cell is still uncertain but opinion favours classification in the monocyte-macrophage lineage, the problems with cell-mediated immunity presumably arising because of defects in antigen presentation or macrophage microbicidal activity. The events which lead to these immunological deficiencies are still obscure but it seems as though the malignant cells interfere with the development of the corresponding normal cells, almost as though they were producing some cell-specific chalone or transfecting suppressor factor.

The malignant cells bear the surface markers one would expect of normal lymphocytes reaching the stage at which maturation had been arrested. Thus, chronic lymphocytic leukaemia cells resemble mature B-cells in expressing surface Ia and Ig, albeit of a single idiotype in a given patient. Using the Tdt enzyme and antisera directed against Ia, Ig and specific antigens on cortical thymocytes, mature T-cells and non-T, non-B acute lymphoblastic leukaemia cells, it has been possible to classify the lymphoid malignancies in terms of the phenotype of the equivalent normal cell (figure 4.23). This is proving to be of great value in the diagnosis, prognosis and treatment of many of these conditions. For example, whereas T-ALL and B-ALL cases have a poor prognosis, the non-T, non-B ALL patients who include most childhood leukaemias, belong to a prognostically favourable group, many of whom are curable with current therapies.

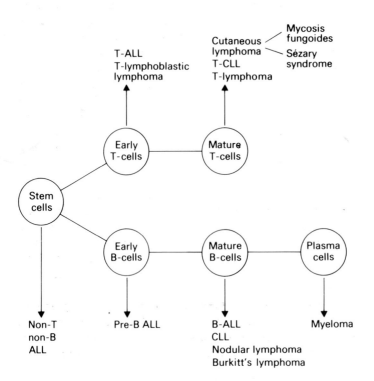

Figure 4.23. Cellular phenotype of human lymphoid malignancies. ALL, acute lymphoblastic leukaemia; CLL, chronic lymphocytic leukaemia. (After Greaves M.F. & Janossy G.)

Phylogeny of the immune response

It has long been known that natural defence mechanisms such as phagocytosis occur in invertebrates. More recently it has become clear that bactericidins may be induced in the haemolymph of species like the lobster by infection with different Gram negative and positive bacteria. The bactericidins can reach a maximum in one to two days with peak titres of $1:100$ or more. They show broad reactivity in that they can kill bacteria antigenically unrelated to the inducing organism; characterization of these molecules to see if they are related in any way to vertebrate immunoglobulins is awaited with interest. With respect to cell-mediated immune reactions, there are now reports that the earthworm can develop transplantation immunity to tissues of the same or other species while permanently accepting autografts (i.e. grafts of its own tissue). An understanding of the nature of these cellular and humoral responses will surely provide some insight into whether the cellular reaction is really the most primitive in evolutionary terms.

All vertebrates are capable of generating an immunological response on antigenic stimulation. Both B- and T-cell responses can be elicited even in the lowliest vertebrate studied, the California hagfish. This unpleasant cyclostome (which preys upon moribund fish by entering their mouths and eating the flesh from the inside) was originally considered 'the negative hero of the phylogeny of immunity' since unlike the lamprey, a more advanced cyclostome, it appeared incapable of reacting immunologically. It now transpires that hagfish can make antibodies to haemocyanin and reject allografts, provided they are maintained at temperatures approaching $20°$ (in general poikilotherms make antibodies better at higher temperatures). The antibodies were present in a $28S$ macroglobulin fraction, but further up the evolutionary scale in the cartilaginous fishes, well-defined $18S$ and $7S$ immunoglobulins with heavy and light chains have now been defined.

It is worthy of note that the thymus is lymphoid in the bony and cartilaginous fishes but in the lamprey there is no clear indication of a lymphoid thymus although a primitive epithelial organ has been recognized. So far there has been no definite evidence of thymus tissue in the hagfish although a small round cell with a thin rim of basophilic cytoplasm found in peripheral blood may be a candidate for an 'early lymphocyte'.

One could imagine the way in which immunoglobulins might have evolved from enzymes. Take, for example, an enzyme which has as its substrate a sugar common to the surface of many types of bacterium. The enzyme will bind to the substrate molecule on the bacterial surface using the same forces which are involved in antigen-antibody interactions. If mutation in the enzyme molecule were to produce a configuration capable of binding to a structure on the surface of a phagocyte (or if mutation changed the phagocyte so that it could bind the enzyme), we would have a bacterium-binding protein cytophilic for phagocytes which would thereby act as an opsonin to increase the rate of bacterial phagocytosis (cf. p. 189). Gene duplication and further mutations would lead to variations in the substrate (antigen)-recognizing portion and in the phagocyte-binding region giving molecules with different recognition specificities and a variety of biological functions.

Summary

Antibody-forming cells can be recognized by immunofluorescence or plaque techniques. Ig peptide chains are synthesized as a single unit starting at the N-terminal end. In myeloma, the monoclonal protein shows as a sharp 'M' band on paper electrophoresis or a 'bump' on the precipitin arc in immunoelectrophoresis; in some cases heavy chains with a central deletion are excreted in the urine. Myeloma light chain dimers appear as Bence–Jones protein in the urine and the variable regions can polymerize to form amyloid deposits. Immortal cell lines making monoclonal antibodies provide powerful new immunological reagents. IgM antibody responses reach an early peak and decline; IgG levels are quantitatively much higher and more persistent and dominate the secondary response. Some Ig classes are particularly thymus dependent. Freund's adjuvant which stimulates T-cell activity only improves the response to thymus-dependent antigens.

Approximately ten genes control the overall antibody response to complex antigens: some affect macrophage antigen handling and some the rate of proliferation of differentiating B-cells. Genes coding for antibodies of given specificities may be inherited together with (i.e. linked to) genetic markers for the heavy chain. Immune response genes linked to the major histocompatibility locus define products (with Ia specificities) on the T- and B-cells and macrophages which control the interactions required for T-B collaboration.

Regulation of the antibody response is strongly influenced by antigen concentration; since the response is largely antigen-driven, as effective antigen levels fall through catabolism and antibody feedback, the synthesis of antibody wanes. T-cells regulate B-lymphocyte responses not only through co-operative help but also by T-cell suppressor activity. Lymphocytes can interact with the idiotypes on the receptors of other lymphocytes to form a network (Jerne). Idiotypes which occur frequently and are shared by a multiplicity of antibodies (public or cross-reacting Id) are targets for regulation by anti-idiotypes in the network thus providing a further mechanism for control of the immune response. The network offers the potential for therapeutic intervention to manipulate immunity.

Immunological tolerance can be induced by exposure to antigens in neonatal and (less readily) in adult life. T-cells are more readily tolerized than B-cells leaving T-dependent B-cells 'helpless'. Elimination of specific cells or generation of T-suppressors may occur, while unresponsiveness to some self-components results from immunological 'silence'.

Multipotent haemopoietic stem cells from the bone marrow differentiate within the thymus to become immunocompetent T-cells. In mammals the bone marrow itself provides the microenvironment for differentiation of B-cells. In man, maternal IgG is the only class to cross the placenta.

Lymphoid cells may become malignant and proliferate clonally, sometimes differentiating further before maturation arrest. The surface phenotype is of diagnostic value.

Primitive lymphoid tissue and separate B- and T-cell adaptive immune responses are associated phylogenetically with the appearance of the lowliest vertebrates.

Further reading

Beer A.E. & Billingham R.E. (1976) *The Immunobiology of Mammalian Reproduction*. Prentice-Hall, New Jersey.

Bevan M.J., Parkhouse R.M.R., Williamson A.R. & Askonas B.A. (1972) Biosynthesis of immunoglobulins. *Progress in Biophysics & Mol.Biol.* **25**, 131.

Brenner R., Hijmans W. & Haaijman J.J. (1981) The bone marrow: the major source of serum Ig, but still a neglected site of antibody formation. *Clin. Exp. Immunol.* **46**, 1.

Dresser D.W. (ed.) (1976) Immunological tolerance. *Brit.Med.Bull.* **32**, No. 2.

Greaves M.J. & Janossy G. (1978) Patterns of gene expression and the cellular origins of human leukaemias. *Biochim. Biophys. Acta* **516**, 193–230.

Hammerling G.J., Hammerling U. & Kearney J.F. (eds) (1981) *Research Monographs in Immunology*. Vol. 3. Monoclonal antibodies and T-cell hybridomas. Elsevier, Amsterdam.

Henry K. & Farrer-Brown G. (1981) *Colour Atlas of Thymus and Lymph Node Histology with Ultrastructure*. Wolfe Medical Publications, London.

Jerne N.K. (1973) The immune system (Network theory). *Scientific American* **229**(1), 52.

Marchalonis J.J. (ed.) (1976) *Comparative Immunology*. Blackwell Scientific Publications, Oxford.

Milstein C. *et al.* (1979) Monoclonal antibodies and cell surface antigens. In *Human Genetics, Possibilities and Realities*. p. 251. Ciba Foundation Series 66 (Excerpta Medica).

Moller E. (ed.) (1978) Acquisition of the T cell repertoire. *Immunol.Rev.* **42**.

Moller E. (ed.) (1978) Role of macrophages in the immune response. *Immunol.Rev.* **40**.

Paul W.E., Fathman C.G. & Metzger H. (eds) (1983) *Ann. Rev. Immunol.* **1**. (Several chapters.)

Pick E. (ed.) *Lymphokines—A Forum for Immunoregulatory Cell Products* (Series). Academic Press, London.

Porter R. & Knight J. (1972) *Ontogeny of Acquired Immunity.* Ciba Foundation Symposium. Elsevier, Amsterdam.

Quesenberry P. & Levitt L. (1979) Haemopoietic stem cells. *N. Engl. J. Med.*, **301**, 755, 819 & 868.

Rheinherry E. & Schlossman S. (1982) Human T-lymphocyte differentiation (colour chart). *Immunol. Today* **3**, No. 9.

Strober W., Hanson L.A. & Sell K.W. (eds) (1982) *Recent Advances in Mucosal Immunity.* Raven Press, New York.

Watson J., Trenkner E. & Cohn M. (1973) The use of bacterial lipopolysaccharides to show that two signals are required for the induction of antibody synthesis. *J.Exp.Med.* **138**, 699. (Note that these authors do not consider cross-linking of receptors to be a necessary condition for induction.)

Yamamura T. & Tada T. (1984) *Progress in Immunology V.* Academic Press, Tokyo.

Zucker-Franklin D., Greaves M.F., Grossi C.E. & Marmont A.M. (1980) *Atlas of Blood Cells. Function and Pathology.* Edi. Ermes, Milan and Lea & Febiger, Philadelphia.

5

The Immune Response III—Theoretical Aspects

Instructive theory

The ability of animals to synthesize antibodies directed against determinants such as dinitrobenzene and sulphanilic acid, which were so unlikely to occur in nature, made it difficult to accept the idea based on Ehrlich's earlier views that the body has preformed antibodies whose production is further stimulated by the entry of antigen. Instead attention turned to theories in which the antigen acted instructively as a template around which a standard unfolded γ-globulin chain could be moulded to provide the appropriate complementary shape. The molecule would be stabilized in this configuration by disulphide linkages, hydrogen bonds and so forth; on separation from the template the molecule would now have a specific combining site for antigen (figure 5.1).

Selective theory

An alternative view holds that the information required for the synthesis of the different antibodies is already present in the genetic apparatus. The gene which codes for a specific antibody is selected and 'switched on' by contact of antigen with the cell, and through transcription and translation of the appropriate messenger RNA, immunoglobulin peptide chains with corresponding individual primary amino acid sequences are synthesized; based on the sequence, these chains then fold spontaneously to a preferred globular configuration which possesses the specific antigen-combining sites (figure 5.1).

An analogy may help in the comparison of these two theories. If we consider the purchase of a suit, two courses of action are open. We may *instruct* the tailor to make the suit to measure, in which case we act as a template for the suit to be made on. Alternatively the tailor may be an enterprising fellow who has already made up 10^8 different suits, one of which is almost certain to fit any intending purchaser; all we have to do is *select* the best fit for ourselves. Although in both cases the know-how of making suits (cf. protein

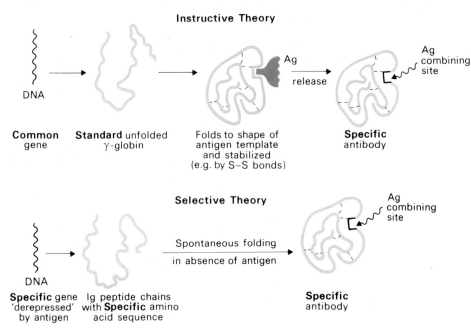

Instructive Theory

DNA → Standard unfolded γ-globin → Folds to shape of antigen template and stabilized (e.g. by S–S bonds) — Ag release → Specific antibody — Ag combining site

Common gene   Standard unfolded γ-globin   Folds to shape of antigen template and stabilized (e.g. by S–S bonds)   Specific antibody

Selective Theory

DNA → Ig peptide chains with **Specific** amino acid sequence — Spontaneous folding in absence of antigen → Specific antibody — Ag combining site

Specific gene 'derepressed' by antigen   Ig peptide chains with **Specific** amino acid sequence   Specific antibody

Figure 5.1. Comparison of instructive and selective theories for generating specific antigen-combining site.

synthesis) is there, in the first instance we provide essential information for the final shape (as the antigen does), whereas in the second situation the tailor himself had the foresight to make a whole variety of differently shaped suits (information already in the DNA) before seeing the customer (antigen).

Evidence for a selective theory

It is generally held that the evidence favours selective theories unequivocally. No antigen capable of acting as a template can be detected in antibody-forming cells. Antibody molecules which have been unfolded by reduction of inter-chain disulphide bonds and treatment with guanidine, spontaneously refold and largely recover their antigen-binding activity showing that the primary amino acid sequences determine the correct tertiary structure of the binding site. Most convincingly, purified antibodies show differences in amino acid sequence, particularly in the hypervariable regions which bind antigen. These reflect differences in DNA nucleotide sequence thereby strongly implicating genetic control of specificity, a view supported by the observation that the capacity to express a given public idiotype (i.e. a hypervariable region shape) is inherited in a simple Mendelian fashion and may be linked to the possession of an Ig heavy chain allele (allotype).

Clonal selection model

The evidence clearly favours a genetic theory and we should now examine how this can be expressed in cellular terms. Clonal selection, based to a considerable extent on the ideas elaborated by Burnet, is generally regarded as an acceptable working model for antibody synthesis.

It is envisaged that each lymphocyte is genetically programmed to make one particular antibody and molecules of that antibody are built into the cell-surface membrane as receptors. Different lymphocytes make different antibodies so that all the body lymphocytes between them present antibodies with a wide spectrum of specificities. Antigen will combine with those lymphocytes carrying antibody on their surface which is a good fit, and these cells will be stimulated by the reaction on the plasma membrane to differentiate and divide to form a clone of cells synthesizing antibody with the same specificity as that on the surface of the parent lymphocyte (figure 5.2). Some of the progeny revert to small lymphocytes and become memory cells.

Figure 5.2. Clonal selection model. Each lymphocyte expresses the genes coding for one specific antibody, several molecules of which are built into the surface membrane to act as receptors. In the diagram, the antigen combines with the cell capable of making the complementary antibody and this reaction at the cell surface leads to the formation of a clone of daughter cells making and exporting that specific antibody.

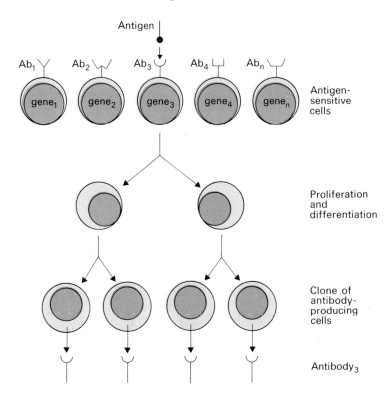

129

Evidence for clonal selection model

ONE CELL/ONE IMMUNOGLOBULIN

With immunofluorescent techniques, immunoglobulin-producing cells can be stained for either κ- or λ-chains but not both, and in the heterozygous rabbit, for the maternal allotypic marker or the paternal but never both together (*allelic exclusion*). Furthermore, plasma cell tumours only produce one, and not more than one, myeloma protein. Similar restrictions apply to the staining of surface Ig on B-lymphocytes described in the previous chapter (p. 63).

That these surface immunoglobulins can behave as antibodies is suggested by the ability of a small percentage of lymphocytes to bind specific antigens such as sheep cells (forming 'rosettes') or radioactive salmonella flagellin. This binding can be blocked by anti-immunoglobulin sera. Humphrey has further shown that the percentage of cells binding antigen is increased in primed and decreased in tolerant animals.

When a soluble antigen like polymerized flagellin binds to a specific cell it causes patching and capping of the surface Ig in just the same way as an anti-Ig serum (cf. p. 64). If the antigen-capped cells are now stained with fluorescent anti-Ig, all the Ig is found in the cap, there being none on the remainder of the lymphocyte surface, i.e. when antigen reacts with a cell, all the Ig molecules on the cell surface combine with the antigen showing that they have similar specificity. In summary, the surface Ig of each B-lymphocyte represents the product of only one of the two chromosomes which code for each Ig chain and behaves as antibody of a single specificity.

RELATION OF SURFACE ANTIBODY TO
FUTURE PERFORMANCE

When cells are taken from an animal which has given a primary response to both ovalbumin and bovine serum albumin (BSA) and are passed down a column of glass beads coated with BSA, they retain the ability to give a secondary antibody response to ovalbumin but are unresponsive to BSA. Thus the BSA-responsive cells have anti-BSA receptors on their surface which cause them to stick to the BSA-coated beads (figure 5.3).

Other investigations have shown that cells primed for a humoral secondary response can be inhibited if treated with anti-immunoglobulin serum before the second contact with antigen. One may conclude that the surface antibody plays a key role in the recognition of antigen for the triggering of the lymphocyte response.

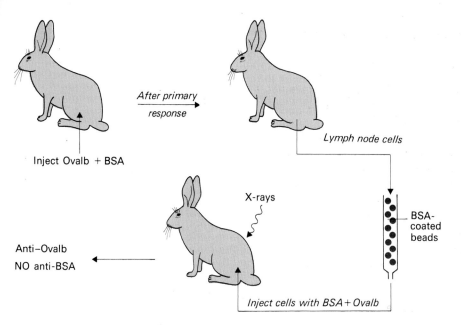

Figure 5.3. Absorption of antibody-forming cell precursors on antigen-coated column. Lymph node cells primed to ovalbumin (ovalb) and bovine serum albumin (BSA) are run down a column of BSA-coated glass beads and injected into an irradiated recipient. On secondary challenge anti-ovalb but no anti-BSA is produced showing that the cells destined to make anti-BSA were bound to the column presumably through their specific anti-BSA receptors on the surface. (Based upon the work of Wigzell H. & Anderson B. (1969) *J.Exp.Med.* **129**, 23.)

Validity of the clonal selection model

Antibody affinity and antigen dosage

The combination of antigen and antibody is reversible and the complex may readily dissociate, depending upon the strength of binding. This can be defined broadly through the equilibrium constant of the reaction:

$$Ag + Ab \rightleftharpoons AgAb$$

and the reactants will behave according to the laws of mass action (cf. Chapter 1, p. 12). If the antigen and antibody fit together very closely, the equilibrium will lie well over to the right; we refer to such antibodies which bind strongly to the antigen as *high-affinity antibodies* (strictly *high avidity* in the case of multivalent antigens, cf. p. 13). Experimentally it is found that injection of *small* amounts of antigen leads to the production of *high*-affinity antibodies whereas *larger* amounts of antigen give more antibody of *lower* affinity. How can we account for this on the clonal selection model?

It may be supposed that when an appropriate number of antigen molecules are bound to the antibody receptors on the cell surface, the lymphocyte will be stimulated to develop into an antibody-producing clone. When only small amounts of antigen are present, only those lymphocytes with high-affinity antibody receptors will be able to bind sufficient antigen for stimulation to occur and their daughter cells will, of course, also produce high-affinity antibody. Consideration of the antigen–antibody equilibrium equation will show that as the concentration of antigen is increased, even antibodies with relatively low affinity will bind more antigen; therefore at high doses of antigen the lymphocytes with lower affinity antibody receptors will also be stimulated and, as may be seen from figure 5.4, these are more abundant than those with receptors of high affinity.

Figure 5.4. Antigen concentration in relation to affinity of surface antibody receptors on lymphocytes which are stimulated. A certain antigen concentration $[Ag]_1$ will lead to binding of sufficient antigen molecules to lymphocytes bearing receptors of affinity 10^6 litres/mole and higher to cause stimulation; assuming the cells will synthesize the same antibody as that present on their surface, the antibodies so produced will thus have affinity of 10^6 litres/mole and higher. At a much higher antigen concentration $[Ag]_2$, lower affinity receptors will now be capable of binding the requisite number of antigen molecules to be triggered. Thus the antibodies produced will now be of affinity 10^4 litres/mole and higher, but as the cell distribution curve shows that the number of cells capable of synthesizing the low-affinity antibodies is much greater, the resulting antiserum will consist predominantly of these low-affinity immunoglobulins.

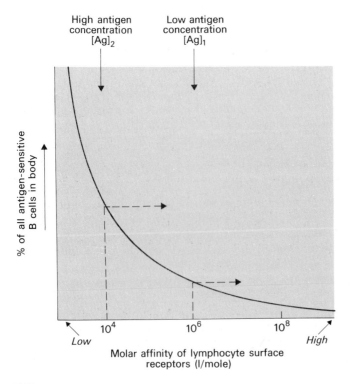

Molar affinity of lymphocyte surface
receptors (l/mole)

Feedback inhibition of antibody synthesis

It was mentioned earlier (p. 101) that the injection of pre-formed antibody could inhibit an immune response to antigen and that this suggests a possible negative feedback model for control of antibody synthesis *in vivo*. The higher the affinity of the injected IgG antibody used to inhibit the immune response, the more effective it is. On the basis of the clonal selection model it may be argued that there will be a competition between injected antibody and the lymphocyte receptors for antigen and only cells with receptors of higher affinity than the administered antibody will be triggered. The higher the affinity of the antibody, the smaller will be the percentage of the total cells available (cf. figure 5.4).

Increase of affinity during immunization

As immunization proceeds, only lymphocytes with higher and higher affinity receptors can be triggered because the concentration of available antigen steadily falls. In addition, feedback inhibition by synthesized antibody will 'turn off' cells with equal or lower affinity receptors. Furthermore, if somatic mutation in the Ig hypervariable regions occurs during an immune response, antigen will selectively bind and trigger those lymphocytes in which the mutant gene codes for receptors with higher affinity.

Hapten inhibition of antibody synthesis

Mitchison has found that if lymphoid cells are taken from a mouse primed with a hapten-carrier complex, treated *in vitro* with excess of free hapten and then transferred to an irradiated recipient, they fail to give a secondary response to the hapten-carrier injected simultaneously. This inhibition by free hapten is ascribed to its binding to lymphocyte surface receptors so making them unavailable for reaction with the antigen hapten-carrier complex. When a cross-reacting hapten is used for the inhibition step, the final antiserum produced gives reasonably good binding with the homologous hapten but very poor cross-reaction, i.e. the hapten used for inhibition had selectively suppressed the reactivity of those cells with which it was best able to combine.

Effect of net charge of the antigen

Rabbit IgG antibodies can be separated by ion exchange chromatography into two major fractions, in one of which the proteins have a greater net positive charge than in the other. Antigens with a net negative charge favour the synthe-

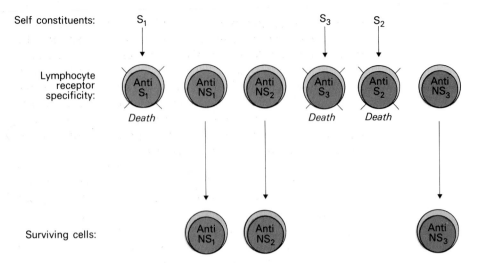

Self constituents: S_1 S_3 S_2

Lymphocyte receptor specificity:

Anti S_1 — Death   Anti NS_1 Anti NS_2 Anti S_3 — Death   Anti S_2 — Death   Anti NS_3

Surviving cells: Anti NS_1 Anti NS_2 Anti NS_3

Figure 5.5. Induction of tolerance to self-constituents (S_1–S_3) by selective elimination of lymphocytes with self-reacting surface receptors. These cells are either killed or inactivated or inhibited by specific T suppressors. Surviving cells are able to react only with non-self (NS) foreign antigens of specificity NS_1, NS_2, NS_3, etc.

sis of the more positively charged antibodies and *vice versa* (Sela & Mozes). This would be fully consistent with the preferential binding of antigens to cells with surface receptors of opposite charge, other factors being equal.

Immunological tolerance

The clonal selection model readily provides a basis for the mechanism of tolerance induction. It has only to be postulated that under the conditions known to cause unresponsiveness, contact with antigen causes death or long-term inactivation of the antigen-sensitive cell rather than its stimulation. Although we are uncertain of the mechanism, the idea that deletion or inactivation of specific clones is responsible for tolerance induction is attractive. For example, it can account for the development of self-tolerance since all lymphocytes having receptors capable of reacting with circulating or accessible self-components would be eliminated or suppressed leaving only those cells with receptors for non-self determinants in the immunological armamentarium (figure 5.5).

Genetic theories of antibody variability

The variation in primary amino acid sequence of different antibodies, the differences between animal strains in their immunological responsiveness to selected synthetic and viral antigens and the plausibility of the clonal selection model all speak for a genetic basis underlying antibody variability. Similarities in amino acid sequence (homology) between the loops formed by intrachain disulphide bonds in the constant parts of heavy and light chains (figure 2.13) and to some extent between variable and constant parts, suggest that the existing genes controlling immunoglobulin structure are derived from a primitive smaller gene—coding for a peptide half the length of a light chain—by a process of duplication and translocation with early divergence of V genes.

Rough estimates place the total repertoire of different antibody molecules which can be synthesized by a given individual at around 10^8 or perhaps even more. To help us understand the genetic basis for this quite remarkable diversity, we should first review the current status of our knowledge concerning the form and number of inherited (i.e. germ line) genes encoding antibody molecules.

GENES CODING FOR ANTIBODY

These fall into three clusters on three different chromosomes coding for κ, λ and heavy chains respectively. There appears to be only one variable region (V) gene for mouse λ chain and the genetic basis for the synthesis of this peptide is illustrated in figure 5.6. In common with other eukaryotic proteins, the chain is encoded in multiple distinct gene segments separated by intervening nucleotide sequences, *introns*, which are removed either by DNA translocation or by excision of the corresponding mRNA sequence. There is a leader sequence required for passage of the peptide through the endoplasmic reticulum, a V_λ segment coding for amino acid residues 1 to 98, a joining segment (J—not to be confused with the J peptide in IgM and IgA) encoding the remaining 11 amino acids of the variable region, and a C_λ gene segment giving rise to the constant region. As a lymphocyte undergoes differentiation to become an immunocompetent cell capable of synthesizing λ chains, there is a rearrangement or translocation of the DNA bringing the L, V_λ and J segments together but still separated from the C_λ by an intron of 1250 nucleotides. Splicing of the transcribed RNA in the nucleus produces an mRNA which can now be used for the synthesis of a continuous λ chain peptide.

The same general principles apply to the arrangement of κ and heavy chain genes although they exist in far greater variety (figure 5.7). The V_κ genes occur as a series of 50–100 clusters or sets each containing 6–8 closely related individual genes. Although the genes within a given set show some framework and hypervariable diversity, they resemble each other far more than they do V_κ genes in other sets. There are 5 different J segments but just a single constant region gene.

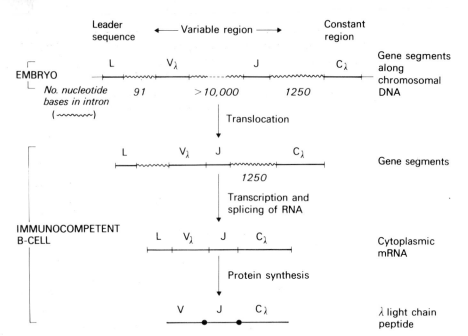

Figure 5.6. Genetic basis for synthesis of mouse λ chain. As the cell becomes immunocompetent, the variable region is formed by the combination of V_λ with the joining segment J, a process facilitated by base sequences in the intron following the 3′ end of the V_κ segment pairing up with sequences in the intron 5′ to J. This variable region V_κ J segment is separate from the gene encoding the constant region as originally predicted by Dreyer and Bennett. The final joining occurs when the intervening sequence is spliced out of the mRNA transcript. In the human, the V_λ genes are more complex (cf. V_κ genes below).

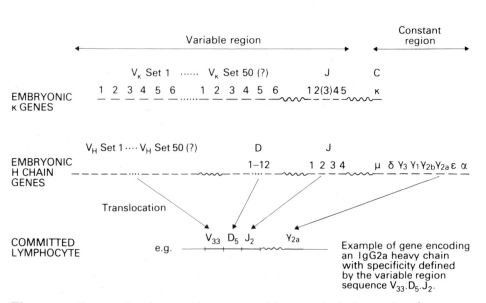

Figure 5.7. Genes coding for κ and heavy chain peptides in the mouse. The sequence of C_H genes in the human is μ, δ, γ_1, γ_2, γ_3, γ_4, ε, α_1 and α_2.

The heavy chain constellation shows additional features: the subclass constant region genes form a single cluster and there is a group of 12 highly variable D segments inserted between the V and J regions. The D and J segments together encode almost the entire third hypervariable region which forms one side of the combining site groove (figure 2.10).

Allelic exclusion

Since each cell has chromosome complements derived from each parent, the differentiating B-cell has 4 light and 2 heavy chain gene clusters to choose from. Once the V.D.J DNA rearrangement has occurred within one light and one heavy chain cluster, the V genes on the other 4 chromosomes are held by some mechanism in the embryonic state so that the cell is able to express *only one light and one heavy chain*. As we have discussed above, this so-called allelic exclusion is essential for clonal selection to work since the cell is then only programmed to make the one antibody it uses as a cell surface receptor to recognize antigen. Furthermore, this gene exclusion mechanism prevents the formation of molecules containing two different light or two different heavy chains which would have non-identical combining sites and therefore be functionally monovalent with respect to the majority of antigens; such antibodies would be non-agglutinating and would tend to have low avidity because the bonus effect of multivalency could not operate.

Antibody class switch

The arrangement of heavy chain genes permits a given V.D.J variable region to associate sequentially with different constant region genes so accounting for class switch during the antibody response (figure 5.8). The co-existence of IgM and IgD bearing the same idiotype on the surface of a given B-lymphocyte prior to its maturation as an antibody-forming cell (p. 119) is probably due to differential splicing of a large $\mu + \delta$ RNA transcript to yield separate μ and δ mRNAs with identical variable regions.

T-cell receptor

The ability of T-cell clones and hybridomas to discriminate finely between closely related antigens implies possession of antigen-specific receptors. After many years of searching, the nature of these receptors is now becoming clearer. Unlike Ig antibodies, the T-cell has the job of recognizing an MHC

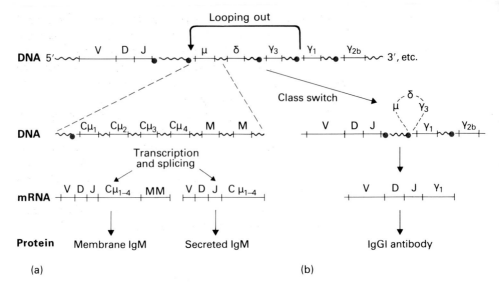

Figure 5.8. Immunoglobulin heavy chain genes and the mechanisms for their involvement in: (a) synthesis of membrane-bound IgM, which functions as a receptor anchored in the membrane by the hydrophobic sequence encoded by the gene segments M–M, and the secreted form which lacks this sequence, (b) class switching to transfer a given variable region to a different heavy chain isotype (in this example from IgM to IgG1) based on a 'looping out' process which utilizes the specialized switch sequences (•) and leads to a loss of the intervening DNA (μ, δ and $\gamma3$). Rare examples of mutant clones expressing an isotypic gene 5′ of the parent heavy chain gene suggest that switching to constant region genes on the sister chromatid may sometimes occur.

molecule in addition to the antigen (an issue discussed further on p. 292). Antisera or monoclonals specific for the antigen recognition unit of T-cell clones immunoprecipitate a membrane molecule consisting of two peptides of 40K and 43K in the mouse and 43 and 49K in the human. Examination of T-lymphomas, clones or hybridomas with appropriate cDNA probes showed there to be no functional rearrangement of the conventional Ig genes characteristic of the B-cell (cf. figures 5.6 and 5.7). However, using the mRNA from T-cell lines and hybridomas, it has now been possible to isolate cDNA clones which selectively recognize mRNA from T- as distinct from B-cell lines and which hybridize to a region of the genome in these T-cells that has undergone rearrangement of the kind seen with Ig genes. Sequence studies on such clones derived from human and mouse sources show that they code for an unglycosylated peptide of around 35K which has a structure analogous with the V, J and constant regions of Ig peptides. Partial sequences on other similar cDNA clones (at the time of writing) showed close similarity in the carboxy terminal section but considerable diversity in the putative variable region. Assuming that the peptide proves to be a component of the T-cell receptor, it seems likely that this sequence diversity will be much greater than that of the Ig V domains which are relatively highly conserved outside the hyper-variable complementarity regions which make up the antigen combining site. If the combining site of the T-cell receptor is considerably larger than that of Ig antibody, it might accommodate both foreign antigen plus the associated MHC molecule. Thus, in addition to the three Ig variable gene clusters (V_H, V_κ, V_λ) already known on three different chromosomes, we must add a fourth (and presumably soon a fifth) cluster coding for the once elusive T-cell receptor.

THE GENERATION OF DIVERSITY

The problem of generating 10^8 or more different antibody molecules is now seen as a problem of generating 10^8 or more different combining sites since the variable genes in any cluster can all link with the same constant region segment and it is therefore only necessary to have single C region genes. Several mechanisms have evolved to achieve this goal, and in discussing these we will concern ourselves just with the mouse since most information is available for this species.

Inheritance of germ-line V region genes

Starting with the germ-line gene segments present in the embryonic cells which are the building blocks from which our universe of binding sites must be created, it is estimated that the numbers of V genes encoding heavy and κ-light chains (V_H and V_κ genes) are both of the order of 2×10^2. To these must be added the small number of D and J segments (figure 5.7).

Intra-chain amplification

During the combinatorial events which join V, D and J segments as the B cell differentiates, $V_\kappa \rightarrow J_\kappa$, $V_H \rightarrow D$ and $D \rightarrow J_H$ associations are entirely random. This will generate approximately 10^3 ($2 \times 10^2 V \times 4J$) different light chain and 10^4 ($2 \times 10^2 V \times 12D \times 4J$) heavy chain variable regions.

Some rearranged D genes are longer than their germ-line counterparts, suggesting that unusual joining may occur among D segments to form new D-D segments. Another ploy to squeeze even more variation out of the germ-line repertoire involves *variable boundary* recombination of V_κ and J_κ, and V_H, D and J_H in which the segments are joined at different points in their DNA sequences, producing hybrid codons as well as codon insertions or deletions. These further mechanisms would be expected to push up the total of light chain variable gene recombinants to around 5×10^3 and of heavy chain variable regions to 10^5. It is worth noting that these recombination events between V, D and J segments greatly amplify the diversity of the third hypervariable region in both heavy and light chains.

Inter-chain amplification

The immune system took a further ingenious step forward when heavy and light chains evolved separately. When one heavy chain is paired with different light chains the specificity of the final antibody is altered; for example, pairing of a heavy chain containing the T15 idiotype with three different light chains produced antibodies with different affinities for phosphorylcholine. Thus random association between 5×10^3 light and 10^5 heavy chains could generate a total of 5×10^8 ($5 \times 10^3 \times 10^5$) specificities. Not a bad score considering that we started with something of the order of 400 germ-line genes! But we go even further.

Somatic mutation

There is inescapable evidence that V region genes can undergo significant somatic mutation. Analysis of 18 murine λ myelomas revealed 12 with identical structure, 4 showing just one amino acid change, 1 with 2 changes and 1 with 4 changes, all within the hypervariable regions and indicative of somatic mutation of the single mouse λ germ-line gene. In another study, following immunization with pneumococcal antigen, a single germ-line T15 V_H gene gave rise by mutation to several different V_H genes all encoding phosphorylcholine antibodies (figure 5.9).

A number of features of this somatic diversification phenomenon deserve mention. The mutations are the result of single nucleotide substitutions, they are restricted to the variable as distinct from the constant region and occur in both framework and hypervariable regions. The mutation rate calculated by dividing the substitutions by the nucleotide bases sequenced is remarkably high, between 2 and 4% for V_H genes as compared with a figure of less than 0.0001% for a non-immunological lymphocyte gene. In addition, the mutational mechanism is bound up in some way with class switch since mutations are more frequent in IgG and IgA than in IgM antibodies, affecting both heavy (figure 5.9) and light chains.

140

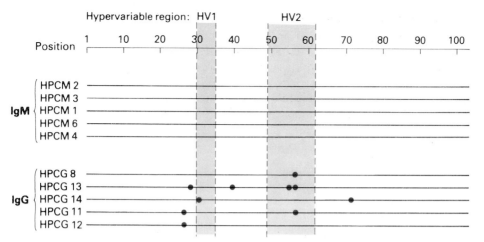

Figure 5.9. Mutations in a germ-line gene. The amino acid sequences of the V_H regions of five IgM and five IgG monoclonal phosphorylcholine antibodies generated during an anti-pneumococcal response in a single mouse are compared with the primary structure of the T15 germ-line sequence. A line indicates identity with the T15 prototype and a red circle (•) a single amino acid difference. Mutations have only occurred in the IgG molecules and are seen in both hypervariable and framework segments (after Gearhart P.J. (1982) *Immunol. Today* **3**, 107).

Conclusions

The total number of antibody specificities which can be generated by the immune system is thus seen to be breathtakingly high, but this is an essential feature of the defensive strategy since we are surrounded by myriads of microorganisms with the capacity to evolve into shapes which do not at present exist. We must be capable of producing antibodies of reasonable affinity to fit any conceivable molecular shape, just like our prescient tailor at the beginning of the chapter who was always one jump ahead because he made so many different suits, they would fit any possible future customer. Even if the initial lymphocytes triggered are of low affinity, the multivalence of IgM will ensure acceptable avidity for multideterminant microbial antigens, and in the case of proteins which are essentially univalent with respect to each epitope (cf. p. 71), T-cell help will induce classswitching and an attendant mutational mechanism which will lead to maturation of affinity through positive selection by antigen (cf. p. 133).

How is the complex of germ-line genes protected from genetic drift? With a library of say 400 V genes, selection would act only weakly on any single gene which had been functionally crippled by mutation and this implies that a major part of the library could be lost before evolutionary forces operated. One idea is that each set of six to eight related V genes (figure 5.7) contains a prototype coding for an antibody which is indispensable for protection against some common pathogen so that mutation in this gene would put the host at a disadvantage and would therefore be selected against. If any of the other closely related genes in its set become defective through mutation, this indispensable gene could repair them by gene conversion, a mechanism known to act on families of genes to maintain a degree of sequence homogeneity, and in which two genes interact in such a way that the nucleotide sequence of part or all of one becomes identical to that of the other.

Summary

Antigen does not act as a template for antibody production; the complete information for antibody synthesis is already in the genome. Folding of the antibody molecule, and hence specificity, depends upon the primary amino acid structure and differences in amino acid sequence between different antibodies reflect differences in DNA nucleotide sequence. Immune responsiveness is genetically controlled.

The clonal selection model assumes that each immuno-competent lymphocyte is programmed to synthesize one immunoglobulin which is inserted into the plasma membrane as a surface receptor. An antigen which reacts strongly with this surface antibody will be bound selectively, trigger the cell and cause clonal amplification and differentiation to provide a large population of cells all making antibody of the required specificity plus an expanded population of memory cells. The model accounts for the inverse relation between antigen dose and antibody affinity, the greater effectiveness of high affinity antibody in feedback inhibition of the immune response and the increase in affinity with immunization; it envisages immunological tolerance in terms of deletion or inactivation of specific clones.

There are three distinct clusters of genes coding for κ, λ and heavy Ig peptide chains. In the mouse, the germ-line contains approximately 2×10^2 V_κ and 4J (joining) segments encoding the variable region of κ light chains, and around 2×10^2 V_H, 12D and $4J_H$ segments encoding heavy chain variable regions. Only single genes encode each Ig constant region isotype. As the lymphocyte differentiates to become a committed cell, random combinations between V and J segments on the light chain and V, D and J elements on the heavy chain probably generate roughly 5×10^3 genes coding for light chain and 10^5 for heavy chain variable regions. Additional amplification occurs through random association of heavy and light chains producing a potential of 5×10^8 different antigen-combining sites. Somatic mutation, particularly in the IgG and IgA classes increases this variation even further. In the secreting cell, coupling between the V(D)J and the constant region is effected by splicing the nuclear mRNA; a switch to coupling with another C_H gene leads to production of antibody with the same specificity but different class or subclass. The T-cell receptor consists of two peptides of molecular weight of the order of 40K which do not involve the Ig gene clusters. Preliminary sequence data on one of the peptides reveals a structure similar to an Ig peptide but with a much larger hypervariable region possibly related to the need to recognize antigen plus MHC. This incredible diversity in potential specificities protects the individual from the myriads of existing and future microorganisms.

Further reading

Edelman G.M. (ed.) (1974) *Cellular Selection and Regulation in the Immune Response.* Society of General Physiologists Series, Vol 29. Raven Press, New York.

Fudenberg H.H., Pink J.R.L., Stites D.P. & Wang A.-C. (1977) *Basic Immunogenetics,* 2nd edn. Oxford University Press, New York.

Honjo T. (1983) Immunoglobulin genes. *Ann. Rev. Immunol.* **1**, 499.

Schilling J., Clevinger B., Davie J.M. & Hood L. (1980) Amino acid sequence of homogeneous antibodies to dextran and DNA rearrangements in heavy chain V-region gene segments. *Nature* **283**, 35.

Siskind G.W. & Benacerraf B. (1969) Cell selection by antigen in the immune response. *Adv. Immunol.* **10**, 1.

Williams A.F. (1984) The T-lymphocyte antigen receptor—elusive no more. (Editorial) *Nature* **308**, 108.

6 Interaction of Antigen and Antibody

The primary interaction between an antigenic determinant and the combining site of an antibody, governed by the affinity, gives rise to a number of secondary phenomena such as precipitation, agglutination, phagocytosis, cytolysis, neutralization and so on. In this chapter we consider the practical implications of this interaction and begin to explore its consequences.

Precipitation

Multivalent antigens mixed with bivalent antibodies in solution can combine to form complexes which aggregate and precipitate. As described in Chapter 1 (p. 5) the amount of precipitate varies with the proportions of the reagents and, generally speaking, insoluble complexes are formed in *antibody excess* while the complexes generated in *antigen excess* tend to be soluble. A variety of techniques depend upon visualization of the precipitation reaction in gels.

PRECIPITATION IN GELS

In the double diffusion method of Ouchterlony, antigen and antibody placed in wells cut in agar gel diffuse towards each other and precipitate to form an opaque line in the region where they meet in optimal proportions. A preparation containing several antigens will give rise to multiple lines. The immunological relationship between two antigens can be assessed by setting up the precipitation reactions in adjacent wells; the lines formed by each antigen may be completely confluent indicating immunological identity, they may show a 'spur' as in the case of partially related antigens, or they may cross, indicative of unrelated antigens (figure 6.1). The origins of these patterns are explained in figure 6.2. It should be emphasized that even in the case of confluent lines this can only indicate immunological identity in terms of the antiserum used, not necessarily molecular identity. For example, purified antibodies to the dinitrobenzene hapten would give a line of confluence when set up against dinitrobenzene–

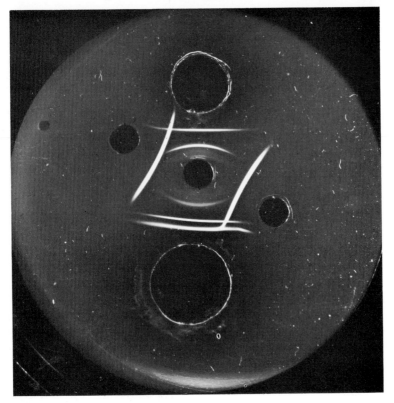

Antiserum in centre well

Figure 6.1. Multiple lines formed in the Ouchterlony test (double-diffusion precipitation) when rabbit antiserum (centre well) reacts in agar gel with four different antigen preparations (peripheral wells). Non-identity and partial identity of antigens are shown respectively by crossing over and spur formation between precipitin lines.

Figure 6.2. (a) Line of confluence obtained with two antigens which cannot be distinguished by the antiserum used.

(b) Spur formation by partially related antigens having a common determinant a but individual determinants b and c reacting with a mixture of antibodies directed against a and b. The antigen with determinants a and c can only precipitate antibodies directed to a. The remaining antibodies (Ab_b) cross the precipitin line to react with the antigen from the adjacent well which has determinant b giving rise to a 'spur' over the precipitin line.

(c) Crossing over of lines formed with unrelated antigens.

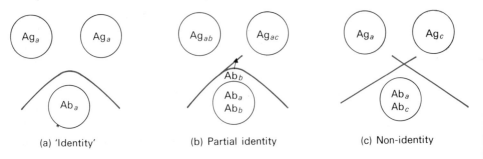

(a) 'Identity'   (b) Partial identity   (c) Non-identity

ovalbumin and dinitro-benzene–serum albumin conjugates placed in adjacent wells.

Where reagents are present in balanced proportions, the line formed will generally be concave to the well containing the reactant of higher molecular weight, be it antigen or antibody. This is a consequence of the usually slower diffusion rate of larger sized molecules.

The gel precipitation method can be made more sensitive by incorporating the antiserum in the agar and allowing the antigen to diffuse into it; up to 90% serum in agar may be employed (Feinberg). This method of single radial immunodiffusion is used for the quantitative estimation of antigens.

SINGLE RADIAL IMMUNODIFFUSION (SRID)

When antigen diffuses from a well into agar containing suitably diluted antiserum, initially it is present in a relatively high concentration and forms soluble complexes; as the antigen diffuses further the concentration continuously falls until the point is reached at which the reactants are nearer optimal proportions and a ring of precipitate is formed. The higher the concentration of antigen, the greater the diameter of this ring (figure 6.3). By incorporating, say, three standards of known antigen concentration in the plate, a calibration curve can be obtained and used to determine the amount of antigen in the unknown samples tested (figure 6.4). The method is used routinely in clinical immunology, particularly for immunoglobulin determinations, and also for substances such as the third component of complement, transferrin, C-reactive protein and the embryonic protein, α-fetoprotein, which is associated with certain liver tumours.

IMMUNOELECTROPHORESIS

The principle of this has been described earlier (p. 26). The method is of value for the identification of antigens by their electrophoretic mobility, particularly when other antigens are also present. In clinical immunology, semiquantitative information regarding immunoglobulin concentrations and identification of myeloma proteins is provided by this technique.

There have been some felicitous developments of the principle combining electrophoresis with immunoprecipitation in which movement in an electric field drives the antigen directly into contact with antibody. *Countercurrent immunoelectrophoresis* may be applied to antigens which migrate towards the positive pole in agar (see figure 6.5). This qualitative technique is much faster and considerably more sensitive than double diffusion (Ouchterlony) and is used for the detection of hepatitis B antigen or antibody, DNA antibodies

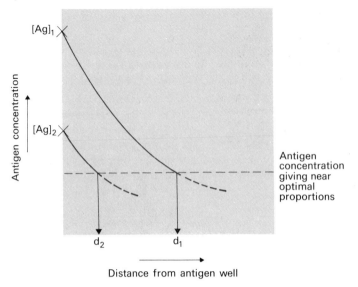

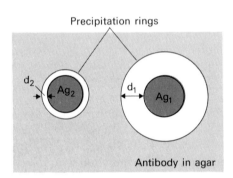

Precipitation rings

Antibody in agar

Figure 6.3. Single radial immunodiffusion: relation of antigen concentration to size of precipitation ring formed. Antigen at higher concentrations diffuses further from the well before it falls to the level giving precipitation with antibody near optimal proportions.

in SLE (p. 315), autoantibodies to soluble nuclear antigens in mixed connective tissue disease, and *Aspergillus* precipitins in cases with allergic bronchopulmonary aspergillosis. *Rocket electrophoresis* is a quantitative method which involves electrophoresis of antigen into a gel containing antibody. The precipitation arc has the appearance of a rocket, the length of which is related to antigen concentration (figure 6.6). Like countercurrent electrophoresis this is a rapid method but again the antigen must move to the positive pole on electrophoresis; it is therefore suitable for proteins such as albumin, transferrin and caeruloplasmin but immunoglobulins are more conveniently quantitated by single radial immunodiffusion. One powerful variant of the rocket system, Laurell's *two-dimensional immunoelectrophoresis*, involves a preliminary electrophoretic separation of an antigen mixture in a direction perpendicular to that of the final 'rocket-stage'

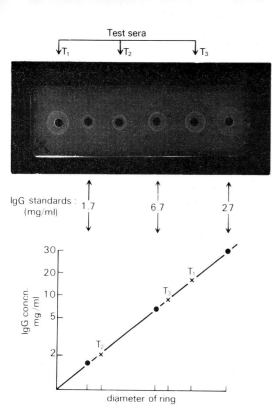

Figure 6.4. Measurement of IgG concentration in serum by single radial immunodiffusion. The diameter of the standards (●) enables a calibration curve to be drawn and the concentration of IgG in the sera under test can be read off:

T$_1$—serum from patient with IgG
  myeloma; 15 mg/ml
T$_2$—serum from patient with hypo-
  gammaglobulinaemia; 2.6 mg/ml
T$_3$—normal serum; 9.6 mg/ml.
(Courtesy of Dr F.C. Hay.)

Figure 6.5. Countercurrent immuno-electrophoresis. Antibody moves 'backwards' in the gel on electrophoresis due to endosmosis; an antigen which is negatively charged at the pH employed will move towards the positive pole and precipitate on contact with antibody. ˙

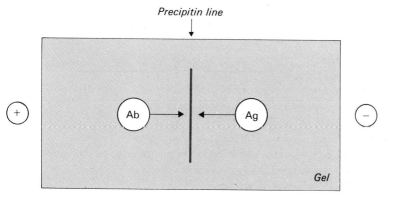

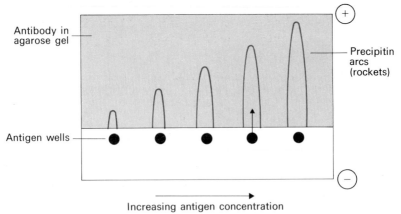

Antibody in agarose gel

Precipitin arcs (rockets)

Antigen wells

Increasing antigen concentration

Figure 6.6. Rocket electrophoresis. Antigen is electrophoresed into gel containing antibody. The distance from the starting well to the front of the rocket-shaped arc is related to antigen concentration.

(figure 6.7a). In this way one can quantitate each of several antigens in a mixture. One straightforward example is the estimation of the degree of conversion of the third component of complement (C3) to the inactive form C3c (cf. pp. 168 and 257) which may occur in the serum of patients with

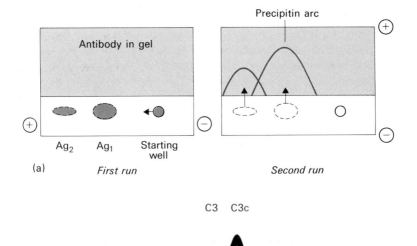

Precipitin arc

Antibody in gel

Ag_2 Ag_1 Starting well

(a)   *First run*   *Second run*

C3   C3c

(b)   Direction of first run ⟶

Figure 6.7. Two-dimensional immunoelectrophoresis. (a) Antigens are separated on the basis of electrophoretic mobility. The second run at right angles to the first drives the antigens into the antiserum-containing gel to form precipitin peaks; the area under the peak is related to the concentration of antigen. (b) Actual run showing C3 conversion (C3 → C3c) in serum. In this case the arcs interact because of common antigenic determinants. (Courtesy of Dr C. Loveday.)

active SLE or the synovial fluid of affected joints in active rheumatoid arthritis, to give but two examples (figure 6.7b).

QUANTIFICATION BY NEPHELOMETRY

The small aggregates formed when dilute solutions of antigen and antibody are mixed creates a cloudiness or turbidity which can be measured by the scattering of an incident light source (nephelometry). Greater sensitivity can be obtained by using monochromatic light from a laser and by adding polyethylene glycol to the solution so that aggregate size is increased. In favoured laboratories which can sport the appropriate equipment, this method is replacing single radial immunodiffusion for the estimation of immunoglobulins, C3, C-reactive protein, etc.

Radioactive binding techniques

MEASUREMENT OF ANTIBODY

These methods assess antibody level either by determining the capacity of an antiserum to complex with radioactive antigen or by measuring the amount of immunoglobulin binding to an insoluble antigen preparation. Perhaps the point should be made that it is not possible to define the *absolute* concentration of antibody in a given serum because each serum contains immunoglobulins with a range of binding affinities and the estimation of the amount of antigen bound to antibody depends upon the concentration and affinities of the antibodies as well as the nature and sensitivity of the test. With this proviso, the quantitative tests described do give a measure of the antibody content of a serum which is of practical value.

Using radioactive antigen

The two methods to be considered involve the addition of excess radio-labelled antigen to the antiserum followed by assessment of the amount of antigen which has been complexed with antibody (this being the antigen binding capacity). This is achieved either by:

1 *The Farr technique* in which complexed antigen is separated from that in the free form by precipitation with 50% ammonium sulphate (only applicable to those antigens soluble at this salt concentration), or

2 *The antiglobulin coprecipitation technique* in which the antigen bound to antibody is precipitated together with the rest of the immunoglobulin by an antiglobulin serum, leaving

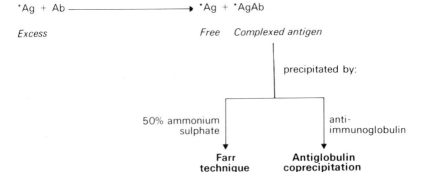

Excess   Free   Complexed antigen

Figure 6.8. Determination of antigen-binding capacity. After addition of excess radioactive antigen (*Ag), that part bound to antibody as a complex is precipitated either by ammonium sulphate (Farr) or by an antiglobulin (antiglobulin coprecipitation).

free antigen in the supernatant (figure 6.8). By using antibodies to different immunoglobulin classes and subclasses as the antiglobulin reagent, it is possible to determine the distribution of antibody activity among the classes. For example, addition of a radioactive antigen to human serum followed by a precipitating rabbit antihuman IgA would indicate how much antigen had been bound to the serum IgA.

Using insoluble antigen

The antibody content of a serum can be assessed by the ability to bind to antigen which has been insolubilized either by coupling to an immunoadsorbent or by physical adsorption to a plastic tube; the bound immunoglobulin may then be estimated by addition of a radio-labelled anti-Ig raised in another species (figure 6.9). Consider, for example, the determination of DNA autoantibodies in systemic lupus erythematosus (cf. p. 315). When a patient's serum is added to a plastic tube coated with antigen (in this case DNA), the autoantibodies will bind to the tube and remaining serum proteins can be readily washed away. Bound antibody can now be estimated by addition of ^{125}I-labelled purified rabbit anti-human IgG; after rinsing out excess unbound reagent, the radioactivity of the tube will clearly be a measure of the autoantibody content of the patient's serum. The distribution of antibody in different classes can obviously be determined by using specific antisera. Take the radioallergosorbent test (RAST) for IgE antibodies in allergic patients. The allergen (e.g. pollen extract) is covalently coupled to a paper disc which is then treated with patient's serum. The amount of specific IgE bound to the paper is then estimated by addition of labelled anti-IgE.

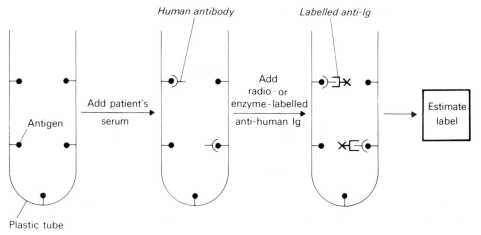

Figure 6.9. The solid phase 'tube test' for quantitative determination of antibody.

MEASUREMENT OF ANTIGEN

Radioimmunoassay

The binding of radioactively labelled antigen to a limited fixed amount of antibody can be partially inhibited by addition of unlabelled antigen and the extent of this inhibition can be used as a measure of the unlabelled material added. The principle of this form of saturation analysis is explained in figure 6.10. Methods vary in the means used to separate free antigen from that bound to antibody: some use copre-

Figure 6.10. Principle of radioimmuno-assay (simplified by assuming a very highly avid antibody and one combining site per antibody molecule).

(a) If we add 150 mol of radio-labelled Ag to 100 mol of Ab, 50 mol of Ag will be free and 100 bound to Ab. The ratio of the counts of free to bound will be 1 : 2.

(b) If we now add 150 mol of unlabelled Ag plus 150 mol radio Ag to the Ab, again only 100 mol of total Ag will be bound, but since the Ab cannot distinguish labelled from unlabelled Ag, half will be radioactive. The remaining antigen will be free and the ratio free : bound radioactivity changes to 2 : 1. This ratio will vary with the amount of unlabelled Ag added and this enables a calibration curve to be constructed.

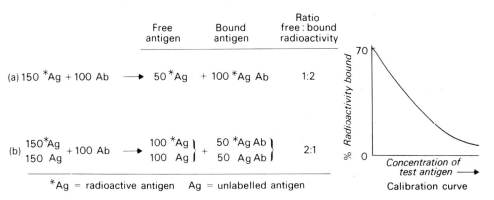

*Ag = radioactive antigen   Ag = unlabelled antigen

153

cipitation of the complex with anti-immunoglobulin sera, others adsorption of free antigen on to charcoal and so on. With the development of methods for labelling antigens to a high specific activity, very low concentrations down to the 10^{-12} g/ml level can be detected and most of the protein hormones can now be assayed with this technique. One disadvantage is that these methods cannot distinguish active protein molecules from biologically inactive fragments which still retain antigenic determinants. Other applications include the assay of carcinoembryonic antigen, hepatitis B (Australia) antigen and smaller molecules such as steroids, prostaglandins and morphine-related drugs (appropriate antibodies are raised by coupling to an immunogenic carrier).

Immunoradiometric assay

This differs from radioimmunoassay in the sense that the labelled reagent is used in excess. For the estimation of antigen, antibodies are coated on to a solid surface such as plastic and the test antigen solution added; after washing, the amount of antigen bound to the plastic can be estimated by adding an excess of radio-labelled antibody. The specificity of the method can be improved by using solid phase and labelled antibodies with specificities for different parts of the antigen:

Solid phase —$\boxed{Ab_1}$—(→ ●—$\boxed{Ag}$—■ ←]—$\boxed{*Ab_2}$

One widely used application is the radioimmunosorbent test (RIST) for IgE. Rabbit anti-IgE is coupled by cyanogen bromide to microcrystalline cellulose and reacted with dilutions of an IgE-containing standard serum or the patient's serum under test. Bound IgE is then measured by addition of labelled anti-IgE.

'Immunoblotting'

After separation from a complex mixture by electrophoresis in a solid phase such as polyacrylamide or agar gel, antigens can be 'blotted' by transverse electrophoresis on to nitrocellulose sheets where they bind non-specifically and can be identified by staining with appropriately labelled antibodies. This technique has been used successfully to identify components of neurofilaments which have been separated in sodium dodecyl sulphate (SDS)-polyacrylamide gels; obviously, such a procedure will not work with antigens which are irreversibly denatured by this detergent. Conversely, the spectrotype of an antiserum can be revealed by isoelectric focusing, blotting and then staining with labelled antigen.

Because of health hazards, the expense of counting equipment and the deterioration of labelled reagents through radiation damage, other types of label have been sought. Enzymes such as peroxidase and phosphatase which give a coloured reaction product have been successfully employed particularly in the ELISA (enzyme-linked immunosorbent assay), an immunometric assay for antibody (figure 6.9) or antigen. Chemiluminescent and new fluorescent tags are under active scrutiny but almost the ultimate in sensitivity (around 10^3 molecules of antigen) is claimed for a method combining enzyme label with radioactive substrate.

Immunohistochemistry

IMMUNOFLUORESCENCE

Fluorescent dyes such as fluorescein and rhodamine can be coupled to antibodies without destroying their specificity. Coons showed that such conjugates would combine with antigen present in a tissue section and that the bound antibody could be visualized in the fluorescence microscope. In this way the distribution of antigen throughout a tissue and within cells can be demonstrated. Looked at another way, the method can also be used for the detection of antibodies directed against antigens already known to be present in a given tissue section or cell preparation. There are three general ways in which the test is carried out.

1. *Direct test*

The antibody to the tissue substrate is itself conjugated with the fluorochrome and applied directly (figure 6.11a). For example, suppose we wished to show the tissue distribution of a gastric autoantigen reacting with the autoantibodies present in the serum of a patient with pernicious anaemia. We would isolate IgG from the patient's serum, conjugate it with fluorescein, and apply it to a section of human gastric mucosa on a slide. When viewed in the fluorescence microscope we would see that the cytoplasm of the parietal cells was brightly stained. By using antisera conjugated to dyes which emit fluorescence at different wavelengths, two different antigens can be identified simultaneously in the same preparation. In figure 3.7h (p. 55), direct staining of fixed plasma cells with a mixture of rhodamine-labelled anti-IgG and fluorescein-conjugated anti-IgM craftily demonstrates that these two classes of antibody are produced by different cells. The technique of coupling biotin to the antiserum and

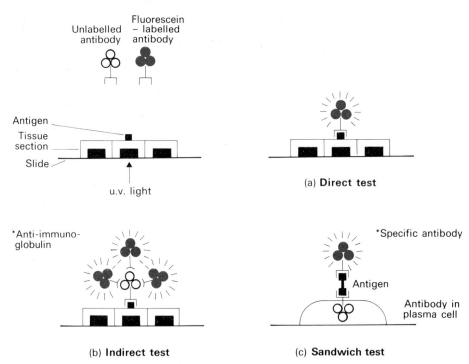

Figure 6.11. Fluorescent antibody tests.
* = fluorescein labelled.

then finally staining with fluorescent avidin is finding increasing favour.

2. *Indirect test*

In this double layer technique, the unlabelled antibody is applied directly to the tissue substrate and visualized by treatment with a fluorochrome-conjugated anti-immuno-globulin serum (figure 6.11b). In this case, in order to find out whether or not the serum of a patient has antibodies to gastric parietal cells, we would first treat a gastric section with the serum, wash well and then apply a fluorescein-labelled rabbit anti-human immunoglobulin; if antibodies were present, there would be staining of the parietal cells (figure 6.12a).

This technique has several advantages. In the first place the fluorescence is brighter than with the direct test since several fluorescent anti-immunoglobulins bind on to each of the antibody molecules present in the first layer (figure 6.11b). Secondly, since the conjugation process is lengthy, much time can be saved when many sera have to be screened for antibody because it is only necessary to prepare a single labelled reagent, viz. the anti-immunoglobulin. Furthermore, the method has great flexibility. For example, by using con-

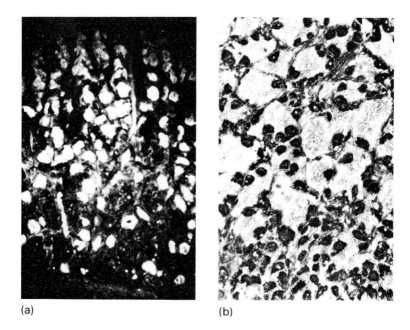

(a)   (b)

Figure 6.12. Staining of gastric parietal cells by (a) fluorescein and (b) peroxidase-linked antibody. The sections were sequentially treated with human parietal cell autoantibodies and then with the conjugated rabbit anti-human IgG. The enzyme was visualized by the peroxidase reaction. (Courtesy of Miss V. Petts.)

jugates of antisera to individual immunoglobulin heavy chains, the distribution of antibodies among the various classes and subclasses can be assessed at least semi-quantitatively. One can also test for complement fixation on the tissue section by adding a mixture of the first antibody plus a source of complement, followed by a fluorescent anti-complement reagent as the second layer. Even greater sensitivity can be attained by using a third layer. Thus, in the example quoted of antibodies to parietal cells, we could treat the stomach section sequentially with the following: patient's serum containing antibodies to parietal cells, then a rabbit anti-human IgG, and finally a fluorescein-conjugated goat anti-rabbit IgG. However, as with most immunological techniques as *sensitivity* is increased, *specificity* becomes progressively reduced and careful controls are essential.

Applications of the indirect test may be seen in figure 6.12a and in Chapter 11 (e.g. figure 11.2, pp. 316–17).

3. *Sandwich test*

This is a double layer procedure designed to visualize specific antibody. If, for example, we wished to see how many cells in a preparation of lymphoid tissue were synthesizing antibody to pneumococcus polysaccharide, we would first fix the cells with ethanol to prevent the antibody being washed away during the test, and then treat with a solution of the polysaccharide antigen. After washing, a fluorescein-labelled antibody to the polysaccharide would then be added to locate those cells which had specifically bound the antigen (figure 6.11c). The name of the test derives from the fact that antigen is sandwiched between the antibody present in the cell substrate and that added as the second layer.

OTHER LABELLED ANTIBODY METHODS

In place of fluorescent markers, other workers have evolved methods in which enzymes such as peroxidase or phosphatase are coupled to antibodies and these can be visualized by conventional histochemical methods at both light microscope (figure 6.12b) and electron microscope (figure 6.13) level.

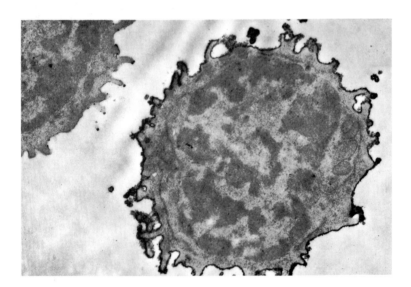

Figure 6.13. Electron microscopic visualization of human IgG on the surface of a B-lymphocyte by treatment of viable cell suspensions with peroxidase-coupled anti-IgG. Note the adjacent unstained lymphocyte. (Courtesy of Miss V. Petts.)

Intracytoplasmic antigens pose certain problems for the latter since the cells must be damaged to allow penetration by the labelled antibody, and in order to avoid morphological degeneration of cellular structures it is necessary to fix the tissue; however, the greater the degree of fixation, the more difficult it is for the antibody to diffuse through the cytoplasm. Technological improvements in this area would not be amiss.

Reactions with cell surface antigens

BINDING OF ANTIBODY

Surface antigens can be detected and localized by the use of labelled antibodies. Because antibodies cannot readily penetrate living cells except by endocytosis, treatment of cells with labelled antibody in the cold (to minimize endocytosis) should lead to staining only of antigens on the surface. Such studies have been carried out using antibodies labelled with peroxidase (figure 6.13) and with fluorescein (figures 3.11 and 6.14). The amount of fluorescent antibody bound to each

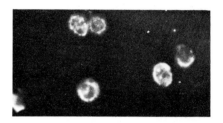

Figure 6.14. Antigens on the surface of viable human thyroid cells as demonstrated with thyroid autoantibodies in the indirect test. Note the patchy distribution. (Courtesy of Mrs H. Lindqvist; after Fagreus A. & Jonsson J.)

cell can be quantified by flow cytofluorography as described earlier (p. 63) and an example of the data which can be generated by these machines is given in figure 6.15.

After combination with antibody, many antigens are removed from the cell surface either through capping and endocytosis, or shedding into the extracellular medium as complexes. This 'stripping' process may have deleterious consequences for the host if it makes virally infected cells or tumours refractory to immunological attack.

Immunochemical analysis of surface antigens is possible if they are radio-labelled either by lactoperoxidase iodination of viable cells, by sequential oxidation of the surface glycoproteins and reduction with tritiated sodium borohydride or by metabolic incorporation of radioactive precursors. The membrane antigens can then be solubilized in a detergent which does not influence antigen–antibody interactions, and precipitated through combination with a specific antibody. The molecular weight of the antigen and its constituent peptides can be determined by running the precipitate in SDS-polyacrylamide gel electrophoresis and looking for the distribution of radioactivity (figure 6.16).

AGGLUTINATION

Whereas the cross-linking of multivalent protein antigens by antibody leads to precipitation, cross-linking of cells or large particles by antibody directed against surface antigens leads

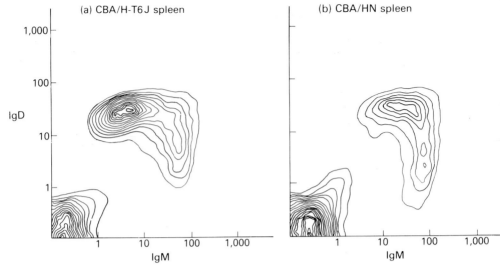

Figure 6.15. Flow cytofluorographic analysis in a fluorescence-activated cell sorter (FACS) of spleen cells from (a) CBA/J and (b) CBA/N mice stained with both fluorescein-labelled anti-IgM and Texas Red conjugated anti-IgD. The axes represent relative fluorescence while the contours give an indication of cell numbers. The CBA/N strain which is defective in its response to type II thymus independent antigens like pneumococcus polysaccharide (cf. p. 71) lacks the population with low surface IgM and high IgD seen in the normally responding strain CBA/J (Parks D.R., Hardy R.R. & Herzenberg L.A. (1983) *Immunol. Today* **4**, 145). Since Texas Red is excited at a different wavelength from fluorescein, the FACS had to be fitted with two lasers to acquire this data; with the advent of newer dyes such as the algal photosynthetic pigment, phycoerythrin, which have fluorescence emission peaks well separated from fluorescein yet can be excited at the same wavelength, comparable results should be obtainable with a single laser. Light scatter measurements in the FACS also provide information on cell size and viability which allows discrimination against dead cells and analysis of fluorescence in relation to cell size.

to agglutination. Since most cells are electrically charged, a reasonable number of antibody links between two cells is required before the mutual repulsion is overcome. Thus agglutination of cells bearing only a small number of determinants may be difficult to achieve unless special methods such as further treatment with an antiglobulin reagent are used. Similarly, the higher avidity of multivalent IgM antibody relative to IgG (cf. p. 38) makes the former more effective as an agglutinating agent, molecule for molecule.

Agglutination reactions are used to identify bacteria and to type red cells; they have been observed with leucocytes and platelets and even with spermatozoa in certain cases of male infertility due to sperm agglutinins. Because of its sensitivity and convenience, the test has been extended to the identification of antibodies to soluble antigens which have been artificially coated on to various types of particle. Red cells have been popular and they can be coated with proteins after first modifying their surface with tannic acid or chromium chlo-

Figure 6.16. Analysis of membrane-bound classical transplantation antigens (cf. p. 273). The membranes from human cells pulsed with ^{35}S-methionine were solubilized and immunoprecipitated with a monoclonal antibody to HLA-A and B molecules. An autoradiograph (A) of the precipitate run in SDS-polyacrylamide gel electrophoresis shows the HLA-A and B chains as a 43,000 molecular weight doublet (the position of a 45,000 marker is arrowed). If membrane vesicles were first digested with Proteinase K before solubilization, a labelled band of molecular weight 39,000 can be detected (B) consistent with a transmembrane orientation of the HLA chain: the 4,000 hydrophilic C-terminal fragment extends into the cytoplasm and the major portion, recognized by the monoclonal antibody and by tissue typing reagents, is present on the cell surface (cf. figure 10.6). (From data and autoradiographs kindly supplied by Dr M.J. Owen.)

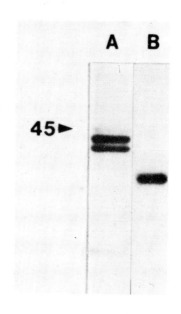

ride, or by direct use of bifunctional cross-linking agents such as bisdiazobenzidine. The large rapidly sedimenting red cells of the turkey are finding increasing favour for this purpose. The tests are usually carried out in the wells of plastic agglutination trays where the settling pattern of the cells on the bottom of the cup may be observed (figure 6.17); this provides a more sensitive indicator than macroscopic clumping. Inert particles such as bentonite and polystyrene latex have also been coated with antigens for agglutination reactions, particularly those used to detect the rheumatoid factors (figure 6.18).

OPSONIC (FC) ADHERENCE

On combination with IgG antibodies, antigens develop an increased adherence to polymorphonuclear leucocytes and macrophages through the specific IgG Fc binding sites on the surface of these cells. To take one example, bacteria coated with antibody become 'opsonized'—i.e. 'ready for the table' or 'tasty for the phagocytes'—and will adhere to phagocytic cells; this in turn facilitates the engulfment and subsequent digestion of the micro-organisms. Opsonic adherence and the related *immune adherence* reactions which involve binding through complement components (see below) are of major importance in the defence against infection. They may also be concerned in the removal of lymphocytes from the circulation by anti-lymphocyte serum and of red cells by the autoantibodies in autoimmune haemolytic

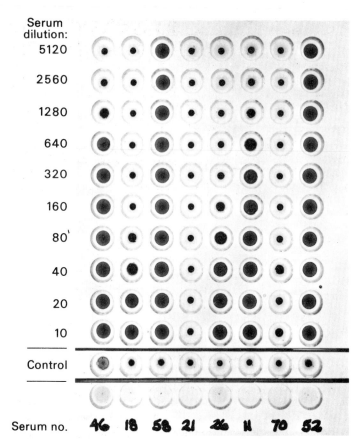

Serum dilution:
5120
2560
1280
640
320
160
80'
40
20
10
Control

Serum no. 46 18 58 21 26 11 70 52

Figure 6.17. Tanned red cell haemagglutination test for thyroglobulin autoantibodies. Thyroglobulin-coated cells were added to dilutions of patients' sera. Uncoated cells were added to a 1 : 10 dilution of serum as a control. In a positive reaction, the cells settle as a carpet over the bottom of the cup. Because of the 'V'-shaped cross-section of these cups, in negative reactions the cells fall into the base of the 'V' forming a small easily recognizable button. The reciprocal of the highest serum dilution giving an unequivocally positive reaction is termed the *titre*. The titres reading from left to right are: 640, 20, > 5,120, neg, 40, 320, neg, > 5,120. The control for serum No. 46 was slightly positive and this serum should be tested again after absorption with uncoated cells.

anaemia. The *extracellular killing* of antibody-coated target cells (cf. p. 242) depends upon adherence to Fc receptors on the effector cell surface. IgE-mediated degranulation of mast cells by antigen which triggers acute inflammatory responses and sometimes anaphylaxis, provides an interesting contrast, since in this case the Ig molecules are already firmly bound to their Fc receptors before the reaction with antigen.

STIMULATION

A quite unexpected phenomenon has been observed in that antibodies to cell-surface components may sometimes lead

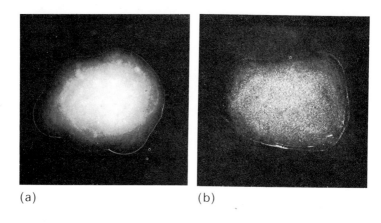

Figure 6.18.
Macroscopic agglutination of latex coated with human IgG by serum from a patient with rheumatoid arthritis. This contains rheumatoid factor, an autoantibody directed against determinants on IgG. (a) Normal serum, (b) patient's serum.

(a)   (b)

not to cytotoxic reactions as discussed below, but to actual stimulation of the cell. This probably occurs if the antibodies are directed against receptors on the surface which can generate a stimulatory signal when triggered by combination with the antibody. Examples are:

1   The transformation and mitosis induced in small lymphocytes by anti-lymphocyte serum and anti-immunoglobulin sera *in vitro*. The latter combine with the immunoglobulin antigen receptors on the cell surface and mimic the changes produced by antigen which activate the cell.

2   Degranulation of human mast cells by anti-IgE serum. The anti-IgE brings about the same sequence of changes as would specific antigen combining with the surface-bound IgE molecules.

3   Stimulation of thyroid cells by autoantibodies present in the serum of patients with thyrotoxicosis.

4   Parthogenetic division of sea-urchin eggs by antibody.

Stimulation may also be observed at the molecular level as in the increase in enzymic activity of certain penicillinase and β-galactosidase variants caused by addition of the appropriate antibodies which induce allosteric changes in the enzyme conformation.

CYTOTOXIC REACTIONS

If antibodies directed against the surface of cells are able to fix certain components present in the extracellular fluids, collectively termed *complement*, a cytotoxic reaction may occur. Historically, complement activity was recognized by Bordet who showed that the lytic activity against red cells of freshly drawn rabbit anti-sheep erythrocyte serum was lost on ageing or heating to 56°C for half-an-hour but could be restored by addition of fresh serum from an unimmunized rabbit. Thus, for haemolysis one requires a relatively heat stable factor, the antibody, plus a heat labile factor, complement, present in all fresh sera.

163

Complement

NATURE OF COMPLEMENT

This classical activity ascribed to complement (C′) depends upon the operation of nine protein components (C1–C9) acting in sequence of which the first consists of three major subfractions termed C1q, C1r and C1s. Some of the characteristics of the three most abundant components are given in table 6.1.

	C1q	C4	C3
Serum concn., $\mu g/ml$	100–200	400	1,200
Molecular weight	400,000	230,000	185,000
Thermolability	+	−	−
Immunoelectrophoresis	γ	β_{1E}	β_{1C}

Table 6.1. Some characteristics of the three most abundant complement components in human serum.

When the first component is activated by an immune complex (e.g. antibody bound to a red cell), it acquires the ability to activate several molecules of the next component in the sequence; each of these is then able to act upon the next component and so on, producing a cascade effect with amplification. In this way, the triggering of one molecule of C1 can lead to the activation of thousands of the later components. At each stage, activation is accompanied by the appearance of a new enzymic activity and since one enzyme molecule can process several substrate molecules, so each complement factor can cause the processing or activation of many molecules of the next component in the sequence (figure 6.19). The terminal components of the complement cascade have the ability to punch a 'functional hole' through the cell membrane on which they are fixed by perturbation of the phospholipid structure, and this leads to cell death. Thus, through this sequential amplification process, the activation of one C1 molecule can lead to a macroscopic event, namely the lysis of a cell. As will be seen later, the interme-

Figure 6.19. Enzymic basis of the amplifying complement cascade. The activated *enzyme₁* splits a peptide fragment from several molecules of *proenzyme₂* which all become active *enzyme₂* molecules capable of splitting *proenzyme₃* and so on.

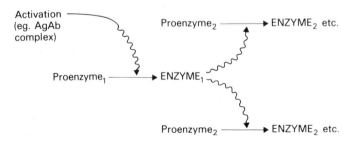

Activation (eg. AgAb complex)

Proenzyme₁ ⟶ ENZYME₁

Proenzyme₂ ⟶ ENZYME₂ etc.

Proenzyme₂ ⟶ ENZYME₂ etc.

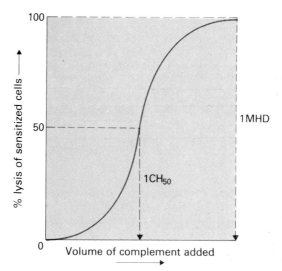

Figure 6.20. Relationship of added complement to percentage lysis of standard suspension of red cells sensitized with antibody. At the 50% lysis point, the curve is steep and the amount of C' giving 50% lysis ($1\ CH_{50}$) can be accurately determined. The curve only gradually reaches 100% lysis and the amount of C' giving 100% lysis (1 Minimum Haemolytic Dose: 1 MHD) is less precisely assessed. The MHD is nonetheless adequate for routine serological purposes but for more accurate work the CH_{50} unit is preferred.

diate stages in the complement sequence also give rise to other biological activities which are of importance in health and disease. Like the blood clotting, kallikrein and fibrinolytic systems which also involve enzyme cascades, the complement components have a complex system of inhibitors to regulate activation.

Complement is measured as an activity as are other enzyme systems and is expressed in terms of the degree of lysis of a standard suspension of antibody-coated sheep red cells produced within a fixed time (figure 6.20).

ACTIVATION OF COMPLEMENT

The activation of C1 is initiated by binding through C1q to C_{H2} sites on IgG or C_{H3} sites on IgM antibodies forming a complex with antigen. Aggregation of immunoglobulin by heating it to 60°C for 20 minutes also leads to the changes in structure which allow complement activation. Different immunoglobulin classes have different Fc structures and only IgG and IgM can bind C1. There are differences even within the IgG subclasses: IgG1 and IgG3 fix complement well, IgG2 modestly and IgG4 poorly, if at all. C1q is polyvalent with respect to IgG binding and consists of a central collagen-like stem branching into six peptide chains each tipped by an IgG binding subunit (resembling the blooms on a bunch of flowers). At least two of these subunits must bind to immunoglobulin C_{H2} sites for activation of C1q. With IgM this is less of a problem since several Fc regions are available within a single molecule, although these only become readily accessible when the F(ab')$_2$ arms bend out of the plane of the inner Fc region on combination with antigen (cf. figure 2.17). On the other hand, IgG antibodies will only fix complement when two or more molecules are bound to closely adjacent sites on the antigen. It is for this reason that IgM antibodies to red cells have a high haemolytic efficiency since a 'single hit' will produce full complement activation and cell death. With IgG antibodies, a far larger number of 'hits' will be required before, by chance, two IgG antibodies are bound at adjacent sites and are then able to initiate the complement sequence.

Complement can be activated by another route, the so-called *alternative pathway* (see below). This can be stimulated by certain cell wall polysaccharides such as bacterial endotoxin and yeast zymosan, by some aggregated immunoglobulins such as human IgA and guinea pig IgG1 known to be ineffective for C1q binding, and, as we shall see later, by a feedback mechanism from the classical pathway.

THE COMPLEMENT SEQUENCE

Classical pathway (figure 6.21)

Let us analyse the sequence of events which takes place when IgM or IgG antibodies combine with the surface membrane of a cell in the presence of complement. C1q is linked in a trimolecular complex through calcium to C1r and C1s. After the binding of C1 to the Fc regions of the immune complex, C1s acquires esterase activity and brings about the activation and transfer to sites on the membrane (or immune complex) of first C4 and then C2 (unfortunately components were numbered before the sequence was established). This complex has 'C3-convertase' activity and splits C3 in solution to produce a small peptide fragment (C3a) and a residual molecule (C3b) which have quite distinct functions:

1   C3a has *anaphylatoxin* activity in that it causes histamine release from mast cells and attracts polymorphonuclear leucocytes largely through release of mast cell chemotactic factor.

2   C3b, like C2 and C4, exposes an internal thioester bond immediately after proteolytic cleavage of the parent C3 which enables it to react with adjacent regions on the membrane. By this means a large number of C3b molecules may be transferred to the surface membrane through the action of the convertase. There are specific receptors for this

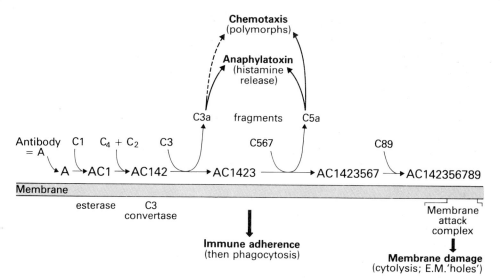

Figure 6.21. Sequence of classical complement activation by membrane-bound antibody showing formation of C3a and C5a fragments chemotactic for polymorphs and with anaphylatoxin activity causing histamine release. Immune adherence through C3 to macrophages, platelets or red cells facilitates phagocytosis. Fixation of C8 and 9 generates cytolytic activity. Fragments released during the activation of C4 and C2 are thought to have chemotactic and kinin-like activity respectively.

membrane-bound C3b on polymorphs and macrophages (all mammalian species studied), platelets (rabbits) and red cells (primates) which allow *immune adherence* of the antigen-antibody-C3b complex to these cells so facilitating subsequent phagocytosis (figure 6.21). The bound C3 presents a new structural configuration not present on the native molecule which can provoke the formation of the autoantibody *immunoconglutinin*.

Control of C3b levels is maintained through the action of a C3b inactivator (Factor I). C3b readily combines with Factor H to form a complex which is broken down by Factor I and loses its haemolytic and immune adherence properties; it then becomes highly susceptible to attack by trypsin-like enzymes present in the body fluids and splits to form the fragments C3c and C3d (figure 6.22; cf. also figure 6.7).

Alternative pathway

In the classical pathway we have just discussed, the active C3b fragment is formed by the action of C142 convertase. Another C3 convertase, $C\overline{3bB}$ (the horizontal bar denotes activation) can be generated by a distinct series of reactions collectively termed the alternative pathway (figure 6.23) which can be triggered by extrinsic agents, in particular microbial polysaccharides such as endotoxin, acting indepen-

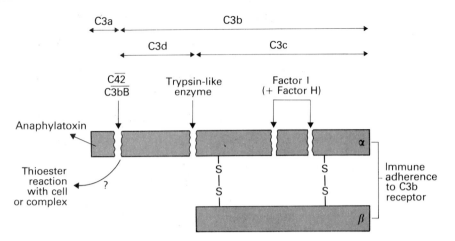

Figure 6.22. The structural basis for the cleavage of C3 by C3 convertases and the inactivation of C3b by successive action of the C3b inactivator, Factor I, and a pro-tease. Factor I was previously termed C3bina and before that KAF; factor H was originally called β_{1H}.

dently of antibody. The convertase is formed by the action of Factor D on a complex of C3b and Factor B. This creates an interesting positive feedback loop in which the product of C3 breakdown helps to form more of the cleavage enzyme.

The present view is that the low concentrations of C3b in plasma formed by proteolysis can give rise to $\overline{C3bB}$ convertase under normal conditions; however, the lability of $\overline{C3bB}$ and the action of C3b inactivator prevent the system from getting out of hand and allow the feedback loop to 'tick over' quietly. Microbial polysaccharides and other initiators of the alternative pathway boost the levels of $\overline{C3bB}$ convertase by providing a surface upon which the enzyme is stabilized (probably with the help of properdin).

Post C3 pathway

The sequence reaches its full amplitude at the C3 stage which represents the essential heart of the complement system. Thereafter C5 is split to give C5a and C5b fragments. C5a is a potent molecule which increases vascular permeability directly and through mast cell degranulation. It is the dominant polymorph chemotactic agent in the complement system and also activates the neutrophil to stimulate a microbicidal oxygen burst, the extracellular release of lysosomal enzymes and the synthesis of leukotriene B4 which prolongs the vascular permeability induced by C5a. Both C3a and C5a are inactivated by a carboxypeptidase which removes the terminal arginine. Meanwhile, the C5b binds as a complex with C6 and 7 to form a thermostable site on the

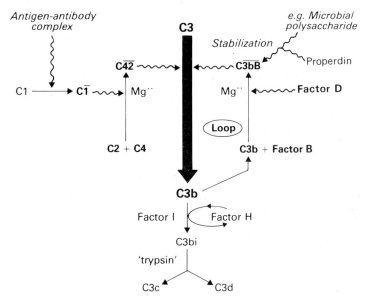

CLASSICAL ACTIVATION — ALTERNATIVE ACTIVATION

Antigen-antibody complex

C3

Stabilization

e.g. Microbial polysaccharide

$\overline{C42}$ — $\overline{C3bB}$ — Properdin

C1 → $\overline{C1}$ → Mg·· — Mg·· → Factor D

Loop

C2 + C4 — C3b + Factor B

C3b

Factor I — Factor H

C3bi

'trypsin'

C3c — C3d

Figure 6.23. The alternative complement pathway showing points of similarity with the classical sequence. Both pathways generate a C3 convertase, $\overline{C42}$ in one case and $\overline{C3bB}$ in the other, which activates C3 to provide the pivotal event in the complement system. The alternative pathway can be studied independently of the classical sequence under circumstances where the latter is inoperative as, for example, in C4-deficient serum or in a serum treated with Mg-EGTA to complex Ca^{2+} and inactivate C1. The C3b inactivator Factor I splits C4b in the same manner as it does C3b. C3 and C4 resemble each other structurally as do C2 and Factor B. The alternative pathway is probably the older of the two in phylogenetic terms and being independent of antibody may be looked upon as a component of the 'innate' defence system. The classical pathway, on the other hand, is linked to the adaptive immune system in its dependence on antibody (linked to antigen) for triggering. ∿➤ represents an activation process. The convention of using a horizontal bar above a complement component to designate its activation is used. The activated components are usually fragments of the original molecules, e.g. the alternative pathway convertase is actually $\overline{C3bBb}$ and the classical convertase $\overline{C4b2b}$, but in the interests of simplicity in a complicated system, such details have been omitted.

membrane which recruits the final components C8 and C9 to generate the 'membrane attack complex'. This is an annular structure inserted into the membrane and projecting from it (figure 6.24a and b) which forms a transmembrane channel fully permeable to electrolytes and water. Due to the high internal colloid osmotic pressure, there is a net influx of Na^+ and water leading to cell lysis.

Yet more complexity is introduced by the phenomenon of *reactive lysis* (Lachmann & Thomson); a proportion of the activated C5b,6,7 complexes formed remain free and not only are they chemotactic for neutrophils but are also able to

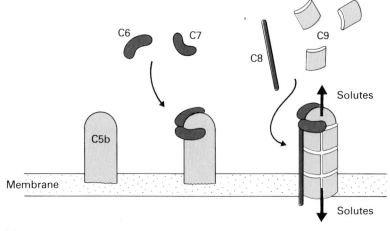

(a)

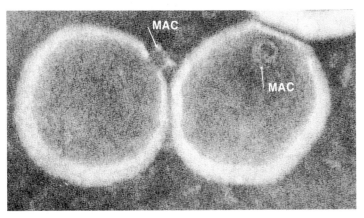

(b)

Figure 6.24. The C5–9 membrane attack complex. (a) After C5b binds to the membrane, the terminal complement components assemble around it to form a transmembrane channel which is permeable to solutes and leads to osmotic lysis of the cell (after D. Male & D.L. Brown). (b) Electron micrograph of a membrane attack complex (MAC) incorporated into liposomal membranes clearly showing the annular structure. The cylindrical attack complex is seen from the side inserted into the membrane of the liposome on the left, and end-on in that on the right (courtesy Prof. J. Tranum-Jensen and Dr S. Bhakdi).

bind to 'innocent' cells in the vicinity. Once fixed to the cell surface they can complete the complement sequence by binding C8, 9 with resultant cytolysis.

ROLE IN DEFENCE

Cytolysis

The full complement system leading to membrane damage can cause bacteriolysis in Gram-negative organisms by

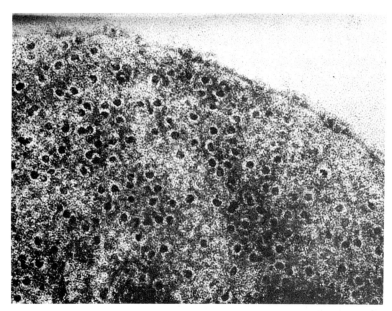

Figure 6.25. Multiple lesions in cell wall of *Escherichia coli* bacterium caused by interaction with IgM antibody and complement. Each lesion is caused by a single IgM molecule and shows as a 'dark pit' due to penetration by the 'negative stain'. This is somewhat of an illusion since in reality these 'pits' are like volcano craters standing proud of the surface, and are each single 'membrane attack' complexes. Comparable results may be obtained in the absence of antibody since the cell wall endotoxin can activate the alternative pathway in the presence of higher concentrations of serum. Magnification × 400,000. (Courtesy of Drs R. Dourmashkin and J.H. Humphrey.)

allowing lysozyme access to the peptidoglycan cell wall (p. 190). Negatively stained preparations in the electron microscope show the 'pits' on the surface (figure 6.25) which correspond with individual membrane attack complexes.

Immune (C3b) adherence

This plays a major role in facilitating the phagocytosis of micro-organisms after coating with antibody and complement or after activation of the alternative pathway. Since many C3 molecules are bound on to the surface at each site of complement activation, adherence to macrophages and polymorphs may operate largely through C3 binding although it should be noted that subsequent phagocytosis is provoked to a greater extent by IgG rather than C3b. Purified C3b has been shown to trigger extracellular release of lysosomal enzymes from macrophages and it is possible, but not yet established, that this could damage adhering micro-organisms.

Immunoconglutinin

This may play a role by agglutinating relatively small complexes containing bound C3 thereby making them more susceptible to phagocytosis.

Acute inflammation

The fragments produced during complement consumption stimulate two helpful features of the acute inflammatory response. First, the chemotactic factors attract phagocytic neutrophil polymorphs to the site of complement activation, and secondly anaphylatoxin, through histamine release, increases vascular permeability and hence the flow of serum antibody and more complement to the infected area.

Solubilization of immune complexes

Deposits of large antigen–antibody aggregates formed during an immune response can provoke hypersensitivity reactions and can sometimes be difficult to digest even when engulfed by macrophages. It is gratifying therefore to know that the complement system can disrupt such aggregates into small soluble complexes. Alternative pathway C3 convertase becomes stabilized on the surface and brings about extensive covalent coupling of C3b to the Ig molecules; this leads to disaggregation presumably by hindering the interactions between Fc regions which are important for precipitate formation (cf. figure 1.4b; p. 6).

Role in the antibody response

Very effective complement depletion can be produced by injection of a cobra venom factor which contains the reptilian equivalent of C3b. This fires the alternative pathway by forming a complex with Factor B but because of its insensitivity to the mammalian C3b inactivator, it persists long enough to discharge the feedback loop to exhaustion and deplete C3 and the terminal components C5–9. During the IgM phase of a primary immune response, the localization of antibody-complexed antigen on dendritic cells in germinal centres does not occur in animals pretreated with cobra venom suggesting a role for C3–9. Failure of antigen localization hampers the development of B-cell memory to T-dependent antigens and late IgG responses.

The presence of C3 receptors and of Factor B on the surface of B-cells would not be inconsistent with a role for C3b in the regulation of the antibody response but no clear picture has yet emerged.

Complement is implicated in disease processes involving cytotoxic and immune-complex mediated hypersensitivities which will be discussed in more detail in Chapter 8. Cytotoxic reactions are seen in nephrotoxic nephritis and autoimmune haemolytic anaemia. Complexes formed in antibody excess giving rise to immune vasculitis of the Arthus type are seen, for example, in Farmer's lung and cryoglobulinaemia with cutaneous vasculitis; soluble complexes formed in antigen excess give 'serum sickness' type reactions with considerable deposition in the kidney glomeruli as found in many forms of chronic glomerulonephritis. Some patients with mesangiocapillary glomerulonephritis and partial lipodystrophy have low complement levels due to the presence in serum of the so-called C3 nephritic factor which appears to be an IgG autoantibody capable of activating the alternative pathway by combining with and stabilizing the $\overline{C3bB}$ convertase.

In paroxysmal nocturnal haemoglobinuria (PNH) the erythrocytes are particularly susceptible to reactive lysis as a result of an unusual, as yet unexplained ability to fix the activated trimolecular complex, C5,6,7. Massive complement activation can lead to disseminated intravascular coagulation. A good model for this is the Shwartzmann reaction produced in rabbits by intravascular endotoxin. This activates the alternative pathway so that the endotoxin becomes coated with C3b and sticks to platelets by immune adherence; the C5,6,7 complexes generated cause platelet destruction by reactive lysis with release of clotting factors. Although in man, C3b adherence reactions involve red cells and leucocytes rather than platelets, somewhat similar mechanisms associated with intense complement consumption underlie the disseminated intravascular coagulation seen in human patients with Gram-negative septicaemia or dengue haemorrhagic shock produced by a substantial viraemia occurring in the second infection of individuals with high titre antibodies.

COMPLEMENT DEFICIENCIES

The importance of complement in defence against infections is emphasized by the occurrence of repeated life-threatening infection with pyogenic bacteria in a patient lacking C3b inactivator. Because of his inability to destroy C3b there is continual activation of the alternative pathway through the feedback loop leading to very low C3 and Factor B levels with normal C1, 4 and 2. On the other hand, permanent deficiencies in C5, C6, C7, C8 and C9 have all been described in man, yet in virtually every case the individuals are healthy and not particularly prone to infection apart from an increased susceptibility to disseminated *Neisseria gonorrhoeae* and *N. meningitis*. Thus full operation of the terminal complement system does not appear to be essential for survival and adequate protection must be largely afforded by opsonizing antibodies and the immune adherence mechanism.

Failure to generate the classical C3-convertase through deficiencies in C1r, C4 and C2 has been reported in a small number of cases associated with an unusually high incidence of SLE-like syndromes (cf. p. 312) perhaps due to a decreased ability to mount an adequate host response to infection with a putative aetiological agent or to eliminate antigen–antibody complexes effectively (cf. p. 255). An inhibitor of active C1 is grossly lacking in hereditary angio-oedema and this can lead to recurring episodes of acute circumscribed non-inflammatory oedema mediated by a vasoactive C2 fragment (figure 6.26). The patients are het-

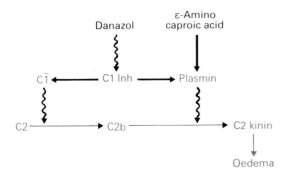

Figure 6.26. C1 inhibitor deficiency and angioedema. C1 inhibitor stoichiometrically inhibits C$\overline{1}$, plasmin, kallikrein and activated Hageman factor and deficiency leads to formation of the vasoactive C2 kinin by the mechanism shown. —▶ = inhibition; ∿▶ = stimulation or activation. The synthesis of C1 inhibitor can be boosted by methyltestosterone or preferably the less masculinizing synthetic steroid, Danazol; alternatively, attacks can be controlled by giving ε-aminocaproic acid to inhibit the plasmin.

erozygotes and synthesize small amounts of the inhibitor which can be raised to useful levels by administration of the synthetic anabolic steroid Danazol or, in critical cases, of the purified inhibitor itself. ε-Aminocaproic acid, which blocks the plasmin-induced liberation of the C2 kinin, provides an alternative treatment.

GENETICS

Multiple allotypic (polymorphic) forms of human C2, C3, C4, C6 and Factor B have been described. The nonfunctional alleles responsible for deficiencies of C4 and C2 map to the major histocompatibility complex and it is now evident that the cluster of genes encoding C4, C2 and Factor B lies close to the HLA-B locus (see p. 303 for further discussion of these class III MHC molecules).

In the mouse, control of C3 levels is linked to H-2 while the Ss region encodes the synthesis of C4 (figure 3.12).

Neutralization of biological activity

To continue our discussion on the interaction of antigen and antibody we may focus attention on a number of biological reactions which can be inhibited by addition of specific antibody. Thus the agglutination of red cells by interaction of influenza virus with receptors on the erythrocyte surface can be blocked by antiviral antibodies and this forms the basis for their serological detection. Neutralization of the growth of hapten-conjugated bacteriophage provides an exquisitely sensitive assay for anti-hapten antibodies. A test for antibodies to salmonella H antigen present on the flagella depends upon their ability to inhibit the motility of the bacteria *in vitro*. Likewise, mycoplasma antibodies can be demonstrated by their inhibitory effect on the metabolism of the organisms in culture. The successful treatment of cases of drug overdose with the Fab fragment of specific antibodies has been described and may become a practical proposition if a range of hybridomas can be assembled. Antibodies to hormones such as insulin and TSH can be used to probe the specificity of biological reactions *in vitro*; for example, the specificity of the insulin-like activity of a serum sample on rat epididymal fat pad can be checked by the neutralizing effect of an antiserum. Such antibodies can be effective *in vivo* and, as part of the world-wide effort to prevent disastrous over-population, attempts are in progress to immunize against chorionic gonadotropin using fragments of the β-chain coupled to appropriate carriers, since this hormone is needed to sustain the implanted ovum.

Summary

The formation of single bands of precipitate when antigen and antibody react in gels can be used qualitatively to study the number of reacting components and the immunological relationship between different antigens (Ouchterlony double diffusion system) and the electrophoretic mobility of the antigens (immunoelectrophoresis). Quantitative measurement of antigen concentration is made by single radial immunodiffusion, 'rocket' electrophoresis and two-dimensional electrophoresis. Laser nephelometry provides a sensitive method for the quantification of antigens in solution.

Radioisotopic techniques for assessing the antibody content of serum include: (a) addition of radio-labelled antigen and determination of the amount bound to antibody by ammonium sulphate or a second antibody precipitation (antigen-binding capacity) and (b) determination of the amount of antibody binding to insoluble antigen by addition of a labelled anti-Ig (e.g. 'tube test'). Radioimmunoassay of antigen is a form of saturation analysis in which the test material competes with labelled antigen for a limited amount of antibody, the amount of label displaced being a measure of the antigen in the test sample. Immunoradiometric tests involve the binding of antigen to solid phase antibody and its estimation by excess labelled antibody.

The localization of antigens in tissues, within cells or on the cell surface can be achieved microscopically using antibodies tagged with fluorescent dyes or enzymes such as peroxidase whose reaction product can be readily visualized. In the direct test, the labelled antibody is applied directly to the tissue; in the indirect test the label is conjugated to an anti-Ig used as a second amplifying antibody. Fluorescent antibody bound to the surface of single cells, e.g. lymphocytes, can be quantified by flow cytofluorography. For ultrastructural studies, antibodies are usually tagged with peroxidase.

Antibodies can be used for the immunochemical analysis of detergent solubilized antigens of the plasma membrane. Reaction of antibody with a cell surface antigen can lead to agglutination, enhancement of phagocytosis or extracellular killing, metabolic stimulation and mitosis, and complement-mediated cytotoxicity.

Complement, like the blood coagulation, fibrinolytic and kallikrein systems, involves a multicomponent enzymic cascade in which the first component, on activation, splits a small peptide from several molecules of the second component each of which is now an active enzyme able to act on the third component, etc.; a small number of initiating events leads to a large effect through this amplification method. The most abundant component, C3, is split by a convertase enzyme generated either by the *classical pathway* (C1,4,2) which is initiated by antigen–antibody complexes, or by the alternative pathway (properdin, Factors B and D) which is initiated in the absence of antibody by material such as bacterial polysaccharides. One split product, C3a, attracts polymorphonuclear leucocytes and increases vascular permeability through mediator release from mast cells and basophils. The other product, C3b, binds non-specifically to the antigen surface and increases the efficiency of binding to the polymorphs (attracted by C3a) because of C3b receptors on the surface of these phagocytic cells. Next, C5 is cleaved to release C5a which degranulates mast cells like C3a, but also has a powerful direct chemotactic and stimulatory effect on neutrophil polymorphs. The residue, C5b, binds to the membrane and assembles the terminal components, C6–9, into a membrane attack complex; this forms a trans-membrane channel which is freely permeable to solutes and leads to osmotic lysis of the cell bearing the complex. Through these effects complement plays an important role in the defence against infection. It is also concerned in certain hypersensitivity reactions involving combination of antibody with surfaces (e.g. nephrotoxic nephritis) and immune complexes (e.g. Farmer's lung, chronic glomerulonephritis). Massive activation of complement by microbial products can lead to disseminated intravascular coagulation. Deficiency in early complement components of the classical pathway predisposes to the development of SLE. Like the blood clotting system, inhibitors play a crucial role and if they are defective, disease may result, e.g. hereditary angioedema (C1 inhibitor) or repeated infection (C3b inactivator).

Antigens with biological activity, e.g. hormones such as human chorionic gonadotropin, may be neutralized *in vivo* by antibody.

Further reading

Clausen J. (1969) *Immunochemical Techniques for the Identification and Estimation of Macromolecules.* North-Holland, Amsterdam.

Hudson L. & Hay F.C. (1980) *Practical Immunology*, 2nd edn. Blackwell Scientific Publications, Oxford.

Lachmann P.J. (1980) Complement. In *Clinical Aspects of Immunology*, 4th edn. Lachmann P.J. & Peters D.K. (eds) Blackwell Scientific Publications, Oxford.

Nairn R.C. (1976) *Fluorescent Protein Tracing*, 4th edn. Churchill Livingstone, Edinburgh.

Rose N.R. & Friedman H. (eds) (1976) *Manual of Clinical Immunology.* American Society of Microbiology, Washington, D.C.

Thompson R.A. (1974) *The Practice of Clinical Immunology.* Edward Arnold, London.

Weir D.M. (ed.) (1973) *Handbook of Experimental Immunology*, 2nd edn. Blackwell Scientific Publications, Oxford.

Williams C.A. & Chase M.W. (1967–71) *Methods in Immunology and Immunochemistry*, Vols I–IV. Academic Press, London.

7

Immunity to Infection
I—Mechanisms

We live in a potentially hostile world filled with a bewildering array of infectious agents (figure 7.1) of diverse shape, size, composition and subversive character which would very happily use us as rich sanctuaries for propagating their 'selfish genes' had we not also developed a series of defence mechanisms at least their equal in effectiveness and ingenuity (except in the case of many parasitic infections where the situation is best described as an uneasy and often unsatisfactory truce).

Aside from ill-understood constitutional factors which make one species innately susceptible and another resistant to certain infections, a number of non-specific anti-microbial systems (e.g. phagocytosis) have been recognized which are 'innate' in the sense that they are not intrinsically affected by prior contact with the infectious agent. We shall discuss these systems and examine how, in the state of specific acquired immunity, their effectiveness can be greatly increased by both B- and T-cell activity.

Innate immunity

PREVENTING ENTRY

The simplest way to avoid infection is to prevent the microorganisms from gaining access to the body (figure 7.2). The major line of defence is of course the skin which, when intact, is impermeable to most infectious agents; when there is skin loss, as for example in burns, infection becomes a major problem. Additionally, most bacteria fail to survive for long on the skin because of the direct inhibitory effects of lactic acid and fatty acids in sweat and sebaceous secretions and the low pH which they generate. An exception is *Staphylococcus aureus* which often infects the relatively vulnerable hair follicles and glands.

Mucus, secreted by the membranes lining the inner surfaces of the body, acts as a protective barrier to block the adherence of bacteria to epithelial cells. Microbial and other foreign particles trapped within the adhesive mucus are

179

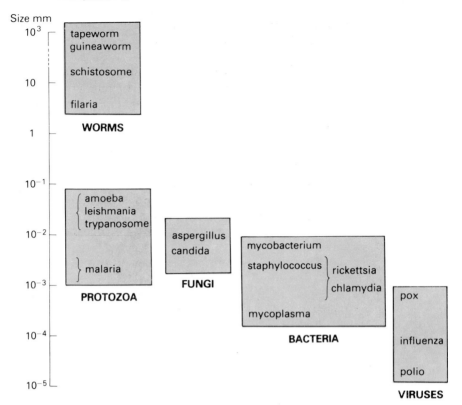

Figure 7.1. The formidable range of infectious agents which confront the immune system. Although not normally classified as such because of their lack of a cell wall, the mycoplasmas are included under bacteria for convenience. Fungi adopt many forms and approximate values for some of the smallest forms are given.

removed by mechanical stratagems such as ciliary movement, coughing and sneezing. Among other mechanical factors which help protect the epithelial surfaces, one should also include the washing action of tears, saliva and urine. Many of the secreted body fluids contain bactericidal components,

Figure 7.2. The first lines of defence against infection: protection at the external body surfaces.

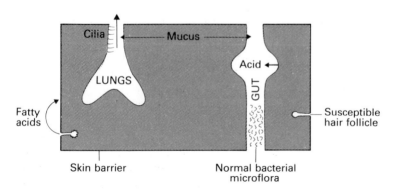

e.g. acid in gastric juice, spermine and zinc in semen, lacto-peroxidase in milk and lysozyme in tears, nasal secretions and saliva.

A totally different mechanism is that of microbial antagonism associated with the normal bacterial flora of the body. These suppress the growth of many potentially pathogenic bacteria and fungi at superficial sites by competition for essential nutrients or by production of inhibitory substances such as colicins or acid. To give one example, pathogen invasion is limited by lactic acid produced by particular species of commensal bacteria which metabolize glycogen secreted by the vaginal epithelium. When protective commensals are disturbed by antibiotics, susceptibility to opportunistic infections by *Candida* and *Clostridium difficile* is increased.

COUNTER-ATTACK AGAINST THE INVADERS

When micro-organisms do penetrate the body, two main defensive operations come into play, the destructive effect of soluble chemical factors such as bactericidal enzymes and the mechanism of phagocytosis—literally 'eating' by the cell.

Humoral factors

Of the soluble bactericidal substances elaborated by the body, perhaps the most abundant and widespread is the enzyme lysozyme, a muramidase which splits the exposed peptidoglycan wall of susceptible bacteria (cf. figure 7.7). A number of plasma components, C-reactive protein (CRP), α_1 anti-trypsin, α_2-macroglobulin, fibrinogen, caeruloplasmin, C9 and Factor B, collectively termed *acute phase proteins*, show a dramatic increase in concentration in response to infection or tissue injury. For example, CRP is released from the liver in response to endogenous pyrogen probably derived from endotoxin stimulated macrophages, and its concentration can rise 1000-fold. This protein has been around the animal kingdom for some time since a closely related homologue, limulin, is present in the haemolymph of the horseshoe crab, not exactly a close relative of *Homo sapiens*. In an aggregated form, CRP can bind to a lymphocyte subset with Fcγ receptors and can trigger platelets to release vasoactive mediators. Its major property, and the one by which it was first recognized, is its ability to bind, in a Ca-dependent fashion, to a number of micro-organisms which contain phosphoryl choline in their membranes, the complex having the useful property of activating complement by the classical pathway. We remember, of course, that many microbes activate the alternative pathway directly and we will explore the consequences in more detail below; suffice it to say under this heading that such activation can result in damage to the outer membrane of the infective agent mediated by the terminal components C8 and C9. Tissue injury by bacteria releases enzymes which activate the clotting system and thereby limit the spread of infection.

Lastly we should include the *interferons*, a family of broad spectrum anti-viral agents present in birds, reptiles and fishes as well as the higher animals and first recognized by the phenomenon of viral interference in which an animal infected with one virus resists superinfection by a second unrelated virus. Cells synthesize interferon when infected by a virus and secrete it into the extracellular fluid whence it binds to specific receptors on neighbouring cells which now become incapable of supporting viral replication. This insensitivity to infection will clearly act to limit the spread of virus. The effectiveness of interferon *in vivo* may be inferred from experiments in which mice injected with an antiserum to murine interferons could be killed by several hundred times' less virus than was needed to kill the controls. However, it must be presumed that interferon plays a significant role in the recovery from, as distinct from the prevention of, viral infections. Different species of interferons have been identified: interferon-β (IFNβ) is produced by fibroblasts and probably most other cells, IFNα, of which there are 14 subtypes, is derived from leucocytes, and IFNγ is made by T-cells.

Interferons can heighten the cytotoxic activity of non-specific killer cells (NK; p. 300). Although originally identified through their ability to destroy certain tumour cells in culture spontaneously, it has now been shown that these cells are cytotoxic for cells infected with a number of different viruses. Thus, NK cells, stimulated by interferon released by intracellular virus will actively kill the virally infected target cell and insofar as this task is completed before the virus has had time to replicate, the system forms a nicely integrated innate immune mechanism for combating viral infection.

Phagocytosis

The engulfment and digestion of micro-organisms is assigned to two major cell types recognized by Metchnikoff at the turn of the century as *micro-* and *macrophages*. The smaller polymorphonuclear neutrophil (cf. figures 3.7f; 3.8g, i, j) is a non-dividing short-lived cell with granules containing a wide range of bactericidal factors and glycogen stores which can be utilized by glycolysis under anaerobic conditions. It is the dominant white cell in the bloodstream. Macrophages derive from bone marrow promonocytes which, after differentiation to blood monocytes, finally settle in the tissues as mature

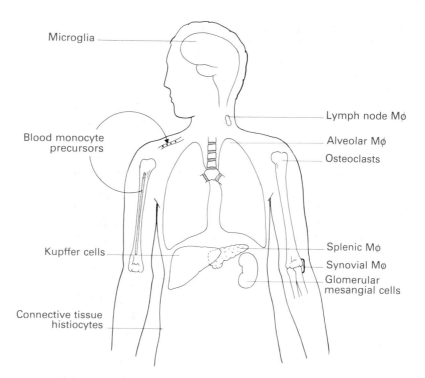

Microglia

Blood monocyte precursors

Kupffer cells

Connective tissue histiocytes

Lymph node Mφ

Alveolar Mφ

Osteoclasts

Splenic Mφ

Synovial Mφ

Glomerular mesangial cells

Figure 7.3. The mononuclear phagocyte system (previously included with endothelial cells and polymorphs under the term 'the reticuloendothelial system' or RES). Promonocyte precursors in the bone marrow develop into circulating blood monocytes which eventually become dis-tributed throughout the body as mature macrophages (Mφ) as shown. The other major phagocytic cell, the polymorphonuclear neutrophil, is largely confined to the bloodstream except when recruited into sites of acute inflammation.

macrophages where they constitute the so-called *reticuloendothelial system* (figure 7.3). They are present throughout the connective tissue and around the basement membrane of small blood vessels and are particularly concentrated in the lung (alveolar macrophages), liver (Kupffer cells), and lining of spleen sinusoids and lymph node medullary sinuses where they are strategically placed to filter off foreign material. Other examples are mesangial cells in the kidney glomerulus, brain microglia and osteoclasts in bone. Unlike the polymorphs, they are long-lived cells with significant rough-surfaced endoplasmic reticulum and mitochondria and whereas the polymorphs provide the major defence against pyogenic (pus-forming) bacteria, as a rough generalization it may be said that macrophages are at their best in combating those bacteria, viruses and protozoa which are capable of living within the cells of the host.

Before phagocytosis can occur, the microbe must first adhere to the surface of the polymorph or macrophage, an event mediated by some rather primitive recognition mecha-

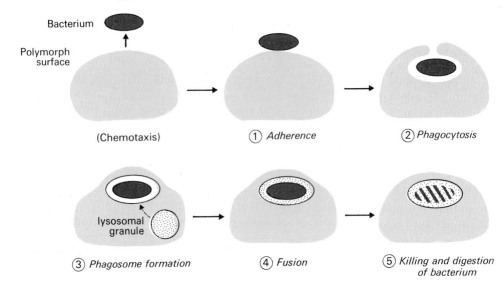

Bacterium

Polymorph
surface

(Chemotaxis)

① *Adherence*

② *Phagocytosis*

lysosomal
granule

③ *Phagosome formation*

④ *Fusion*

⑤ *Killing and digestion
of bacterium*

Figure 7.4. Phagocytosis of bacterium by
neutrophil leucocyte (see also figure 3.8g–j).

nism on the part of the phagocytic cells. Depending upon its
nature, a particle attached to the membrane may initiate the
ingestion phase in which it becomes engulfed by cytoplasmic
processes and comes to lie within a vacuole termed a phagosome (figures 7.4 & 3.8g–j). A lysosomal granule then fuses
with the vacuole to form a phagolysosome in which the
ingested microbe is slaughtered by a battery of mechanisms
(table 7.1). Dominant among these are the oxygen-dependent
systems. Phagocytosis is associated with a dramatic increase
in activity of the hexose monophosphate shunt. This provides NADPH and a burst of oxygen consumption as this is
metabolized by either a plasma membrane NADPH oxidase
or a cytochrome which becomes activated as contact with the
microbe is made during ingestion and continues to function
on the inner surface of the phagolysosome. The oxygen is
converted to superoxide anion, hydrogen peroxide, singlet
oxygen and hydroxyl radicals, all powerful microbicidal
agents. The combination of peroxide, myeloperoxidase and
halide ions constitutes a potent halogenating system capable
of killing both bacteria and viruses. Low pH, lysozyme, lac-
toferrin and the cationic proteins constitute a series of bacte-
riostatic and bactericidal factors which are oxygen-
independent and can therefore function under anaerobic
circumstances. The rich variety of proteolytic and other
hydrolytic enzymes present are concerned in the digestion of
the killed organisms.

   To some extent there is an extracellular release of lysosomal constituents during phagocytosis which may play an
amplifying role. The basic polypeptides, for example, stimu-

Table 7.1. Antimicrobial systems in phagocytic vacuoles.

Oxygen-dependent mechanisms:

$$\text{Glucose} + NADP^+ \xrightarrow[\text{shunt}]{\text{hexose monophosphate}} \text{pentose phosphate} + NADPH$$

$$NADPH + O_2 \xrightarrow{\text{oxidase}} NADP^+ + \mathbf{O_2^-}$$

$$\left. \begin{array}{l} \end{array} \right\} \quad \begin{array}{l} O_2 \text{ burst} + \text{generation} \\ \text{of superoxide anion} \end{array}$$

$$2O_2^- + 2H^+ \xrightarrow[\text{dismutation}]{\text{spontaneous}} \mathbf{H_2O_2} + {}^1\mathbf{O_2}$$

$$O_2^- + H_2O_2 \xrightarrow{} \mathbf{.OH} + OH^- + {}^1\mathbf{O_2}$$

$$\left. \begin{array}{l} \end{array} \right\} \quad \begin{array}{l} \text{Spontaneous formation} \\ \text{of further} \\ \text{microbicidal agents} \end{array}$$

$$H_2O_2 + Cl^- \xrightarrow{\text{myeloperoxidase}} \mathbf{OCl^-} + H_2O$$

$$OCl^- + H_2O \xrightarrow{} {}^1\mathbf{O_2} + Cl^- + H_2O$$

$$\left. \begin{array}{l} \end{array} \right\} \quad \begin{array}{l} \text{Myeloperoxidase} \\ \text{generation of micro-} \\ \text{bicidal molecules} \end{array}$$

$$2O_2^- + 2H^+ \xrightarrow[\text{dismutase}]{\text{superoxide}} O_2 + H_2O_2$$

$$2H_2O_2 \xrightarrow{\text{catalase}} 2H_2O + O_2$$

$$\left. \begin{array}{l} \end{array} \right\} \quad \begin{array}{l} \text{Protective mechanisms} \\ \text{used by host} + \\ \text{many microbes} \end{array}$$

Oxygen-independent mechanisms:

Low pH (lactic acid formation)	Not a microbial paradise
Lysozyme	Splits mucopeptide in bacterial cell wall
Lactoferrin	Deprives proliferating bacteria of iron
Cationic proteins (leukin, phagocytin)	**Damage to microbial membranes
Proteolytic enzymes (including elastase) Variety of other hydrolytic enzymes	Digestion of killed organisms

*Microbicidal species in bold letters.
O_2^-, superoxide anion; ${}^1O_2$, singlet (activated) oxygen; $.OH$, hydroxyl free radical.
**There is a transient rise in pH to allow the cationic proteins to function optimally; thereafter the pH falls so that the acid hydrolases can act.

late an acute inflammatory reaction with increased vascular permeability, transudation of serum proteins and egress of leucocytes from blood vessels by diapedesis. The release of an endogenous pyrogen from the polymorphs may explain, in part at least, the fever which often accompanies an infection and the output of acute phase proteins from liver.

It is clear then, that the phagocytic cells possess an impressive anti-microbial potential, but when an infectious agent gains access to the body, this formidable array of weaponry is useless until some way is found to enable the phagocyte to 'home on to' the micro-organism. The body has solved this problem with the effortless ease that comes with a few million years of evolution by developing the complement system.

As we argued in Chapter 6, the surface carbohydrates of many microbial species are able to activate the alternative pathway thereby generating C3 convertase activity. The convertase now splits C3 to give C3b which binds to the surface of the microbe, and the small peptide C3a which provides the answer we need through its ability to attract polymorphs mainly by releasing a chemotactic factor from the mast cell (a later product of the sequence C5a, has similar properties but is an even more powerful chemoattractant in its own right; cf. p. 168). The polymorphs move up the chemotactic gradient until suddenly they come face to face with the C3b-coated micro-organisms to which they become attached by virtue of their surface C3b receptors so thoughtfully placed there by the subtle processes of evolution.

The degranulation of mast cells by C3a and C5a (the anaphylatoxins) has further ramifications through the release of histamine which causes transudation of complement components and movement of polymorphs from the local blood vessels into the surrounding tissue providing the ingredients of an acute inflammatory reaction (figure 7.5).

Adherence to the surface of the phagocyte having been achieved, it remains only for the cell to be stimulated by its contact with the micro-organism for the ingestion phase to be initiated. How splendid—but what happens if the micro-organism should be of such physical and chemical constitution that it lacks the decency either (a) to activate the

Figure 7.5. The role of complement in the defence against infection showing the consequences of activation of the alternative pathway by a bacterium with splitting of C3 and generation of an *acute inflammatory reaction* involving increased vascular permeability through separation of capillary endothelial cells and an influx of polymorphs. The next component, C5a, is a powerful chemotactic and vasoactive peptide and the terminal components C8 and C9 may be lytic.

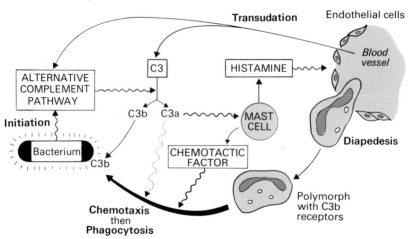

alternative complement pathway or (b) to be able to stimulate phagocytic ingestion? Once again the body has produced an ingenious solution: it has devised a variable adaptor molecule.

Acquired immunity

Looking at the problem teleologically (which usually gives the right answer for the wrong reasons), the body had to develop a molecule with the intrinsic ability to activate complement and phagocytosis but which could be adapted to stick on to any one of a host of different micro-organisms so that each would then become susceptible to the combined complement—phagocyte defence system. And lo and behold, it came to pass, and we marvelled and called it— ANTIBODY! An immunoglobulin of the appropriate class, e.g. human IgG1, activates complement by a separate pathway (classical) through binding C1q to its C_{H2} domain thereby generating a C3 convertase; the C_{H3} domain binds to specific Fc receptors on the phagocyte and through them initiates ingestion. The whole molecule is attached to the foreign invader through the antigen binding region of the variable domains, the body making sure of its defences by manufacturing antibody molecules with a wide range of combining specificities (figure 7.6).

The B-lymphocyte system developed in order to produce antibodies, and by allowing each lymphocyte to synthesize only one type of antibody, great flexibility could be introduced. Although there are sufficient lymphocytes to produce a wide range of different antibodies, it would be wasteful to maintain large numbers of lymphocytes capable of reacting with antigens which the body did not encounter. The system of clonal triggering and formation of memory cells ensures

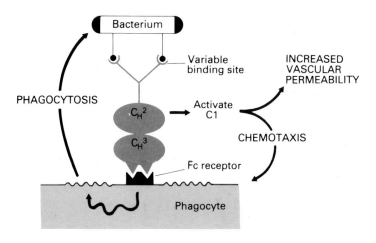

Figure 7.6. Stylized representation of the variable adaptor molecule, alias antibody, developed to activate the host defences against a variety of infectious agents (cf. figure 2.13, p. 33).

that the body only concentrates its main energies on antigens which it actually meets while retaining the potential to react against some obscure microbe which might infect the body at any time in the future. The ability to respond specifically to a particular infection and to generate memory cells is, of course, the basis of *acquired* as distinct from *innate* immunity but it should be perfectly plain that antibody, as one agent of acquired immunity, acts to enhance the mechanisms of innate immunity.

Immunity to bacterial infection

ROLE OF HUMORAL ANTIBODY

Destruction of bacteria

The outer surface of the bacterium is invariably the site at which the defence mechanisms leading to bacterial cell death are initiated. The cell walls of bacteria are multifarious (figure 7.7) and in some cases are resistant to a number of microbicidal agents while many virulent forms escape phago-cytosis by coating themselves with capsules which do not adhere readily to phagocytic cells or which possess anti-phagocytic properties. Other strains secrete substances which frustrate the phagocytic process and in some instances are even directly toxic to the phagocytes themselves. Antibodies can defeat these devious attempts to avoid engulfment by

Figure 7.7. The structure of bacterial cell walls. All types have an inner cell membrane and a peptidoglycan wall which can be cleaved by lysozyme and lysosomal enzymes. The outer lipid bilayer of Gram-negative bacteria which is susceptible to the action of complement or cationic proteins, sometimes contains lipopolysaccharide (LPS; also known as endotoxin; composed of O-specific oligosaccharide side-chains attached to a basal core polysaccharide, itself linked to the mitogenic moiety, lipid A; 148 O antigen variants of *Escherichia coli* are known). The mycobacterial cell wall is highly resistant to breakdown. When present, capsules may protect the bacteria from phagocytosis.

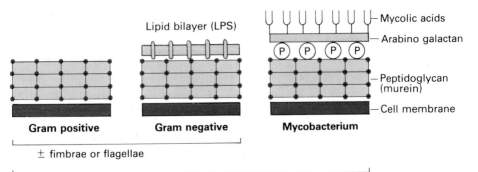

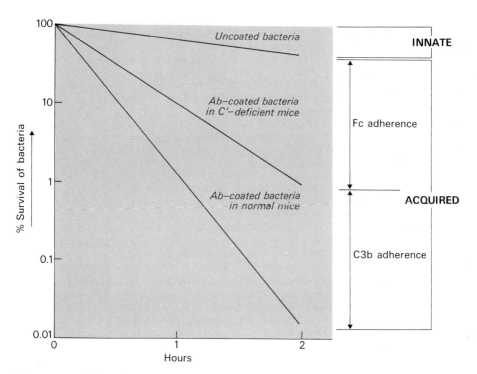

Figure 7.8. Effect of opsonizing antibody and complement on rate of clearance of virulent bacteria from the blood. The uncoated bacteria are phagocytosed rather slowly (*innate immunity*) but on coating with antibody, adherence to phagocytes is increased many-fold (*acquired immunity*). The adherence is somewhat less effective in animals temporarily depleted of complement.

neutralizing the anti-phagocytic molecules and by binding to the surface of the organisms so 'opsonizing' them for ingestion by polymorphs and macrophages. Thus, antibody has a dramatic effect on phagocytosis and the rate of clearance of organisms from the bloodstream is strikingly enhanced when they are coated with specific Ig (figure 7.8). The less effective removal of coated bacteria in complement-depleted animals emphasizes the synergism between antibody and complement for opsonization (cf. pp. 161 and 171) which is mediated through specific high affinity receptors for IgG and C3b on the phagocyte surface (figure 7.9). It is clearly advantageous that the subclasses which bind strongly to these Fc receptors (e.g. IgG1 and 3 in the human) also fix complement well.

Bacteria may also be captured by antibody already fixed to the Fc receptor site (cytophilic antibody) but it is probable that adherence is mediated more through opsonization than through the prior binding of cytophilic antibody to the phagocyte. Complexes containing C3 may show immune adherence to primate red cells and rabbit platelets to provide phagocytosable aggregates.

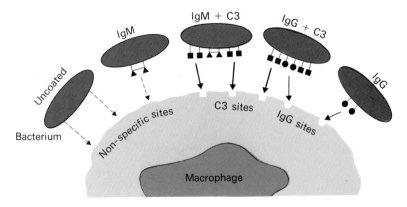

Figure 7.9. Immunoglobulin and complement coats greatly increase the adherence of bacteria (and other antigens) to macrophages and polymorphs. Uncoated or IgM (⊢⊣) coated bacteria adhere relatively weakly to non-specific sites but there are specific receptors for IgG (Fc) (●) and C3 (■) on the macrophage surface which considerably enhance the strength of binding. The augmenting effect of complement is due to the fact that two adjacent IgG molecules can fix many C3 molecules thereby increasing the number of links to the macrophage (cf. 'bonus' effect of multivalency; p. 13). Although IgM does not bind specifically to the macrophage, it promotes adherence through complement fixation.

Some strains of Gram-negative bacteria which have a lipoprotein outer wall resembling mammalian surface membranes in structure are susceptible to the bactericidal action of fresh serum containing antibody. The antibody initiates the development of a complement-mediated lesion producing similar 'holes' to those caused by complement in mammalian cells (cf. figure 6.25); this is said to allow access of serum lysozyme to the inner peptidoglycan wall of the bacterium with eventual cell death. Activation of complement through union of antibody and bacterium will also generate the C3a and C5a anaphylatoxins leading to extensive transudation of serum components including more antibody, and to the chemotactic attraction of polymorphs to aid in phagocytosis. In other words the series of events described in figure 7.5 can be entirely recreated by substituting the antibody-initiated classical complement sequence in place of the alternative pathway.

Protecting external surfaces

Adherence to the epithelial cells of the mucous membranes is essential for viral infection and bacterial colonization. IgA antibodies afford protection in the external body fluids, tears, saliva, nasal secretions and those bathing the surfaces of the intestine (so-called 'coproantibodies') and lung, by coating bacteria and viruses and preventing such adherence to mucosal surfaces. It might be anticipated that in order to fulfil this function, secretory IgA molecules would themselves have very little innate adhesiveness for cells, and certainly no high affinity Fc receptors for this Ig class have yet been described. If an infectious agent succeeds in penetrating the IgA barrier, it comes up against the next line of defence of the MALT system (p. 81) which is manned by IgE. It is worth noting that most serum IgE arises from plasma cells in mucosal tissues and in the lymph nodes that drain them. Although present in low concentration, IgE is bound very firmly to the Fc receptors of the mast cell (p. 234) and contact with antigen leads to the release of mediators which effectively recruit agents of the immune response. Thus histamine, by increasing vascular permeability, causes the transudation of IgG and complement into the area while chemotactic factors for neutrophils and eosinophils attract the effector cells needed to dispose of the infectious organism coated with specific IgG and C3b (figure 7.10). Where the

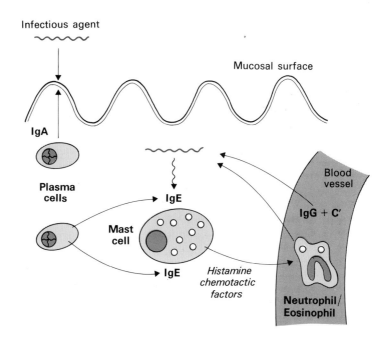

Figure 7.10.
Defence of the mucosal surfaces. IgA prevents adherence of organisms to the mucosa. IgE recruits agents of the immune response by firing the release of mediators from mast cells.

opsonized organism is too large for phagocytosis, these cells can kill by an extracellular mechanism after attachment by their Fcγ receptors. This phenomenon, termed antibody-dependent cell-mediated cytotoxicity (ADCC) is discussed further in the following chapter but there is evidence for its involvement in parasitic infections (p. 195). There are obvious parallels between the ways in which complement-derived anaphylatoxins and IgE utilize the mast cell to cause local amplification of the immune defences.

Toxin neutralization

In addition to their role in removal of microbes, circulating antibodies act to neutralize the soluble exotoxins (e.g. phospholipase C of *Clostridium welchii*) released by bacteria. Combination near the biologically active site of the toxin would stereochemically block reaction with the substrate, particularly if it were macromolecular; combination distant from the active site may also cause inhibition through allosteric conformational changes. In its complex with antibody, the toxin may be unable to diffuse away rapidly and will be susceptible to phagocytosis, especially if the complex can be increased in size by the action of naturally occurring antibodies to altered IgG (antiglobulin factors) and altered C3 (immunoconglutinin).

Specific organisms

Let us see how these considerations apply to the defence against infection by common organisms such as streptococci and staphylococci. β-Haemolytic streptococci were classified by Lancefield according to their carbohydrate antigen and the most important from the standpoint of human disease are those belonging to group A. However, the most immunogenic surface component is the M-protein (variants of which form the basis of the Griffith typing). This protein inhibits phagocytosis and the protection afforded by antibodies to the M-component is attributable to the striking increase in phagocytosis which they induce. High titred antibodies to the streptolysin O exotoxin (ASO) are indicative of recent streptococcal infection. The erythrogenic toxin elaborated by strains which give rise to scarlet fever is neutralized by antibody and the erythematous intradermal reaction to the injected toxin is only seen in individuals lacking antibody (Dick reaction). Antibody also neutralizes bacterial enzymes like hyaluronidase which act to spread the infection.

A growing body of evidence is tending to incriminate *Streptococcus mutans* as an important cause of dental caries. The organism has a constitutive enzyme, glucosyltransferase, able to convert sucrose to dextran which is utilized for adhesion to the tooth surface. Passive transfer of IgG, but not IgA or IgM, antibodies to *S. mutans* in monkeys conferred protection against caries. It is thought that IgG antibody and complement in the gingival crevicular fluid bathing the tooth opsonize the bacteria to facilitate phagocytosis and killing by polymorphonuclear leucocytes.

Virulent forms of staphylococci, of which *S. aureus* is perhaps the most common, resist phagocytosis. This may be due partly to capsule formation *in vivo* and partly to the elaboration of factors such as protein A which combines with the Fc portion of IgG (except for subclass IgG3) and inhibits binding to the polymorph Fc receptor. *S. aureus* is readily phagocytosed in the presence of adequate amounts of antibody but a small proportion of the ingested bacteria survives and they are difficult organisms to eliminate completely. Where the infection is inadequately controlled, severe lesions may occur in the immunized host as a consequence of type IV delayed hypersensitivity reactions. Thus, staphylococci were found to be avirulent when injected into mice passively immunized with antibody but caused extensive tissue damage in animals previously given sensitized T-cells (Glynn).

Other examples where antibodies are required to overcome the inherently anti-phagocytic properties of bacterial capsules are seen in immunity to infection by pneumococci, meningococci and *Haemophilus influenzae*. *Bacillus anthrax* possesses an anti-phagocytic capsule composed of a gamma polypeptide of D-glutamic acid but although anti-capsular antibodies effectively promote uptake by polymorphs, the exotoxin is so potent that vaccines are inadequate unless they also stimulate anti-toxin immunity.

IgA produced in genital secretions in response to gonococcal infection appears to be capable of inhibiting the attachment of the organisms, through their pili, to mucosal cells. Nonetheless, such antibody does not protect against reinfection, perhaps due to the ability of gonococcal protease to split IgA1 dimers, or to the existence of multiple non-crossreacting serotypes. Interestingly, the destruction of gonococci by serum containing antibody depends upon activation of the terminal lytic complement components C8 and 9.

Cholera is caused by the colonization of the small intestine by *Vibrio cholerae* and the subsequent action of its enterotoxin. The B subunits of the toxin bind to specific GM1 monosialoganglioside receptors and translocate the A subunit across the membrane where it activates adenyl cyclase. The increased cAMP then causes fluid loss by inhibiting uptake of sodium chloride and stimulating active Cl^- secretion by intestinal epithelial cells. Locally synthesized IgA antibodies against *V. cholerae* lipopolysaccharide and the toxin provide independent protection against cholera, the first by inhibiting bacterial adherence to the intestinal wall, the second by blocking attachment of the toxin to its receptor. In accord with this analysis is the epidemiological data showing that children who drink milk with high titres of IgA antibodies

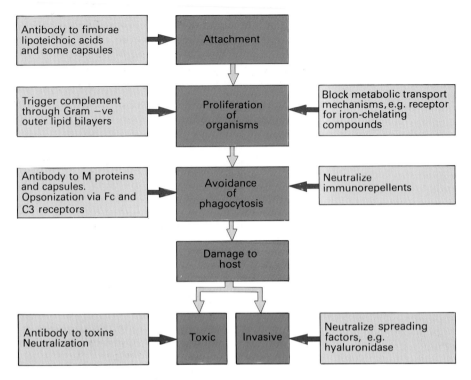

Antibody to fimbrae lipoteichoic acids and some capsules	→ Attachment	
Trigger complement through Gram −ve outer lipid bilayers	→ Proliferation of organisms ←	Block metabolic transport mechanisms, e.g. receptor for iron-chelating compounds
Antibody to M proteins and capsules. Opsonization via Fc and C3 receptors	→ Avoidance of phagocytosis ←	Neutralize immunorepellents
	Damage to host	
Antibody to toxins Neutralization	→ Toxic Invasive ←	Neutralize spreading factors, e.g. hyaluronidase

Figure 7.11. Antibody defences against bacterial invasion.

specific for either of these antigens are less likely to develop clinical cholera.

I thought it might be helpful to summarize the ways in which antibody can parry the different facets of bacterial invasion (figure 7.11).

ROLE OF CELL-MEDIATED IMMUNITY (CMI)

Immunity to intracellular bacteria

Some strains of bacteria such as the tubercle and leprosy bacilli, and listeria and brucella organisms, are able to live and continue their growth within the cytoplasm of macro-phages after their uptake by phagocytosis. In an elegant series of experiments, Mackaness has demonstrated the importance of CMI reactions for the killing of these intracellular facultative parasites and the establishment of an immune state. Animals infected with moderate doses of *M. tuberculosis* overcome the infection and are immune to subsequent challenge with the bacillus. Surprisingly, if they are given an unrelated organism such as *Listeria monocytogenes at the same time* as the second infection with tubercle bacillus, they are resistant and can kill the listeria which have been

194

engulfed by macrophages. Without the prior immunity to *M. tuberculosis* or the second challenge with this organism, the animal would have succumbed to listeria infection. In the same way, an animal immune to listeria can rapidly kill tubercle bacilli given at the same time as a second infection with listeria (table 7.2). Thus the triggering of a specific

Table 7.2. Induction of non-specific immunity by a CMI reaction.

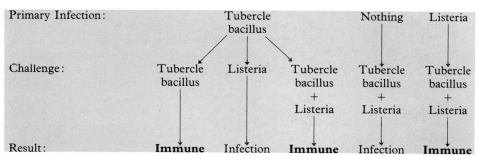

Primary Infection:			Tubercle bacillus			Nothing	Listeria
Challenge:	Tubercle bacillus	Listeria		Tubercle bacillus + Listeria		Tubercle bacillus + Listeria	Tubercle bacillus + Listeria
Result:	**Immune**	Infection		**Immune**		Infection	**Immune**

secondary immune response to one organism may endow the animal with a simultaneous but transient non-specific resistance to unrelated microbes of similar growth habits.

This immunity—both specific and non-specific—can be transferred to a normal recipient with T-lymphocytes but not macrophages or serum from an immune animal (figure 7.12). In support of this view that the specific immunity is mediated by T-cells is the greater susceptibility to infection with tubercle and leprosy bacilli of mice in which the T-lymphocytes have been depressed by thymectomy plus anti-lymphocyte serum. In human leprosy, the disease presents as a spectrum ranging from the *tuberculoid* form with few viable organisms, to the *lepromatous* form characterized by an abundance of *Mycobacterium leprae* within the macrophages. As Turk has emphasized, the tuberculoid state is associated with an active T-lymphocyte system giving good PHA transformation of lymphocytes and cell-mediated dermal hypersensitivity responses, although still not good enough to completely eradicate the bacilli. In the lepromatous form, there is poor T-cell reactivity and the paracortical areas in the lymph nodes are depleted of lymphocytes although there are numerous plasma cells which contribute to a high level of circulating antibody. Clearly CMI rather than humoral immunity is important for the control of the leprosy bacillus.

Macrophage activation

The intracellular organisms survive because they are able to thwart the killing mechanisms of the host macrophage, some-

195

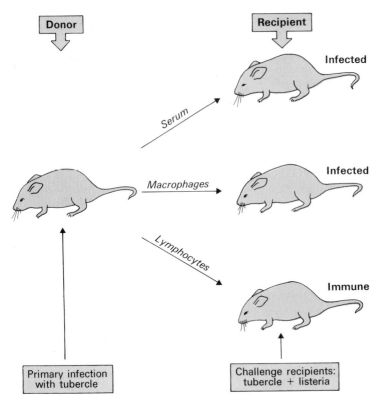

Figure 7.12. Transfer of specific and non-specific immunity by lymphocytes from an immune animal. The syngeneic recipient of the lymphocytes resisted simultaneous challenge with tubercle and listeria organisms. The recipients were not immune to listeria given without the tubercle. The lympho-cytes lost their power to confer passive immunity on the recipients if treated with a cytotoxic anti-T cell serum plus complement prior to injection. Serum or macrophages were ineffective in transferring immunity (after Mackaness).

times by preventing fusion of the lysosomes with the phagosomes (*Mycobacterium tuberculosis*), in some instances by inhibiting the respiratory burst (*Legionella*) and in other cases by escape from the phagosome into the cytoplasm where they are safe from lysosome attack (*Trypanosoma cruzi*). However, if macrophages are activated, especially by the T-cell lymphokine macrophage activating factor (MAF), they acquire the ability to overcome these microbial stratagems and destroy the ingested organisms.

The activation of macrophages (Mø) proceeds through several stages:

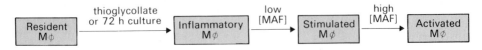

Striking changes on surface components accompany activation. In mouse macrophages there is an increase in Ia

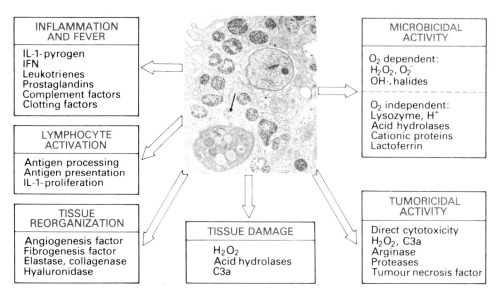

INFLAMMATION AND FEVER		MICROBICIDAL ACTIVITY
IL-1-pyrogen IFN Leukotrienes Prostaglandins Complement factors Clotting factors		O_2 dependent: H_2O_2, O_2^- $OH\cdot$, halides --- O_2 independent: Lysozyme, H^+ Acid hydrolases Cationic proteins Lactoferrin

LYMPHOCYTE ACTIVATION

Antigen processing
Antigen presentation
IL-1-proliferation

TISSUE REORGANIZATION

Angiogenesis factor
Fibrogenesis factor
Elastase, collagenase
Hyaluronidase

TISSUE DAMAGE

H_2O_2
Acid hydrolases
C3a

TUMORICIDAL ACTIVITY

Direct cytotoxicity
H_2O_2, C3a
Arginase
Proteases
Tumour necrosis factor

Figure 7.13. The role of the activated macrophage in the initiation and mediation of chronic inflammation with concomitant tissue repair, and in the killing of microbes (cf. table 7.1) and tumour cells. The electron-micrograph shows a highly activated macrophage with many lysosomal structures one of which (arrowed) is fusing with a phagosome containing a *Toxoplasma gondii* organism (courtesy of Prof. C. Jones).

(dramatic), Fc receptors for IgG2b, and binding sites for tumour cells with acquisition of an activation antigen MB1 (recognized by a monoclonal Ab); the mannose receptor, the F4/80 marker and IgG2a receptors all decline while the Mac-I component, probably part of the C3bi receptor remains unchanged. The activated macrophage has heightened microbicidal powers dominant among which are those based on oxygen radicals. It is undeniably a remarkable and formidable cell, capable of secreting the 60-odd substances which are concerned in chronic inflammatory reactions (figure 7.13)—not the sort to meet in an alley on a dark night!

The mechanism of the Mackaness phenomenon now becomes clear. The specificity of the CMI reaction lies at the level of the initial reaction of the T-cell with its antigen, releasing macrophage activating lymphokines; the non-specific immunity arises from the newly acquired ability of the activated macrophage to kill almost *any* organism it has phagocytosed (figure 7.14). Similar phenomena have been induced in ordinary macrophage cultures treated with lymphokine preparations obtained by incubating sensitized T-cells with antigen.

Where the host has difficulty in effectively eliminating such organisms, the chronic CMI response to locally released antigen leads to the accumulation of densely packed macrophages which release fibrogenic factors and stimulate the for-

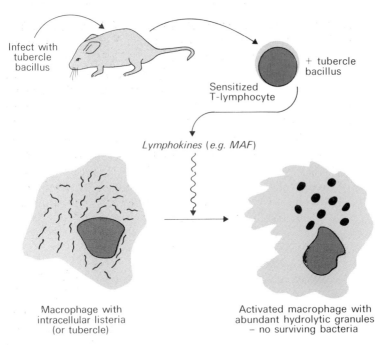

Infect with
tubercle
bacillus

Sensitized
T-lymphocyte

+ tubercle
bacillus

Lymphokines (e.g. MAF)

Macrophage with
intracellular listeria
(or tubercle)

Activated macrophage with
abundant hydrolytic granules
– no surviving bacteria

Figure 7.14. The 'lymphokine connec- intracellular bacteria triggered by a specific
tion': non-specific macrophage killing of cell-mediated immunity reaction.

mation of granulation tissue and ultimately fibrosis. The
resulting structure, termed a granuloma, represents an
attempt by the body to isolate a site of persistent infection.

Immunity to viral infection

Genetically controlled constitutional factors which render a
host or certain of his cells non-permissive (i.e. resistant to
takeover of their replicative machinery by virus) play a
dominant role in influencing the vulnerability of a given
individual to infection. Macrophages may readily take up
viruses non-specifically and kill them. However, in some
instances the macrophages allow replication and if the virus
is capable of producing cytopathic effects in various organs,
the infection may be lethal; with non-cytopathic agents such
as lymphocytic choriomeningitis, Aleutian mink disease and
equine infectious anaemia viruses, a persistent infection will
result.

ANTIGENIC DRIFT AND SHIFT

In the course of their constant duel with the immune system,
viruses are continually changing the structure of their surface
antigens. They do so by processes termed 'antigenic drift'
and 'antigenic shift', the nature of which may be made more

apparent by consideration of different influenza strains. The surface of the influenza virus contains a haemagglutinin by which it adheres to cells prior to infection, and a neuraminidase which releases newly formed virus from the surface sialic acid of the infected cell; of these the haemagglutinin is the more important for the establishment of protective immunity. Minor changes in antigenicity of the haemagglutinin occur through point mutations in the viral genome (drift) but major changes arise through wholesale swapping of genetic material with reservoirs of different viruses in other animal hosts (shift). When alterations in the haemagglutinin are sufficient to render previous immunity ineffective, new influenza epidemics break out (figure 7.15).

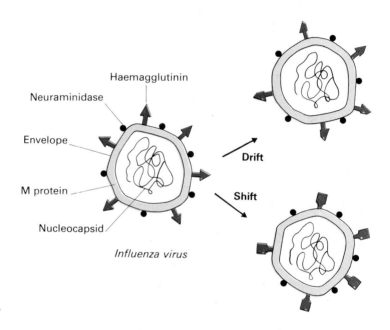

Figure 7.15. Antigenic drift and shift in influenza virus. The changes in haemagglutinin structure caused by drift may be small enough to allow protection by immunity to earlier strains. This may not happen with radical changes in the antigen associated with antigenic shift and so new virus epidemics break out.

Over the last 50 years epidemics have been associated with the emergence by antigenic shift of the A/PR8 strain in 1933 with the structure H_0N_1 (the official nomenclature assigns numbers to each haemagglutinin and neuraminidase major variant), A/FMI in 1947 (H_1N_1), A/Singapore in 1957 (H_2N_2) and A/Hong Kong in 1968 (H_3N_2); note that each new epidemic was associated with a fundamental change in the haemagglutinin.

PROTECTION BY SERUM ANTIBODY

The antibody molecule can neutralize viruses by a variety of means. It may stereochemically inhibit combination with the receptor site on cells, thereby preventing penetration and subsequent intracellular multiplication, the protective effect of antibodies to influenza viral haemagglutinin providing a good example. Similarly, antibodies to the measles haemagglutinin prevent entry into the cell but spread of virus from cell to cell is stopped by antibodies to the fusion antigen. Antibody may destroy a virus particle directly through activation of the classical complement pathway or produce aggregation, enhanced phagocytosis and intracellular death by mechanisms already discussed.

Relatively low concentrations of circulating antibody can be effective and one is familiar with the protection afforded by poliomyelitis antibodies, and by human γ-globulin given prophylactically to individuals exposed to measles. The most clear-cut protection is seen in diseases with long incubation times where the virus has to travel through the bloodstream before it reaches the tissue which it finally infects. For example, in poliomyelitis the virus gains access to the body via the gastro-intestinal tract and eventually passes through the circulation to reach the brain cells which become infected. Within the blood, the virus is neutralized by quite low levels of specific antibody while the prolonged period before the virus infects the brain allows time for a secondary immune response in a primed host.

LOCAL FACTORS

With other viral diseases, such as influenza and the common cold, there is a short incubation time related to the fact that the final target organ for the virus is the same as the portal of entry and no intermediate stage involving passage through the body occurs. There is little time for a primary antibody response to be mounted and in all likelihood the rapid production of interferon is the most significant mechanism used to counter the viral infection. Experimental studies certainly indicate that after an early peak of interferon production, there is a rapid fall in the titre of live virus in the lungs of mice infected with influenza (figure 7.16). Antibody, as assessed by the *serum* titre, seems to arrive on the scene much too late to be of value in aiding recovery. However, recent investigations have shown that antibody levels may be elevated in the *local* fluids bathing the infected surfaces, e.g. nasal mucosa and lung, despite low serum titres and it is the production of antiviral antibody (most prominently IgA) by locally deployed immunologically primed cells which may prove to be of great importance for the *prevention* of subsequent infection. Unfortunately, in so far as the common cold is concerned, a subsequent infection is likely to involve an antigenically unrelated virus so that general immunity to colds is difficult to achieve.

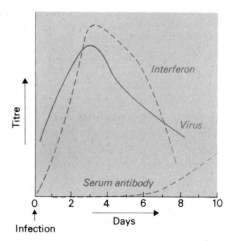

Figure 7.16. Appearance of interferon and serum antibody in relation to recovery from influenza virus infection of the lungs of mice (from Isaacs A. (1961) *New Scientist* **11**, 81).

CELL-MEDIATED IMMUNITY

Local or systemic antibodies can block the spread of cytolytic viruses but alone they are usually inadequate to control those viruses which modify the antigens of the cell membrane and bud off from the surface as infectious particles. Included in this group are: oncorna (= oncogenic RNA virus, e.g. murine leukaemogenic), orthomyxo (influenza), paramyxo (mumps, measles), toga (dengue), rhabdo (rabies), arena (lymphocytic choriomeningitis), adeno, herpes (simplex, varicella zoster, cytomegalo, Epstein–Barr, Marek's disease), pox (vaccinia), papova (SV40, polyoma) and rubella viruses. The importance of cell-mediated immunity for recovery from infection with these agents is underlined by the inability of children with primary T-cell immunodeficiency to cope with such viruses, whereas patients with Ig deficiency but intact cell-mediated immunity are not troubled in this way.

T-lymphocytes from a sensitized host are directly cytotoxic to cells infected with viruses from this group, the new surface antigens on the target cells being recognized by specific receptors on the aggressor lymphocytes. Cytotoxic T-cells are less strain-specific, i.e. show broader cross-reaction, than antibody and strikingly, they do not attack cells infected with the same virus but carrying different class I major histocompatibility antigens (cf. figure 10.17, p. 293). The sensitized T-cells must therefore recognize (a) virally modified histocompatibility antigen, (b) a complex of histocompatibility antigen with virally associated antigen, or (c) *both* virally associated *and* self-histocompatibility antigens.

That cytolytic T-cells may be important in viral infection in the human is suggested by studies on volunteers showing that high levels of cytotoxic activity before challenge with live influenza correlated with low or absent shedding of virus. This direct attack on the cell will effectively limit the infection if the surface antigen changes appear before full replication of the virus, otherwise the organism will spread by two major routes. The first, involving free infectious viral particles released by budding from the surface, can normally be checked by humoral antibody. The second, which depends upon the passage of virus from one cell to another across intercellular junctions, cannot be influenced by antibody but is countered by cell-mediated immunity. Macrophages, attracted to the site by chemotactic factors released by the interaction of T-cells with virally associated antigen, appear to discourage the formation of these intercellular bridges, a capability which may be enhanced by other T-cell lymphokines such as macrophage-activating factor (IFNγ). Furthermore, this interferon and presumably also that produced by the lymphokine-stimulated macrophage will render the contiguous cells non-permissive for the replication of any virus acquired by intercellular transfer (figure 7.17). It may

Figure 7.17. Control of infection by 'budding' viruses. Cytotoxic T-cells kill virally infected targets directly after recognition of new surface antigen (● ● ● ●). Interaction with a separate subpopulation of T-cells releases lymphokines which attract macrophages to inhibit intercellular virus transfer and prime contiguous cells with interferon to make them resistant to viral infection. Free virus released by budding from the cell surface is neutralized by antibody (which is usually thymus-dependent pointing to yet another contribution by the T-cell to viral immunity).

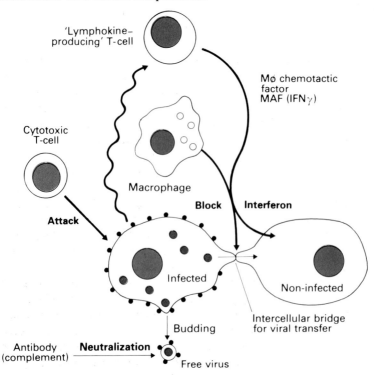

'Lymphokine–producing' T-cell

Mϕ chemotactic factor
MAF (IFNγ)

Cytotoxic T-cell

Macrophage

Block   Interferon

Attack

Infected

Non-infected

Intercellular bridge for viral transfer

Budding

Antibody (complement)   **Neutralization**

Free virus

also increase the non-specific cytotoxicity of NK cells (p. 300) for infected cells. This generation of 'immune interferon' (IFNγ) in response to non-nucleic acid viral components provides a valuable back-up mechanism when dealing with viruses which are intrinsically poor stimulators of interferon synthesis.

The neutralization of free virus particles by antibody is relatively straightforward but the interaction with infected cells is rather more complex. Access to the surface antigens by T-cells would be denied were they blocked by coating with antibody. Nonetheless, these antibodies should be able to initiate type II hypersensitivity killing reactions. Antibody-dependent cell-mediated cytotoxicity (ADCC; p. 242) has been reported with herpes, vaccinia and mumps-infected target cells while Oldstone has described the complement-mediated killing of measles-infected cells by F(ab')$_2$ antibody fragments via the alternative pathway. Antibody may play a different tune, however, since in the case of measles-infected cells, although 10^6 antibody molecules per cell permit complement-mediated cytotoxicity, 10^5 molecules do not kill but cause capping and shedding of surface antigen (cf. p. 64) leaving the cell resistant to attack by any immunological mechanism.

Immunity to parasitic infections

PROTOZOA

The diverse organisms responsible for the major parasitic diseases are listed in figure 7.18. The numbers affected are truly horrifying and the sum of misery they engender is too large to comprehend. To be successful, a parasite must avoid wholesale killing of the human host and yet at the same time escape destruction by the immune system. In practice, each type of parasite is virtually a world unto itself in the complexity of the mechanisms by which this is achieved.

After recovery from parasitic infection, the organisms may be completely eradicated and the host remain solidly immune to reinfection: we speak of a *sterile immunity*. Often the parasites are not completely eliminated but small numbers continue to be harboured even though the host is able to resist superinfection; this state is referred to by parasitologists as *premunition*. Although the precise immunological mechanisms which operate in premunition are still not completely understood the relative roles of humoral antibody and cell-mediated immunity are becoming more clearly established in relation to the defence against protozoal parasites. The generalization may be made that a humoral response develops when the organisms invade the bloodstream (malaria, trypanosomiasis) whereas parasites which grow within the

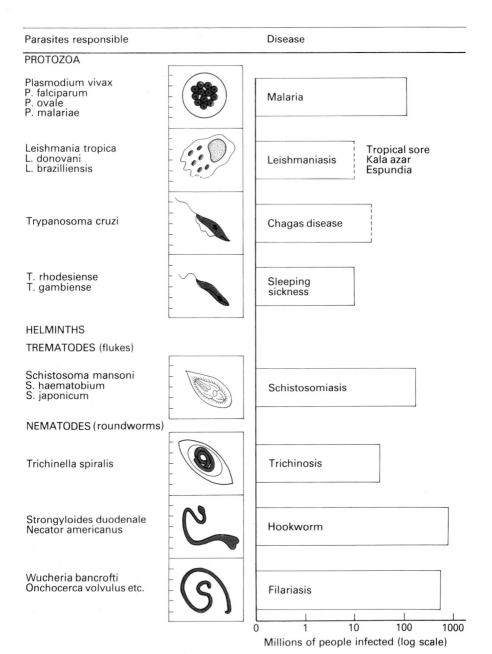

Parasites responsible		Disease

PROTOZOA

Plasmodium vivax
P. falciparum
P. ovale
P. malariae — Malaria

Leishmania tropica
L. donovani
L. brazilliensis — Leishmaniasis — Tropical sore / Kala azar / Espundia

Trypanosoma cruzi — Chagas disease

T. rhodesiense
T. gambiense — Sleeping sickness

HELMINTHS

TREMATODES (flukes)

Schistosoma mansoni
S. haematobium
S. japonicum — Schistosomiasis

NEMATODES (roundworms)

Trichinella spiralis — Trichinosis

Strongyloides duodenale
Necator americanus — Hookworm

Wucheria bancrofti
Onchocerca volvulus etc. — Filariasis

0   1   10   100   1000

Millions of people infected (log scale)

Figure 7.18. The major parasites in man and the sheer enormity of the numbers of people infected.

tissues (e.g. cutaneous leishmaniasis) usually elicit cell-mediated immunity (table 7.3).

Humoral immunity

Circulating antibodies have often been shown to offer protection against the blood-borne forms but the parasites can be

Table 7.3. The relative importance of antibody and cell-mediated responses in protozoal infections.

Parasite	Trypanosoma brucei	Plasmodium	Trypanosoma cruzi	Leishmania
Habitat	Free in blood	Inside red cell	Inside macrophage	Inside macrophage
ANTIBODY				
Importance	+ + + +	+ + +	+ +	+
Mechanism	Lysis with complement. Opsonizes for phagocytosis	Blocks invasion. Opsonizes for phagocytosis	Limits spread in acute infection	Limits spread
Means of evasion	Antigenic variation	Intracellular habitat	Intracellular habitat	Intracellular habitat
CELL MEDIATED				
Importance	–	+ (?)	+ + + (Chronic phase)	+ + + +
Mechanism	–	Direct and lymphokine mediated macrophage activation	Macrophage activation by lymphokines and killing by metabolites of O_2	

wily. Thus in toxoplasmosis, although antibody is protective it cannot eliminate the cystic stage; as a result, the overt clinical disease is rare but subclinical infection is relatively frequent. In trypanosomiasis and malaria, the parasites escape from the cytocidal action of humoral antibody on their cycling blood forms by the ingenious trick of altering their antigenic constitution. Figure 7.19 illustrates how the trypanosome continues to infect the host, even after fully protective antibodies appear, by *antigenic variation* to a form which these antibodies cannot inactivate; as antibodies to the new antigens are synthesized, the parasite escapes again by changing to yet a further variant and so on. This may explain why in hyperendemic areas, children are subjected to repeated attacks of malaria for their first few years and are then solidly immune to further infection. Immunity must presumably be developed against all the antigenic variants before full protection can be attained, and indeed it is known that IgG from individuals with solid immunity can effectively terminate malaria infections in young children. Despite this problem of antigenic variation, recent experiments with

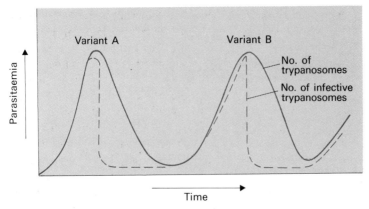

Figure 7.19. Antigenic variation during chronic trypanosome infection. As antibody to the initial variant A is formed, the blood trypanosomes become complexed prior to phagocytosis and are no longer infective, leaving a small number of viable parasites which have acquired a new antigenic constitution. This new variant (B) now multiplies until it, too, is neutralized by the primary antibody response and is succeeded by variant C (after A.R. Gray, see further reading list).

monkeys have raised hopes that a human malaria vaccine may be a real possibility.

Cell-mediated immunity

Trypanosoma cruzi, the organism producing Chagas' disease, may survive after ingestion by macrophages; activation of the macrophages by lymphokines stimulates the formation of hydrogen peroxide and leads to intracellular execution within 48 hours. Cell-mediated immunity is directly concerned in the recovery from certain forms of leishmaniasis but studies on laboratory models have not so far defined all the factors involved. For example, cultured guinea pig macrophages activated by the Mackaness phenomenon so that they non-specifically kill ingested listeria (cf. p. 195), take up *Leishmania enrietti* and allow the organisms to grow. Similarly, activated mouse macrophages which have ingested *Toxoplasma gondii* allow growth through a failure to effect lysosome fusion with the phagosome containing the organism. Almost certainly a further antigen-specific factor, probably antibody, is required to help the macrophage deal with the parasite; in other words the simple idea that a non-specifically activated macrophage will always kill *any* organism growing within its cytoplasm needs some amendment.

HELMINTHS

A marked feature of the immune reaction to helminthic infections such as *Trichinella spiralis* in man and *Nippos-*

trongylus brasiliensis in the rat is the high level of homo-cytotropic (reaginic) antibody produced. In man serum levels of IgE can rise from normal values of around 100 ng/ml to as high as 10,000 ng/ml. This exceptional increase has encouraged the view that IgE represents an important line of defence. One suggestion is that histamine released by contact of antigen with IgE-coated mast cells can aid the expulsion of the worm from the gut. Another view is that such a local anaphylactic reaction may lead to exudation of serum proteins known to contain high concentrations of protective antibodies in all the major immunoglobulin classes. Certainly IgE-mediated release of eosinophil chemotactic factor (cf. figure 7.10) would attract these cells which are known to bind to antibody-coated nematodes. Transfer studies in rats (Ogilvie) have shown that although antibody produces some damage to the worms, T-cells from *immune* donors are required for vigorous expulsion which is probably achieved through lymphokine activation of intestinal goblet cells (figure 7.20).

In connection with IgE-mediated inflammatory reactions, it is of interest that schistosomules, the early immature form of the schistosome, have been killed in cultures containing both specific IgG and eosinophils, which are acting as effec-

Figure 7.20. The expulsion of nematode worms from the gut. The parasite is first damaged by IgG antibody passing into the gut lumen possibly as a consequence of IgE-mediated inflammation and possibly aided by accessory ADCC cells. Lympho-kines released by antigen-specific triggering of T-cells stimulate proliferation of goblet cells and secretion of materials which coat the damaged worm and facilitate its expulsion from the body.

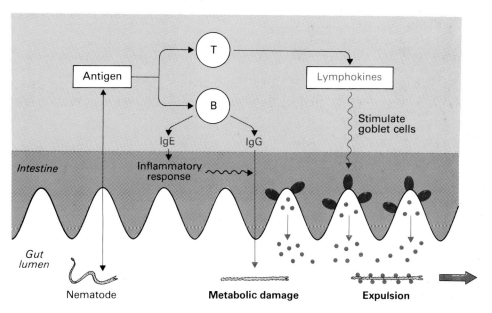

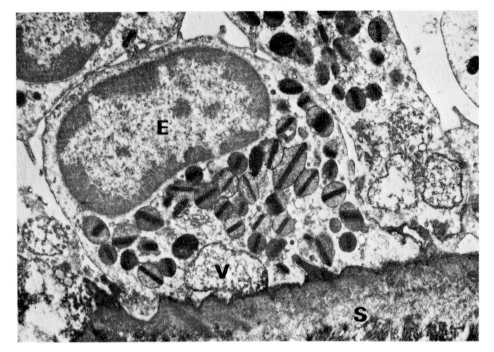

Figure 7.21. Electron micrograph showing an eosinophil (E) attached to the surface of a schistosomulum (S) in the presence of specific antibody. The cell develops large vacuoles (V) which appear to release their contents on to the parasite (× 16,500). (Courtesy of Drs D.J. McLaren & C.D. Mackenzie.)

tors in a form of antibody-dependent cell-mediated cytotoxicity (figure 7.21); after 12 hours or so, the major basic protein forming the electron-dense core of the eosinophilic granules is released on to the parasite and brings about its destruction. Further evidence for an involvement of this cell comes from the experiment in which the protection afforded by passive transfer of antiserum *in vivo* was blocked by pretreatment of the recipient with an anti-eosinophil serum.

Schistosomiasis presents another intriguing feature. The adult worm lives permanently within the mesenteric vessels of the host, despite the fact that the blood which bathes it contains antibodies which can prevent a second infection. Smithers and Terry have shown that the parasites make themselves resistant to these immune processes by disguising themselves with an outer coat of the host's red cell antigens, either by direct acquisition or possibly through synthesis by the parasite itself as a form of antigenic 'mimicry'.

Further reading

See references at end of Chapter 8.

8

Immunity to Infection II—Prophylaxis and Immunodeficiency

Prophylaxis

The control of infection is approached from several directions. One method of breaking the chain of infection has been achieved in the U.K. with rabies and psittacosis by controlling the importation of dogs and parrots respectively. Improvements in public health—water supply, sewage systems, education in personal hygiene—prevent the spread of cholera and many other diseases. And of course when other measures fail we can fall back on the induction of immunity.

PASSIVELY ACQUIRED IMMUNITY

Temporary protection against infection can be established by giving preformed antibody from another individual of the same or a different species. As the acquired antibodies are utilized by combination with antigen or catabolized in the normal way, this protection is gradually lost.

Homologous antibodies

Maternal In the first few months of life while the baby's own lymphoid system is slowly getting under way, protection is afforded by maternally derived antibodies acquired by placental transfer and by intestinal absorption of colostral immunoglobulins. The major immunoglobulin in milk is secretory IgA and this is not absorbed by the baby but remains in the intestine to protect the mucosal surfaces. It is quite striking that the sIgA antibodies are directed against bacterial and viral antigens often present in the intestine, and it is presumed that IgA-producing cells responding to gut antigens, migrate and colonize breast tissue (as part of the MALT system; p. 81) where they secrete their antibodies into the milk.

γ-Globulin Preparations of pooled human adult γ-globulin are of value to modify the effects of chicken pox or measles, particularly in individuals with defective immune responses such as premature infants, children with primary immuno-deficiency or protein malnutrition or patients on steroid treatment. Contacts with cases of infectious hepatitis and smallpox may also be afforded protection by γ-globulin, especially when in the latter case the material is derived from the serum of individuals vaccinated some weeks previously. Human anti-tetanus immunoglobulin is preferable to horse antitoxin which can cause serum reactions.

Isolated γ-globulin preparations tend to form small aggregates spontaneously and these can lead to severe anaphylactic reactions when administered intravenously on account of their ability to aggregate platelets and to activate complement and generate C3a and C5a anaphylatoxins. For this reason the material is always injected intramuscularly. Preparations free of aggregates would be welcome as would separate pools with raised antibody titres to selected organisms such as vaccinia, *Herpes zoster*, tetanus and perhaps rubella. This need will ultimately be satisfied when it becomes possible to produce human monoclonal antibodies on demand.

Heterologous antibodies

Horse globulins containing anti-tetanus and anti-diphtheria toxins have been extensively employed prophylactically, but at the present time the practice is more restricted because of the complication of serum sickness developing in response to the foreign protein. This is more likely to occur in subjects already sensitized by previous contact with horse globulin; thus individuals who have been given horse anti-tetanus (e.g. for immediate protection after receiving a wound out in the open) are later advised to undergo a course of active immunization to obviate the need for further injections of horse protein in any subsequent emergency.

VACCINATION

In the case of tetanus, active immunization is of benefit to the individual but not to the community since it will not eliminate the organism which is formed in the faeces of domestic animals and persists in the soil as highly resistant spores. Where a disease depends on human transmission, immunity in just a proportion of the population can help the whole community if it leads to a fall in the reproduction rate (i.e. the number of further cases produced by each infected individual) to less than one; under these circumstances the disease will die out, witness for example the disappearance of diphtheria from communities in which around 75% of the children have been immunized (figure 8.1). In contrast, focal

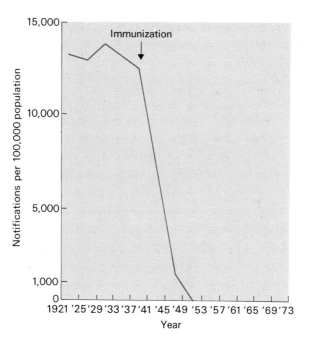

Figure 8.1. Notifications of diphtheria in England and Wales per 100,000 population showing dramatic fall after immunization. (Reproduced from *Immunisation* by G. Dick, 1978, Update Books; with kind permission of author and publishers.)

outbreaks of poliomyelitis have occurred in communities which object to immunization on religious grounds.

The objective of vaccination is to provide effective immunity by establishing adequate levels of antibody and a primed population of cells which can rapidly expand on renewed contact with antigen. The first contact with antigen during vaccination obviously should not be injurious and the manoeuvre is to avoid the pathogenic effect while maintaining protective antigens.

Killed organisms

Parasitic worms and, to a lesser extent, protozoa are extremely difficult to grow up in bulk to manufacture killed vaccines. This problem does not arise for many bacteria and viruses and, in these cases, the inactivated micro-organisms have generally provided safe antigens for immunization. Examples are typhoid (in combination with the relatively ineffective paratyphoid A and B), cholera and killed poliomyelitis (Salk) vaccines. The success of the Salk vaccine was slightly marred by a small rise in the incidence of deaths from poliomyelitis in 1960–61 (figure 8.2) but this has now been attributed to poor antigenicity of one of the three different strains of virus used and present-day vaccines are far more potent. Care has to be taken to ensure that important protective antigens are not destroyed in the inactivation process. During the production of an early killed measles vaccine, the fusion antigen which permits cellular spread of

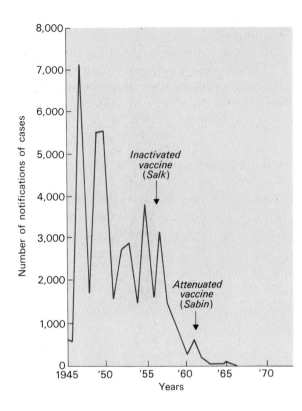

Figure 8.2.
Notifications
of paralytic polio-
myelitis in England
and Wales showing
the beneficial
effects of com-
munity immuniza-
tion with killed and
live vaccines.
(Reproduced from
Immunisation by G.
Dick, 1978, Update
Books; with kind
permission of
author and publi-
shers.)

virus was inactivated; as a result, incomplete immunity was produced and this left the individual susceptible to the development of immunopathological complications on subsequent natural infection. The dangers of incomplete immunity are especially worrying in areas where measles is endemic and the immune response is relatively enfeebled due to protein malnutrition. Since the widespread correction of this dietary deficiency is unlikely in the near future, it is worth considering whether non-specific stimulation by immunopotentiating drugs or thymus hormones at the time of vaccination might provide a feasible solution.

This idea of supplementing a deficient adaptive immune response with some synergistic treatment has surfaced in other contexts. Thus, the antibiotic polymyxin B is too toxic for normal use; however, if certain end groups are removed, the molecule loses its toxicity but still retains its ability to disturb the outer wall of Gram-negative bacteria thereby allowing potentially lytic antibodies and complement to reach previously inaccessible bacterial inner membranes. Another curious phenomenon which might be exploited is the finding that the amoeba *Entamoeba histolytica*, which is resistant to lysis by antibody and complement, shows greatly increased susceptibility if treated with an otherwise non-toxic protein inhibitor.

Attenuated organisms

In many instances, the immunity conferred by killed vaccines, even when given with adjuvant (see below), is often inferior to that resulting from infection with live organisms. This must be partly because the replication of the living microbes confronts the host with a larger and more sustained dose of antigen and that, with budding viruses, infected cells are required for the establishment of good cytotoxic T-cell memory. Another significant advantage is that the immune response takes place largely at the site of the natural infection. This is well illustrated by the nasopharyngeal IgA response to immunization with polio vaccine. In contrast with the ineffectiveness of parenteral injection of killed vaccine, intranasal administration evoked a good local antibody response; but whereas this declined over a period of 2 months or so, per oral immunization with *live attenuated* virus established a persistently high IgA antibody level (figure 8.3).

The objective of attenuation, that of producing an organism which causes only a very mild form of the natural disease, can be equally well attained by using strains which are virulent for another species, but avirulent in man. The best example of this was Jenner's remarkable demonstration that cowpox would protect against smallpox (Latin *vacca*, cow; hence *vaccination*). Since then, a global effort by the World Health Organisation combining extensive vaccination and selective epidemiological control methods, has eradicated the human disease.

Attenuation itself can be achieved by modifying the condi-

Figure 8.3. Local IgA response to polio vaccine. Local secretory antibody synthesis is confined to the specific anatomical sites which have been directly stimulated by contact with antigen. (Data from Ogra P.L. *et al.* (1975) In *Viral Immunology and Immunopathology*, p. 67. Notkins A.L. (ed.). Academic Press, New York.)

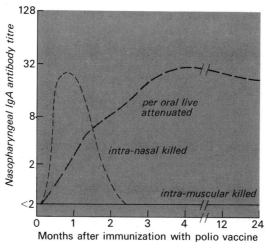

tions under which an organism grows, or by direct genetic modification. Pasteur first achieved the production of live but non-virulent forms of chicken cholera bacillus and anthrax by such artifices as culture at higher temperatures and under anaerobic conditions, and was able to confer immunity by infection with the attenuated organisms. A virulent strain of *Mycobacterium tuberculosis* became attenuated by chance in 1908 when Calmette and Guérin at the Institut Pasteur, Lille, added bile to the culture medium in an attempt to achieve dispersed growth. After 13 years of culture in bile-containing medium, the strain remained attenuated and was used successfully to vaccinate children against tuberculosis. The same organism, BCG (Bacille, Calmette, Guérin), is widely used today for immunization of tuberculin-negative individuals; it may also bestow a reasonable degree of protection against *Mycobacterium leprae* but the circumstances in which this can be achieved have not been fully identified. Attenuation by cold adaptation of influenza and other respiratory viruses seems hopeful; the organism can grow at the lower temperatures (32–34°) of the upper respiratory tract, but fails to produce clinical disease because of its inability to replicate in the lower respiratory tract (37°).

The technique of genetic recombination is being used to generate various attenuated strains of influenza virus with lower virulence for man and some with an increased multiplication rate in eggs (enabling newly endemic strains of influenza to be adapted for rapid vaccine production). A new approach termed 'infection-permissive immunization' utilizes parenteral administration of a recombinant virus which bears the relevant neuraminidase but an irrelevant haemagglutinin: the partial immunity so produced still permits natural infection but prevents the development of disease, and it is anticipated that this process will establish an effective resistance to subsequent contact with the virus. An ingenious trick is to use a virus as a 'piggy-back' for genes from another virus that cannot be grown successfully. The gene encoding hepatitis virus surface antigen (HBsAg) can be introduced into vaccinia; an infected cell will then secrete both vaccinia virus and HBsAg which will then immunize the host.

Attenuated vaccines for poliomyelitis (Sabin), measles and rubella have gained general acceptance. Nonetheless with certain vaccines there is a very small, but still real, risk of developing complications such as the encephalitis which can occur following measles immunization; note, however, that the natural infection carries a far greater risk of encephalitis (ca 1 : 2,000)! With live viral vaccines there is a possibility that the nucleic acid might be incorporated into the host's genome or that there may be reversion to a virulent form, although this will be unlikely if the attenuated strains contain several mutations. Another disadvantage of attenuated strains is the difficulty and expense of maintaining appropriate cold storage facilities especially in out-of-the-way places. In diseases such as viral hepatitis and cancer, the dangers associated with live vaccines would make their use unthinkable. Generally speaking, the risk of complication must be balanced against the expected chance of contracting the disease with its own complications. Where this is minimal some may prefer to avoid general vaccination and to rely upon a crash course backed up if necessary by passive immunization in the localities around isolated outbreaks of infectious disease.

It is important to recognize those children with immunodeficiency before injection of live organisms; a child with impaired T-cell reactivity can become overwhelmed by BCG and die. Perhaps this is only a sick story, but it is said that in one particular country there are no adults with T-cell deficiency. The reason? All children had been immunized with live BCG as part of a community health programme(!) The extent to which children with partial deficiencies are at risk has yet to be assessed. It is also inadvisable to give live vaccines to patients being treated with steroids, immunosuppressive drugs or radiotherapy or who have malignant conditions such as lymphoma and leukaemia; pregnant mothers must also be included here because of the vulnerability of the fetus.

The deviating influence of maternally derived IgG antibody has been discussed in an earlier chapter. Injection of preformed (monoclonal) IgM antibody at the time of immunization with a malaria vaccine seemed to overcome this problem in young mice, but it remains to be seen whether this can be developed into a practical strategy. Preliminary results suggest that infants of 4–6 months can be seroconverted by inhaled aerosol measles vaccine which presumably evades the maternal antibody; this will have singular relevance in endemic measles areas where almost split-second timing is required with conventional immunization as passively acquired antibody wanes.

Individual protective antigens

A whole parasite or bacterium usually contains many antigens which are not concerned in the protective response of the host but may give rise to problems by suppressing the response to protective antigens or by provoking hypersensitivity. Examples of the latter are immune complex glomerulonephritis associated with malaria, cirrhosis resulting from delayed type hypersensitivity to schistosome eggs and

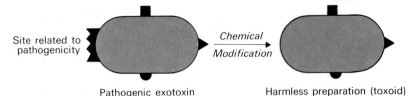

Site related to pathogenicity

Chemical Modification

Pathogenic exotoxin

Harmless preparation (toxoid)

Figure 8.4. Modification of toxin to harmless toxoid without losing many of the antigenic determinants (■ ● ▲). Thus antibodies to the toxoid will react well with the original toxin.

autoimmunity due to cross-reactions between *Trypanosoma cruzi* and components of heart and neural tissue. Vaccination with the isolated protective antigens usually avoids these complications and identification of these antigens then opens up the possibility of producing them synthetically in circumstances where bulk growth of the organism is impractical or isolation of the individual components too expensive.

Identification of protective antigens is greatly facilitated if one has an experimental model. If protection is antibody-mediated, one can try out different monoclonal antibodies and use the successful ones to pull out the antigen. Where antigenic variation is a major factor, desperate attempts are being made to identify some element of constancy which could provide a basis for vaccination, again using monoclonal antibodies with their ability to recognize a single specificity in a highly complex mixture. If protection is based primarily on T-cell activity, the approach would then be through the identification of individual T-cell clones capable of passively transferring protection.

(a) *Purified components* Bacterial exotoxins such as those produced by diphtheria and tetanus bacilli have long been used as immunogens. First, they must of course be detoxified and this is achieved by formaldehyde treatment which fortunately does not destroy the major immunogenic determinants (figure 8.4). Immunization with the *toxoid* will therefore provoke the formation of protective antibodies which neutralize the toxin by stereochemically blocking the active site and encourage removal by phagocytic cells. The toxoid is generally given after adsorption to aluminium hydroxide which acts as an adjuvant and produces higher antibody titres. In the case of cholera, a vaccine which combines the B subunit of cholera toxin with killed vibrios is reported to stimulate gut mucosal antibody formation when given orally, the response being said to equal that seen after clinical cholera. Purified pneumococcal and meningococcal polysaccharide vaccines will probably require coupling to some immunogenic carrier protein since they fail to stimulate T-helpers or induce adequate memory.

(b) *Synthetic peptides* Small peptide sequences corresponding with important epitopes on a microbial antigen can be synthesized readily and economically; long ones are too expensive to manufacture. Naturally, the peptide must be linked to a T-dependent carrier and incorporated into an adjuvant for immunogenicity, the latter in some examples being achieved by direct coupling to muramyl dipeptide (MDP; see below). One might predict that although the synthetic peptide has the correct linear *sequence* of amino acids, its random structure would make it a poor model for the *conformation* of the parent antigen. Curiously this does not always seem to be a serious drawback. The 'loop' peptide of diphtheria toxin, when internally disulphide linked, evokes a good neutralizing response. The same is true for a short peptide derived from the foot and mouth virus-specific protein (VP1). A peptide sequence from polio virus VP1 induced poor neutralizing antibody but did prime the recipient for a good response to the whole organism. It may be that short peptides do not always have the conformation to stimulate adequate B-cell responses, but conceivably they could prime antigen-specific T-cells which are said to recognize the primary sequence rather than the tertiary configuration of a protein; if the primed T-cells enable the host to mount an adequate protective response on subsequent exposure to natural infection, this could prove to be a useful prophylactic strategy.

(c) *Gene cloning* The wonder recombinant DNA technology enables us to make genes encoding part or the whole of a protein peptide chain almost at will, and express them in an appropriate vector. The process can be economical and the potential is vast. Difficulties may arise if the conformation of the peptide is heavily dependent upon the presence of a second peptide, or of a nuclear capsid, or requires carbohydrate residues. However, the latter might be provided by using yeasts with their glycosylation mechanisms as the vector for peptide synthesis.

Idiotype intervention

The association of a germ-line public or cross-reacting idiotype (cf. p. 108) with antibody directed to a given pathogen provides an opportunity for vaccination with monoclonal anti-idiotypes. In general such treatment leads to priming rather than antibody production, and whether this is helpful depends upon the extent to which the boosting effect of a natural infection produces adequate protection. The genetic heterogeneity of human populations could sabotage this approach if the idiotype in question is poorly represented in the immunoglobulin repertoire of many individuals.

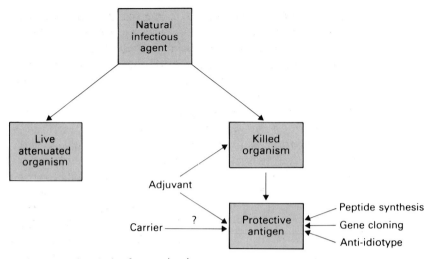

Figure 8.5. Strategies for vaccination.

A vaccine based on monoclonal anti-idiotype which was closely similar in conformation to an epitope on the protective microbial antigen (internal image Id, p. 110) should not suffer from this restriction but should be able to immunize the same individuals who would respond to the antigen itself assuming effective carrier help. Unfortunately, the internal-image set only occurs with very low frequency in the anti-idiotype population and special techniques will probably be necessary to generate these clones.

The overall strategies for vaccination are summarized in figure 8.5.

Adjuvants

For practical and economic reasons, prophylactic immunization should involve the minimum number of injections and the least amount of antigen. We have referred to the undoubted advantages of replicating attenuated organisms in this respect but non-living organisms frequently require an adjuvant which by definition is a substance incorporated into or injected simultaneously with antigen which potentiates the immune response (L. *adjuvare*—to help). The mode of action of adjuvants may be considered under several headings:

1 *Depot effects* Free antigen usually disperses rapidly from the local tissues draining the injection site and an important function of the so-called repository adjuvants is to counteract this by providing a long-lived reservoir of antigen, either at an extracellular location or within macrophages. The most common adjuvants of this type used in man are aluminium

compounds (phosphate and hydroxide) and Freund's incomplete adjuvant (in which the antigen is incorporated in the aqueous phase of a stabilized water in paraffin oil emulsion). Both types increase the antibody response but the emulsions tend to produce higher and far more sustained antibody levels with a broadening of the response to include more of the epitopes in the antigen preparation. Because of the life-long persistence of oil in the tissues and the occasional production of sterile abscesses, attention has been focused on the replacement of incomplete Freund's with a new biodegradable formulation, Adjuvant 65, which contains highly refined peanut oil and chemically pure mannide monooleate and aluminium monostearate as emulsifier and stabilizer respectively. Claims that antibody titres are comparable to those obtained with Freund's and that no long-term adverse effects in man have yet been encountered must be treated with caution.

2 *Macrophage activation* Under the influence of the repository adjuvants, macrophages form granulomata which provide sites for interaction with antibody-forming cells. The maintenance by the depot of consistent antigen concentrations, particularly on the macrophage surface, ensures that as antigen-sensitive cells divide within the granuloma, their progeny are highly likely to be further stimulated by antigen. Virtually all adjuvants stimulate macrophages, the majority probably through direct action, but complete Freund's adjuvant appears to act on the macrophage through the T-cell (cf. p. 96; it will be recalled that complete Freund's is made from the incomplete adjuvant by addition of killed mycobacterium, or more recently the water soluble muramyl dipeptide, MDP, isolated from its active components). The activated macrophages are thought to act by improving immunogenicity through an increase in the amount of antigen on their surface and the efficiency of its presentation to lymphocytes, by the provision of accessory signals to direct lymphocytes towards an immune response rather than tolerance, and by the secretion of soluble stimulatory factors (e.g. interleukin-1) which influence the proliferation of lymphocytes.

3 *Specific effects on lymphocytes* The immunopotentiating and other effects of the mycobacterial component in complete Freund are so striking that their use in man is not normally countenanced; enhancement of T-cell function is seen in helper activity, delayed type hypersensitivity and the production of autoimmune disease. In man, BCG is a potent stimulator of T-, B- and reticuloendothelial cell activity. Levamisole boosts delayed hypersensitivity and isoprinosine is said to overcome the IL-2 defect in autoimmune MRL mice bearing the lymphoproliferative (*lpr*) gene while poly-anions such as poly A : U, and the fungal polysaccharide lentinan, promote T-helper cells. By contrast, bacterial lipopolysaccharide and polyanions such as dextran sulphate are B-cell mitogens with a preferential effect on Bμ cells.

Although the role of modulatory leucocyte mediators such as transfer factor and interferon in these interactions is unclear, it is of interest that polylysine-stabilized poly-I : C, which produces good interferon levels in primates, is said to be an effective adjuvant for immunization to influenza virus.

4   *Anti-tumour action* This will be discussed in Chapter 10 but one may summarize by saying that the major effect is mediated through cytotoxic and cytostatic actions of activated macrophages on tumours, with the stimulation of specific T-cell immunity to the tumour antigens as a further possibility.

Liposomes

Recent interest has centred on the use of small lipid membrane vesicles (liposomes) as agents for the presentation of antigen to the immune system. It may be that the liposome acts as a storage vacuole within the macrophage or perhaps fuses with the macrophage membrane to provide a suitably immunogenic complex. One envisages the possibility of selecting the type of lymphocyte activated by incorporating accessory signalling agents into the liposome membrane, e.g. MDP derivatives, polyanions or levamisole to stimulate T-cells, components of ascaris or *Bordetella pertussis* to exaggerate IgE production, T-cell soluble factors for the triggering of Bγ cells, C3b for homing to lymph node follicles and so on.

Primary immunodeficiency

In accord with the dictum that 'most things that can go wrong, do so', a multiplicity of immunodeficiency states in man have been recognized. These are classified in table 8.1 together with some of the most clear-cut (and correspondingly rare) examples. We have earlier stressed the manner in which the interplay of complement, antibody and phagocytic cells constitutes the basis of a tripartite defence mechanism against pyogenic (pus-forming) infections with bacteria which require prior opsonization before phagocytosis. It is not surprising then, that deficiency in any one of these factors may predispose the individual to repeated infections of this type. Patients with T-cell deficiency of course present

Table 8.1. Classification of immunodeficiency states with examples.

Deficiency	Example	Immune response		Infection	Treatment
		Humoral	Cellular		
Comple-ment	C3 deficiency	Normal	Normal	Pyogenic bacteria	Antibiotics
Myeloid cell	Chronic granulo-matous disease	Normal	Normal	Catalase-positive bacteria	Antibiotics
B-cell	Infantile sex-linked a-γ-globulinaemia (Bruton)	↓↓	Normal	Pyogenic bacteria *Pneumocystis carinii*	γ-Globulin
T-cell	Thymic hypoplasia (DiGeorge)	↓	↓↓	Certain viruses *Candida*	Thymus graft
Stem cell	Severe combined deficiency (Swiss-type)	↓↓	↓↓	All the above	Bone marrow graft

a markedly different pattern of infection, being susceptible to those viruses and moulds which are normally eradicated by cell-mediated immunity.

A relatively high incidence of malignancies, and of auto-antibodies with or without autoimmune disease, has been documented in patients with immunodeficiency but the reason for this association is not yet clear, although failure of T-cell regulation or inability to control key viral infections are among the suggestions canvassed.

Deficiency of innate immunity

In chronic granulomatous disease the monocytes and poly-morphs fail to produce hydrogen peroxide due to a defect in the NADPH oxidase normally activated by phagocytosis. Many bacteria oblige by generating H_2O_2 through their own metabolic processes but if they are catalase positive, the per-oxide is destroyed and the bacteria will survive. Thus, poly-morphs from these patients readily take up catalase positive staphylococci in the presence of antibody and complement but fail to kill them intracellularly. In Chediak–Higashi disease (what a lovely name!), the lysosomes are structurally and functionally abnormal and the patients suffer from pyo-genic infections which can be fatal. Among other rare condi-tions, myeloperoxidase deficiency is associated with susceptibility to systemic candidiasis, while a defective poly-morph response to chemotactic stimuli characterizes the lazy leucocyte syndrome.

Defects in complement, the other major components of the innate immune system, were dealt with in Chapter 6.

B-cell deficiency

In Bruton's congenital a-γ-globulinaemia the production of immunoglobulin in affected males is grossly depressed and there are few lymphoid follicles or plasma cells in lymph node biopsies. The children are subject to repeated infection by pyogenic bacteria—*Staphylococcus aureus, Streptococcus pyogenes* and *pneumoniae, Neisseria meningitidis, Haemophilus influenzae*—and by a rare protozoon, *Pneumocystis carinii*, which produces a strange form of pneumonia. Cell-mediated immune responses are normal and viral infections such as measles and smallpox are readily brought under control. Therapy involves the repeated administration of human γ-globulin to maintain adequate concentrations of circulating immunoglobulin.

IgA deficiency is encountered with relative frequency and these patients often have detectable antibodies to IgA. It is uncertain whether these antibodies prevented development of the IgA system or whether lack of tolerance resulting from an absent IgA system allowed the body to make antibodies to exogenous determinants immunologically related to IgA.

The most common form of immunodeficiency, late onset hypogammaglobulinaemia (also known as common, variable immunodeficiency), is characterized by recurrent pyogenic infections and probably includes many entities. The marrow contains normal numbers of immature B-cells, but a third of the patients lack circulating B-cells with surface Ig and of the remainder, half have subnormal numbers. Where present they are unable to differentiate to plasma cells in some cases or to secrete antibody in others. T-cells are, however, also affected; each lymphocyte has a low surface 5-nucleotidase, the T_M cells lack the characteristic non-specific esterase spot, around 30% have poor responses to PHA and a small proportion have T-cells of phenotype $T8^+Ia^+$ with marked suppressor activity for B-cells. An excess of such cells, revealed by their ability to suppress pokeweed-driven immunoglobulin synthesis by HLA-identical normal lymphocytes, is a feature of the chronic graft-vs-host disease which follows allogeneic bone marrow transplantation in man.

Transient hypogammaglobulinaemia of infancy, characterized by recurrent respiratory infections, is associated with low IgG levels which often return somewhat abruptly to normal by 4 years of age. There is a deficiency in the number of circulating lymphocytes and in their ability to generate help for Ig production by B-cells activated by pokeweed mitogen, but this becomes normal as the disease resolves spontaneously.

Immunoglobulin deficiency occurs naturally in human infants as the maternal IgG level wanes and may become a serious problem in very premature babies.

The DiGeorge and Nezelof syndromes are characterized by a failure of the thymus to develop properly from the third and fourth pharyngeal pouches during embryogenesis (DiGeorge children also lack parathyroids and have severe cardio-vascular abnormalities). Consequently, stem cells cannot differentiate to become T-lymphocytes and the 'thymus dependent' areas in lymphoid tissue are sparsely populated; in contrast lymphoid follicles are seen but even these are poorly developed (figure 8.6). Cell-mediated immune responses are undetectable and although the infants can deal with common bacterial infections they may be overwhelmed by vaccinia or measles, or by BCG if given by mistake. Humoral antibodies can be elicited but the response is sub-normal, presumably reflecting the need for the co-operative involvement of T-cells. (The similarity of this condition to neonatal thymectomy and of B-cell deficiency to neonatal bursectomy in the chicken should not go unmentioned.) Treatment by grafting neonatal thymus leads to restoration of immunocompetence but unless graft and donor are well matched, the thymus is ultimately rejected by the ungrateful host cells it has helped to maturity; in any event, some matching between the major histocompatibility antigens on the non-lymphocytic thymus cells and peripheral cells is essential for the proper functioning of the T-lymphocytes (p. 295).

Complete absence of the thymus is pretty rare and more often one is dealing with a 'partial DiGeorge' in which the T-cells may rise from 6% at birth to around 30% of the total circulating lymphocytes by the end of the first year; antibody responses are adequate. Selective T-cell depression can arise from deficiency in the enzyme, purine nucleoside phosphorylase. The poor T-cell responses make these patients especially susceptible to infection with varicella and vaccinia viruses but despite having less than 10% circulating T-cells, they have normal B-cell immunity suggesting that T-B collaboration can operate at much lower T-cell levels in the human than in the mouse.

Cell-mediated immunity is depressed in immunodeficient patients with ataxia telangiectasia or with thrombocytopenia and eczema (Wiskott–Aldrich syndrome) and it is of great interest that in both conditions about 10% of the patients so far studied have died of malignancies of the lymphoid system or of epithelial tumours. Wiskott–Aldrich is associated with a low IgM and poor antibody responses to many poly-saccharides; evidence that a vital defect in macrophage presentation of antigen underlies the disorder has been presented. The concomitant lack of IgE with IgA may be

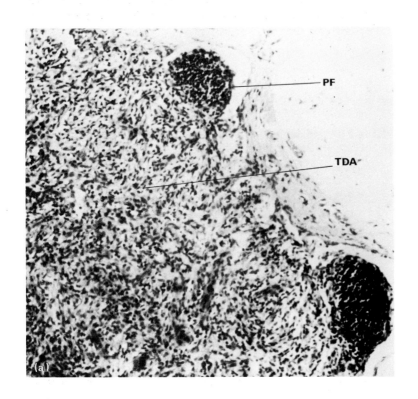

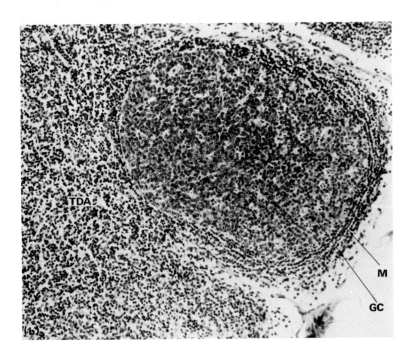

partly responsible for the greater susceptibility to upper respiratory infections in ataxia telangiectasia as compared with individuals deficient in IgA alone. Treatment by injection of transfer factor has been attempted and some success reported.

Isolated cases of T-cell deficiency have been described where the serum contains a lymphocytotoxic antibody which presumably must be selective for T- rather than B-lymphocytes.

T-cells from some patients with mucocutaneous candidiasis are unable to produce MIF when stimulated *in vitro* and it is conceivable that other selective failures of lymphokine synthesis may be uncovered.

Stem-cell deficiency

Without proper differentiation of the common lymphoid stem cell, both T- and B-lymphocytes will fail to develop and there will be a severe combined immunodeficiency of cellular and humoral responses. Normal immune function can be established in the children by grafting with histocompatible bone marrow from a sibling. Cells from other donors too readily initiate a potentially lethal graft-vs-host reaction (cf. p. 277) even when reasonably well-matched, unless steps are first taken to rid the graft of any immunocompetent T-lymphocytes. Some patients lack the enzyme adenosine deaminase which affects both B- and T-cells but predominantly the latter. Half the patients do well on transfusions of normal red cells containing the enzyme whereas others with a longer-standing more severe deficiency which might have affected the thymus epithelium, also require treatment with thymic extracts (thymosin).

The rapidly fatal variant of severe combined immunodeficiency associated with lack of myeloid cell precursors is termed reticular dysgenesis. An attempt has been made to summarize the cellular basis of the various deficiency states in figure 8.7.

Recognition of immunodeficiencies

Defects in immunoglobulins can be assessed by quantitative estimations; levels of 2 g/l arbitrarily define the practical

Figure 8.6. Lymph node cortex. (a) From patient with DiGeorge syndrome showing depleted thymus-dependent area (TDA) and small primary follicles (PF), (b) from normal subject: the populated T-cell area and the well-developed secondary follicle with its mantle of small lymphocytes (M) and pale staining germinal centre (GC) provide a marked contrast. (DiGeorge material kindly supplied by Dr D. Webster; photograph by Mr C.J. Sym.)

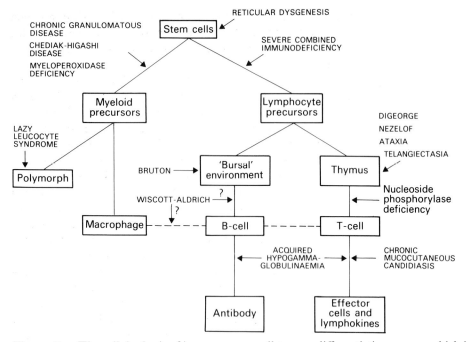

Figure 8.7. The cellular basis of immuno-deficiency states. The arrow indicates the cell type or differentiation process which is defective.

lower limit of normal. The humoral immune response can be examined by first screening the serum for natural antibodies (A and B isohaemagglutinins, hetero-antibody to sheep red cells, bactericidins against *E. coli*) and then attempting to induce active immunization with diphtheria, tetanus, pertussis and killed poliomyelitis—but no live vaccines.

Patients with T-cell deficiency will be hypo- or unreactive in skin tests to such antigens as tuberculin, *Candida*, tricophytin, steptokinase/streptodornase and mumps. Active skin sensitization with dinitrochlorobenzene may be undertaken. The reactivity of peripheral blood mononuclear cells to phytohaemagglutinin is a good indicator of T-lymphocyte reactivity as is also the one-way mixed lymphocyte reaction (see Chapter 10). Enumeration of T-cells is most readily achieved by counting the number of cells forming spontaneous rosettes with sheep erythrocytes or staining with a T3 monoclonal antibody (cf. p. 62).

In vitro tests for complement and for the bactericidal and other functions of polymorphs are available while the reduction of nitroblue tetrazolium (NBT) provides a measure of the oxidative enzymes associated with active phagocytosis.

Secondary immunodeficiency

Immune responsiveness can be depressed non-specifically by many factors. Cell-mediated immunity in particular may be impaired in a state of malnutrition even of the degree which may be encountered in urban areas of the more affluent regions of the world. Iron deficiency is particularly important in this respect.

Viral infections are not infrequently immunosuppressive, and in the case of measles in man, Newcastle disease in chickens and rinderpest in cattle, this has been attributed to a direct cytotoxic effect of virus on the lymphoid cells. In lepromatous leprosy and malarial infection there is evidence for a constraint on immune responsiveness imposed by distortion of the normal lymphoid traffic pathways and additionally, in the latter instance, macrophage function appears to be aberrant. Plasma factors from patients with secondary syphilis which block phytohaemagglutinin transformation of lymphocytes from normal subjects could be responsible for the general reduction in CMI seen in this disease.

Many agents such as X-rays, cytotoxic drugs and corticosteroids, although often used in a non-immunological context, can nonetheless have dire effects on the immune system (p. 285). B-lymphoproliferative disorders like chronic lymphatic leukaemia, myeloma and Waldenström's macroglobulinaemia are associated with varying degrees of hypo-γ-globulinaemia and impaired antibody responses. Their common infections with pyogenic bacteria contrast with the situation in Hodgkin's disease where the patients display all the hallmarks of defective cell-mediated immunity—susceptibility to tubercle bacillus, *Brucella*, *Cryptococcus* and herpes zoster virus.

Acquired immunodeficiency syndrome (AIDS)

AIDS is a particularly unpleasant disease which has leapt into prominence in just the last few years. Over 80% of the cases have occurred in male homosexuals but other groups at risk are intravenous drug users, haemophiliacs receiving Factor-VIII derived from pooled plasma, Haitians (it might be relevant that Haiti is favoured by many homosexuals for holidays) and infants of sexually promiscuous or drug-addicted mothers. In essence, there is a sudden onset of immunodeficiency associated with opportunistic infections involving, most commonly, *Pneumocystis carinii*, but also cytomegalovirus, EB and herpes simplex viruses, fungi such as *Candida*, *Aspergillus* and *Cryptococcus*, and the protozoon *Toxoplasma*; additionally, there is exceptional susceptibility for Kaposi's sarcoma.

Patients with AIDS have lymphopenia, hypergammaglobulinaemia and large numbers of cells which spontaneously secrete Ig in culture. The antibody response to new antigens is poor. The lymphopenia can be largely ascribed to a decrease in the T4 subset which includes the majority of T-helpers; T8$^+$ cells which form the major cytotoxic/suppressor cell subpopulation are normal or increased so giving rise to low T4 : T8 ratios, usually less than 1 and down to 0.1 compared with normal values of 2. *In vitro*, their T-cells respond poorly to antigens or pokeweed mitogen but proliferation induced by concanavalin A or phytohaemagglutinin is virtually normal.

The cause of this marked T-cell deficiency is still a mystery. On epidemiological grounds, a blood-borne transmissible agent would appear to be implicated and cytomegalovirus, T-cell leukaemia virus and 'slow viruses' all have their proponents. Host susceptibility is another factor. This has been linked by some to the recreational use of nitrites by homosexuals or to an immunosuppressive effect of spermatozoa entering the bloodstream through abrasions of the rectal mucosa. In the case of newborn infants, their relative immunodeficiency could make them susceptible hosts for the putative infectious agent.

Summary

Micro-organisms are kept out of the body by the skin, the secretion of mucus, ciliary action, the lavaging action of bactericidal fluids (e.g. tears), gastric acid and microbial antagonism. If penetration occurs, bacteria are destroyed by soluble factors such as lysozyme and by phagocytosis with intracellular digestion. By activating the alternative complement pathway, phagocytic cells are attracted to the bacteria which adhere to the C3b receptors and are engulfed if they activate the surface of the polymorph. Complement activation also causes mast cell release of a further polymorph chemotactic factor together with mediators of vascular permeability which increase the flow of more complement and antibody to the site. The influx of polymorphs and the increase in vascular permeability constitute the potent antimicrobial *acute inflammatory response* (figure 8.8). Primitive recognition mechanisms in the host make the micro-organisms appear to have an adjuvant-like activity in activating this acute inflammatory reaction. The antibody molecule is designed as a flexible adaptor to attach to foreign substances which lack this adjuvant activity and fail to activate the alternative pathway or the surface of the phagocytic cell; the Ig domains fix complement by the classical pathway and stimulate the phagocyte through its Fc receptor.

Humoral immunity to bacteria enhances phagocytosis by this antibody-opsonizing mechanism and by neutralization of the bacterial anti-phagocytic systems; it may also bring about the lysis of cells through the terminal complement com-

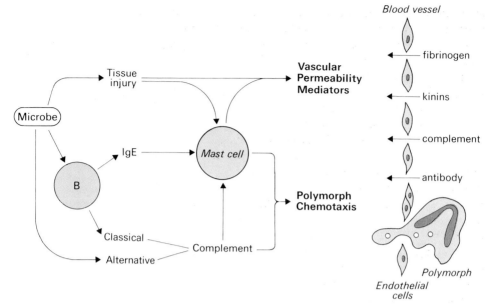

Figure 8.8. Production of a protective acute inflammatory reaction by microbes either (i) through tissue injury (e.g. bacterial toxin) or direct activation of the alternative complement pathway or (ii) by antibody-dependent triggering of the classical complement pathway or mast cell degranulation.

ponents plus lysozyme, and the neutralization of bacterial toxins. The mucosal surfaces are protected by IgA with IgE as a second line of defence. Intracellular facultative parasites such as the tubercle bacillus can grow happily within the macrophage which only becomes able to kill the organisms it harbours if activated by a lymphokine released by the reaction of sensitized T-cells with the antigen: this is one mechanism of cell-mediated immunity.

The innate immunity defences against viruses depend largely on interferon which inhibits intracellular replication of viruses and stimulates the cytotoxic activity of natural killer cells for virally infected targets. Antibodies can neutralize viruses by blocking their combination with cellular receptor sites and by encouraging their destruction by mechanisms similar to those described for bacteria. Antibodies are very effective in *preventing* reinfection with many viruses, serum antibody being important where the virus has to pass through the bloodstream before reaching its target organ and local antibody being essential where the target organ is the same as the portal for entry (e.g. influenza); however, interferon may be more effective in the *recovery* from these infections. Cells infected, with non-cytopathic viruses which 'bud', have altered surface antigens and can be destroyed by cytotoxic T-cells before viral replication occurs. Free 'budded' viral particles can be destroyed by antibody but the other route of intercellular virus spread can only be stopped by the antigen-specific release of T-cell lymphokines which attract and activate macrophages to inhibit multicellular bridges, and which make local cells resistant to infection by bathing them in interferon.

Circulating antibody can offer protection against the

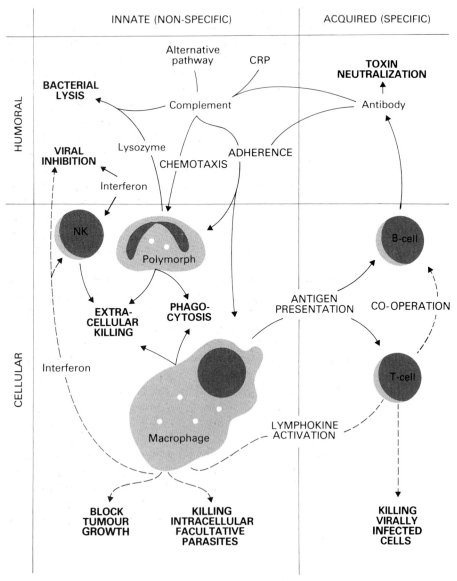

Figure 8.9. Simplified scheme to emphasize the interactions between innate and acquired immunity mechanisms. Reactions influenced by T-cells are indicated by a broken line. T-cell lymphokines include immune interferon (IFNγ). (Developed from Playfair J.H.L. (1974) *Brit. Med. Bull.* **30,** 24.)

blood-borne forms of protozoa, but antigenic variation and suppression of the host's immune response favour survival of the parasites. Organisms such as *Leishmania* and *Toxoplasma*, which prefer an intracellular life, elicit cell-mediated immunity. Helminths provoke a high IgE response which may mediate a cytotoxic attack by eosinophils. Schistosomes protect themselves by mimicking the host.

Generally speaking, the acquired response operates to amplify and enhance innate immune mechanisms; the interactions are summarized in figure 8.9.

Immunity can be acquired passively, from the mother or by injection by preformed antibody, or induced actively either by natural infection or vaccination using killed or live attenuated organisms and toxoids. Live replicating vaccines provide a larger and more potent stimulus in the tissues relevant to the natural infection. Attenuated viral strains are being produced by adaptation to different growth conditions and by genetic recombination. The immunopathological effects of vaccinating with whole organisms can often be avoided by using purified protective antigens; these can be produced by organic synthesis or by gene cloning. Immunogenicity may need to be enhanced by coupling to a carrier and by using adjuvants which act as antigen depots and activate macrophages. The risk of complications attendant upon vaccination must be weighed against the chance of contracting the disease.

Primary immunodeficiency states affecting the complement system, phagocytic cells or antibody synthesis lead to infection by pyogenic bacteria. Children with T-cell deficiency cannot deal adequately with 'budding' viruses (e.g. pox type) and fungi. Severe combined immunodeficiency occurs where there is failure in differentiation of lymphoid stem cells. In many instances replacement therapy is possible: Ig for B-cell, thymus graft for T-cell and bone marrow (stem cells) or adenosine deaminase for severe combined immunodeficiency. Immune deficiency may arise secondarily as a consequence of malnutrition, viral and other infection, cytotoxic drugs, or lymphoproliferative disorders. Acquired immunodeficiency syndrome (AIDS) is characterized by lymphopenia and a low T4 : T8 ratio, susceptibility to opportunistic infections and the development of rapidly progressive Kaposi's sarcoma; the disease appears to occur via a transmissible agent in a susceptible host.

Further reading

Bergsma D., Good R.A., Finstad J. & Paul N.W. (eds) (1975) *Immunodeficiency in Man and Animals* (Birth Defects Series), Vol. 11, No. 1. National Foundation, March of Dimes, New York.

Capron A.R.G. (ed.) (1982) Immunoparasitology. In *Clinics in Immunology & Allergy*. Vol. **2**(3). W.B. Saunders, London.

Cohen S. & Sadun E. (eds) (1976) *Immunology of Parasitic Infections*. Blackwell Scientific Publications, Oxford.

Davis B.D., Dulbecco R., Eisen H.N., Ginsberg H.S. & Wood W.B. (1980) *Microbiology* (including Immunology). 3rd edn. Harper Medical, Lippincott, Philadelphia.

Dick G. (1978) *Immunisation*. Update Books, London.

van Furth R. (ed.) (1975) *Mononuclear Phagocytes in Immunity, Infection and Pathology*. Blackwell Scientific Publications, Oxford.

Gray A.R. (1969) Antigenic variation in trypanosomes. *Bull.World Health Organisation* **41**, 805.

Lachmann P.J. & Peters D.K. (eds) (1982) *Clinical Aspects of Immunology*, 4th edn. Blackwell Scientific Publications, Oxford. See chapters on immunity to infection and immunoprophylaxis.

Mims C.A. (1976) *The Pathogenesis of Infectious Disease*. Academic Press, London.

Notkins A.L. (ed.) (1975) *Viral Immunology and Immunopathology*. Academic Press, New York.

Porter R. & Knight J. (1974) *Parasites in the Immunized Host*. Ciba Foundation Symposium, Elsevier, Amsterdam.

Shvartsman Ya.S. & Zykov M.P. (1976) Secretory anti-influenza immunity. *Adv.Immunol.* **22**, 291.

Taussig M.J. (1984) *Processes in Pathology*. 2nd edn. Blackwell Scientific Publications, Oxford.

WHO (1973) Cell mediated immunity and resistance to infection. *WHO Technical Report Series*, Geneva.

WHO Scientific Group on Immunodeficiency (1983) Primary immunodeficiency disease. *Clin. Immunol. Immunopath.* **28**, 450.

WHO/IUIS Report (1982) Appropriate uses of human Ig in clinical practice. *Bull. World Health Organisation* **60**, 43.

Wilson G.S. (1967) *The Hazards of Immunization*. Athlone Press, London.

Yamamura T. & Tada T. (eds) (1984) *Progress in Immunology V*. Academic Press, Tokyo.

9   Hypersensitivity

When an individual has been immunologically primed, further contact with antigen leads to secondary boosting of the immune response. However, the reaction may be excessive and lead to gross tissue damage (*hypersensitivity*) if the antigen is present in relatively large amounts or if the humoral and cellular immune state is at a heightened level. It should be emphasized that the mechanisms underlying these inappropriate reactions are those normally employed by the body in combating infection as discussed in Chapter 7. We speak of *hypersensitivity reactions* and a state of *hypersensitivity*. Coombs and Gell defined four types of hypersensitivity, to which can be added a fifth, viz. 'stimulatory', which they mention. Types I, II, III and V depend on the interaction of antigen with humoral antibody and tend to be called 'immediate' type reactions although some are more immediate than others! Type IV involves receptors bound to the lymphocyte surface and because of the longer time course this has in the past been referred to as 'delayed-type sensitivity'. The essential basis of these reactions is summarized below and then each is considered separately in more detail.

TYPE I—ANAPHYLACTIC SENSITIVITY

The antigen reacts with antibody bound to mast cells or circulating basophils through a specialized region of the Fc piece. This leads to degranulation of the mast cells and release of vasoactive amines and other mediators (figure 9.1). These antibodies are termed homocytotropic (also referred to as reagins).

TYPE II—ANTIBODY-DEPENDENT CYTOTOXIC HYPERSENSITIVITY

Antibodies binding to an antigen on the cell surface cause (a) phagocytosis of the cell through opsonic (Fc) or immune (C3) adherence, (b) non-phagocytic extracellular cytotoxicity

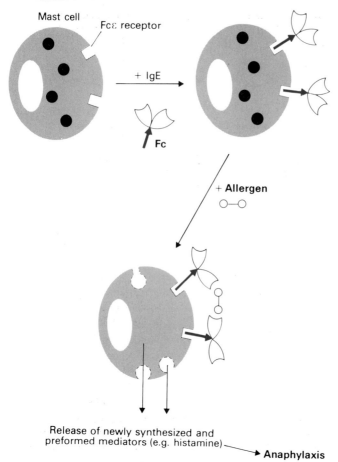

Mast cell

Fcε receptor

+ IgE →

Fc

+ Allergen

Release of newly synthesized and
preformed mediators (e.g. histamine) ——→ **Anaphylaxis**

Figure 9.1. Type I—anaphylactic hypersensitivity. Mast-cell degranulation following interaction of antigen with bound homocytotropic (reaginic) antibodies.

by killer cells with receptors for IgFc, and (c) lysis through the operation of the full complement system up to C8,9 (figure 9.2).

TYPE III—COMPLEX-MEDIATED HYPERSENSITIVITY

The formation of complexes between antigen and humoral antibody can lead to activation of the complement system and to the aggregation of platelets with the consequences listed in figure 9.3.

TYPE IV—CELL-MEDIATED (DELAYED-TYPE) HYPERSENSITIVITY

Thymic-derived T-lymphocytes bearing specific receptors on their surface are stimulated by contact with macrophage-

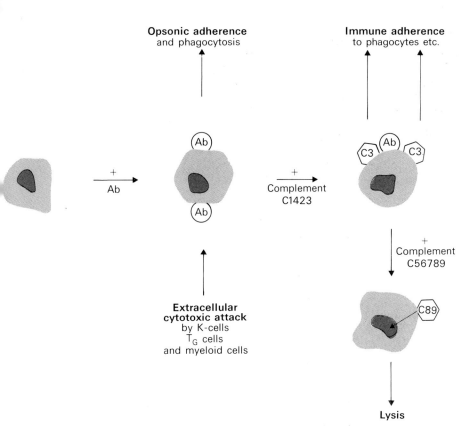

Opsonic adherence
and phagocytosis

Immune adherence
to phagocytes etc.

+
Ab

+
Complement
C1423

(Ab)

(Ab)

(Ab) C3 C3

+
Complement
C56789

Extracellular
cytotoxic attack
by K-cells
T_G cells
and myeloid cells

C89

Lysis

Figure 9.2. Type II—antibody-dependent cytotoxic hypersensitivity. Antibodies directed against cell surface antigens cause cell death not only by C-dependent lysis but also by adherence reactions leading to phagocytosis or through non-phagocytic extracellular killing by certain lymphoreticular cells (antibody-dependent cell-mediated cytotoxicity).

bound antigen to release lymphokines (cf. p. 75) which mediate delayed-type hypersensitivity (e.g. Mantoux test for tuberculin sensitivity); in the reaction against virally infected cells or transplants, the stimulated lymphocytes transform into blast-like cells capable of killing target cells bearing the sensitizing antigens. Failure to eliminate the antigen will cause an accumulation of macrophages and the formation of a granuloma (figure 9.4).

TYPE V—STIMULATORY HYPERSENSITIVITY

Non-complement fixing antibodies directed against certain cell surface components may actually stimulate rather than destroy the cell (figure 9.5). Theoretically stimulation could also occur through the development of antibodies to naturally occurring mitotic inhibitors in the circulation.

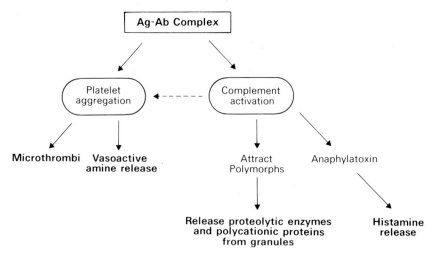

Figure 9.3. Type III—complex-mediated hypersensitivity.

Type I—anaphylactic sensitivity

SYSTEMIC ANAPHYLAXIS

A single injection of 1 mg of an antigen such as egg albumin into a guinea-pig has no obvious effect. However, if the injection is repeated two to three weeks later, the sensitized animal reacts very dramatically with the symptoms of gener-alized anaphylaxis; almost immediately the guinea-pig begins to wheeze and within a few minutes dies from asphyxia. Examination shows intense constriction of the bronchioles

Figure 9.4. Type IV—cell-mediated (delayed-type) hypersensitivity.

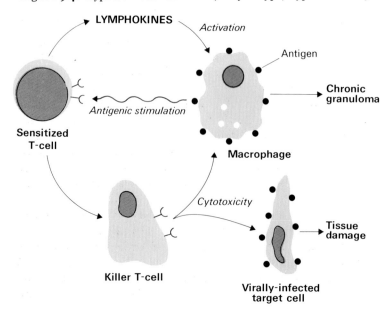

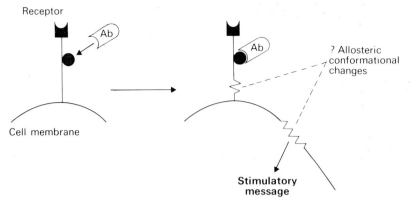

Figure 9.5. Type V—stimulatory hypersensitivity.

and bronchi and generally there is (a) contraction of smooth muscle and (b) dilatation of capillaries.

Similar reactions can occur in human subjects and have been observed following insect bites or injections of penicillin in appropriately sensitive individuals. In many instances only a timely intravenous injection of adrenaline to counter the smooth muscle contraction and capillary dilatation can prevent death.

MECHANISM OF ANAPHYLAXIS

Sir Henry Dale recognized that histamine mimics the systemic changes of anaphylaxis and furthermore that the uterus from a sensitized guinea-pig releases histamine and contracts on exposure to antigen (Schultz–Dale technique). Serum from such an animal can passively sensitize the uterus from a normal guinea-pig so that it, too, will contract on addition of the specific antigen. Contraction is associated with an explosive degranulation of the mast cells (figure 9.6a and b) which is responsible for the release of histamine and, in certain species, of another mediator of anaphylaxis, 5-hydroxytryptamine (serotonin). Other highly active preformed mediators which are released from the granules include platelet activating factor (PAF), heparin, certain enzymes and chemotactic factors for both neutrophils and eosinophils (figure 9.7). Triggering of the mast cell also leads to activation of membrane phospholipase A_2 with release and metabolism of arachidonic acid which produces prostaglandins and thromboxanes via the cyclo-oxygenase pathway and various leukotrienes through the lipoxygenase pathway, possibly in collaboration with accessory cells. Slow-reacting substance (SRS-A) capable of inducing prolonged contraction of certain smooth muscles is now known to be a mixture of leukotrienes C_4 and D_4 (figure 9.7). While extensive mast-

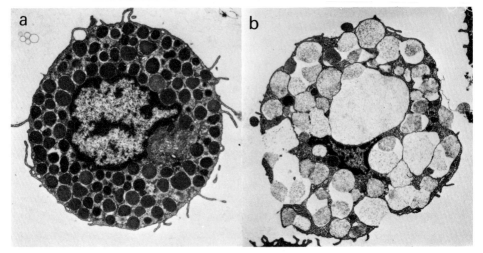

Figure 9.6. The mast cell. (a) An unreleased cell containing many membranebound, histamine-containing granules ($\times$ 5,400). (b) A mast cell degranulated by treatment with anti-Ig for 30 s at 37°. Note that the granules have released their histamine and are morphologically altered, being larger and less electron dense. Although most of the altered granules remain within the circumference of the cell, they are open to the extracellular space ($\times$ 5,400). (By courtesy of Drs D. Lawson, C. Fewtrell, B. Gomperts and M. Raff: from *J. Exp. Med.* 1975, **142**, 391.)

cell degranulation produces serious anaphylactic reactions through the operation of these powerful mediators, it is important to recall that under more balanced conditions, mast cell triggering is a vital component in the defensive acute inflammatory reaction (cf. figure 8.8, p. 229). It is interesting to note that of the cells recruited into such a site, the eosinophil not only has an anti-microbial role, but also can modulate the mast cell mediators; for example, histamine is defused by histaminase and PAF by phospholipase D.

It seems clear that the mast cells become coated by a particular type of antibody whose Fc region can bind specifically to sites on the mast cell surface. The most effective homocytotropic antibodies belong to the IgE class but it is clear that IgG antibodies can also act as reagins although the extent of their contribution to the allergic state in the human is not yet resolved. IgG reagins differ from IgE in their relative insensitivity to mild heat and 2-mercaptoethanol reduction and especially in their lower binding affinity for mast cells; whereas IgE antibodies can be detected at the site of an intradermal injection into a normal individual for several weeks, IgG disperses within a day or so. The technique of *passive cutaneous anaphylaxis* (PCA) introduced by Ovary utilizes this dermal reaction as a highly sensitive indicator for reaginic antibodies. For example, high dilutions of guinea-pig serum containing IgG1 antibodies (different from human IgG1) may be injected into the skin of a normal

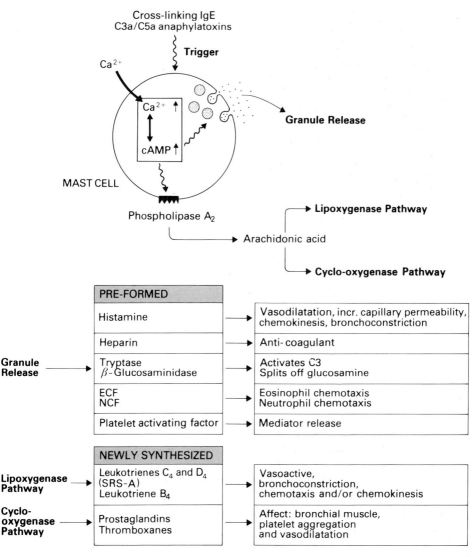

Figure 9.7. Mediators produced by mast-cell triggering (ECF = eosinophil chemo-tactic factor; NCF = neutrophil chemotactic factor).

animal and following the intravenous injection of antigen with a dye such as Evans' Blue, the anaphylactic reaction in the skin will lead to release of vasoactive amines and hence a local 'blueing'.

Degranulation of the mast cell occurs when the bound homocytotropic antibodies are cross-linked either by specific antigen (figure 9.1), by the corresponding divalent anti-immunoglobulin (e.g. anti-IgE or anti-light chain) or by antibodies to the Fcε receptor; univalent (Fab) anti-IgE or anti-Fcε receptor will not cause degranulation. This cross-linking reaction induces a membrane signal which causes an influx of calcium ions and a rapid rise in cAMP concentration; degranulation and phospholipase A_2 activation then follow (figure 9.7).

Nearly 10% of the population suffer to a greater or lesser degree with allergies involving localized anaphylactic reactions to extrinsic allergens such as grass pollens, animal danders, mites in house dust and so on. Contact of the allergen with cell-bound IgE in the bronchial tree, the nasal mucosa and the conjunctival tissues releases mediators of anaphylaxis and produces the symptoms of asthma or hay fever as the case may be. For those unfortunates sensitized to foods such as the strawberry, the price of indulgence may be a generalized urticaria caused by reaction in the skin to materials absorbed from the gut into the bloodstream. Acute anaphylaxis, although rare, may occur in highly sensitive subjects after an insect bite or injections of penicillin or procaine.

Sensitivity is normally assessed by the response to intradermal challenge with antigen. The release of histamine and other mediators rapidly produces a wheal and erythema (figure 9.14a), maximal within 30 minutes and then subsiding. The responsible IgE antibodies can be demonstrated by the ability of patient's serum to passively sensitize the skin of normal humans (Praüsnitz–Kustner or 'P–K' test) or preferably of monkeys. This passive sensitization of human skin can be blocked most effectively by prior injection of a myeloma of IgE rather than of any other class. The interpretation is that the specialized sites on the skin mast cells become fully saturated by binding to the Fc regions of the IgE myeloma globulin which blocks the subsequent attachment of specific IgE antibodies. In some instances, intranasal challenge with allergen provokes a response even though skin tests and the radioallergosorbent test (RAST, p. 152) for specific serum IgE are negative, a phenomenon attributable to local synthesis of IgE antibodies.

The symptoms of atopic allergy are largely but not always completely controllable by anti-histamines. Other effective drugs such as isoprenaline and disodium cromoglycate (Intal) act by preventing mast-cell triggering. Attempts to desensitize patients immunologically by repeated treatment with allergen have at least the merit of a long history and in a significant but as yet unpredictable proportion of patients can lead to worthwhile improvement. It has generally been assumed that the purpose of these inoculations was to boost the synthesis of 'blocking' IgG antibody whose function was to divert the allergen from contact with tissue-bound IgE.

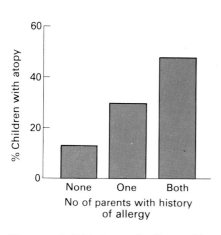

(a) FAMILY HISTORY

% Children with atopy — No of parents with history of allergy: None, One, Both

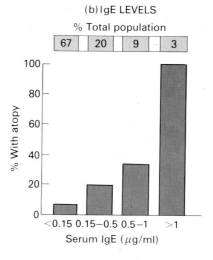

(b) IgE LEVELS

% Total population

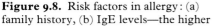

67	20	9	3

% With atopy — Serum IgE (μg/ml): <0.15, 0.15–0.5, 0.5–1, >1

Figure 9.8. Risk factors in allergy: (a) family history, (b) IgE levels—the higher the serum IgE concentration, the greater the chance of developing atopy.

This would be of unquestioned value were the increase in protective antibody (? particularly IgA) to occur locally at the sites vulnerable to allergen exposure. However, if T-lymphocyte co-operation is important for IgE synthesis, the beneficial effects of antigen injection may also be mediated through induction of tolerant or even suppressor T-cells. An especially hopeful finding is the observation that IgE-producing cells or their precursors can be switched off with comparative ease by haptens coupled to thymus-independent carriers such as poly-D-Glu. Lys. or isologous IgG, or by substitution of the allergen by polyethylene glycol. Better results must ultimately be attainable when we understand the rationale of 'hyposensitization' through the use of purified allergens, assessment of T-cell reactivity and quantitative measurement of specific IgG, IgA and IgE antibodies in individuals undergoing treatment. The affinity of these antibodies and their availability at local sites of allergen challenge such as the nasal mucosa are factors which cannot be ignored.

There is a strong familial predisposition to the development of these disorders (figure 9.8a) but although this is linked to inheritance of a given HLA haplotype within any one family, no association with specific HLA types has so far come to light. One factor seems to be the overall ability to synthesize the IgE isotype, the higher the level of IgE in the blood the greater the likelihood of becoming atopic (figure 9.8b). Curiously, it is said that patients with allergy are less likely than their non-atopic counterparts to develop tumours.

Type II—antibody-dependent cytotoxic hypersensitivity

Where an antigen is present on the surface of a cell, combination with antibody will encourage the demise of that cell by promoting contact with phagocytes either by reduction in surface charge, by opsonic adherence directly through the Fc or by immune adherence through bound C3. Cell death may also occur through activation of the full complement system up to C8 and C9 producing direct membrane damage. Although in the case of haemolytic antibodies, the generation of a single active complement site is enough to cause erythrocyte lysis, other cells appear to have repair mechanisms and it is likely that several complement sites need to be recruited in order to overwhelm the cell's defences.

The operation of a quite distinct cytotoxic mechanism is suggested by Perlmann's finding that target cells coated with low concentrations of IgG antibody can be killed 'non-specifically' through an extracellular non-phagocytic mechanism involving non-sensitized lymphoreticular cells which bind to the target by their specific receptors for the $C\gamma2$ and $C\gamma3$ domains of IgG Fc (figure 9.9). This so-called antibody-dependent cell-mediated cytotoxicity (ADCC) may be exhibited by both phagocytic and non-phagocytic myeloid cells (polymorphs and monocytes) and by a weakly glass-adherent cell with Fc receptors dubbed the 'K-cell'. This is almost certainly identical with the natural killer (NK) cell which is cytotoxic for certain tumours and virally infected

Figure 9.9. Killing of antibody-coated target by antibody-dependent cell-mediated cytotoxicity (ADCC). The surface receptors for Ig Fc region bind the effector cell to the target which is then killed by an extracellular mechanism. Several different cell types may display ADCC activity. (a) Diagram of effector and target cells. (b) Electron micrograph of attack on antibody-coated chick red cell by a mouse K-cell showing close apposition of effector and target and vacuolation in the cytoplasm of the latter (courtesy of P. Penfold).

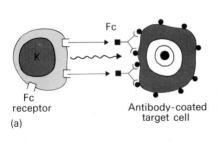

(a)

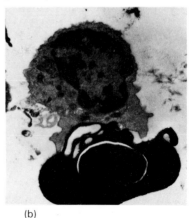

(b)

cells (p. 182); the Fc receptors refine the specificity of this cytotoxic potential by encouraging contact with antibody-coated target cells. Although morphologically similar to a fairly small lymphocyte, the precise lineage of the K-cell is still uncertain. A proportion of human effector cells bear T-markers and therefore belong to the large granular T_G subpopulation. The remainder are 'null' cells in the sense that they lack the presently employed surface markers of mature B- or T-lymphocytes and it will be of interest to see whether they represent stages in the differentiation of lymphoid (or myeloid) lines or belong to an entirely distinct cell type.

Contact between the effector and target cells is essential and activity is inhibited by cytochalasin B which interferes with cell movement, and aggregated IgG which binds firmly to the Fc receptors and blocks their ability to interact with antibody on the surface of the target. ADCC is not affected by inhibitors of protein synthesis and the presence of complement components has not so far been found to be mandatory although Nature would have shown a certain tidiness had the complement system been utilized to provide the cytotoxic effector molecule.

So far, ADCC has been studied exclusively as a phenomenon *in vitro*; to give examples, human K-cells have been shown to be strikingly unpleasant to chicken red cells coated with rabbit antibody, Chang liver cells coated with human antibody and human lymphocytes bearing anti-HLA. Whether ADCC is merely a curiosity of the laboratory test-tube or plays a positive role *in vivo* remains an open question. Functionally, this extracellular cytotoxic mechanism would be expected to be of significance where the target is too large for ingestion by phagocytosis, e.g. large parasites (p. 207) and solid tumours. It could also act as a back-up system for T-cell killing when antibody production might otherwise lead to protection of the target from attack by T-cells through blocking of the surface antigens; the evolution of ADCC mechanisms would ensure that the antibody-coated target was still vulnerable.

ISOIMMUNE REACTIONS

Transfusion reactions

Of the many different polymorphic constituents of the human red cell membrane, ABO blood groups form the dominant system. The antigenic groups A and B are derived from H substance (figure 9.10) by the action of glycosyl transferases encoded by A or B genes respectively. Individuals with both genes (group AB) have the two antigens on

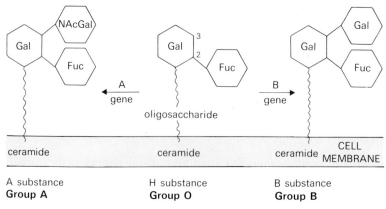

A substance
Group A

H substance
Group O

B substance
Group B

Figure 9.10. The ABO system. The allelic genes A and B code for transferases which add either N-acetylgalactosamine or galactose respectively to H substance. The oligosaccharide is anchored to the cell membrane by coupling to a sphingomyelin called cera-mide. 85% of the population secrete blood group substances in the saliva where the oligosaccharides are present as soluble polypeptide conjugates formed under the action of a secretor (se) gene.

their red cells while those lacking these genes (group O) synthesize H substance only. Antibodies to A or to B occur when the antigen is absent from the red cell surface; thus a person of blood group A will possess anti-B and so on. These *isohaemagglutinins* are usually IgM and are thought to arise through immunization against antigens of the gut flora which are similar to the blood group substances so that the antibodies formed cross-react with the appropriate red cell type. If an individual is blood group A, he will be tolerant to antigens closely similar to A and will only form cross-reacting antibodies capable of agglutinating B red cells; similarly an O individual will make anti-A and anti-B (table 9.1). On transfusion, mismatched red cells will be coated by the isohaemagglutinins and cause severe reactions.

Rhesus incompatibility

The rhesus (Rh) blood groups form the other major antigenic system, the RhD antigen being of the most consequence for isoimmune reactions. A mother with an RhD negative blood group (i.e. dd genotype) can readily be sensitized by red cells

Blood group (Phenotype)	Genotype	Antigen	Serum antibody
A	AA, AO	A	anti-B
B	BB, BO	B	anti-A
AB	AB	A and B	None
O	OO	H	anti-A anti-B

Table 9.1. ABO blood groups and serum antibodies.

244

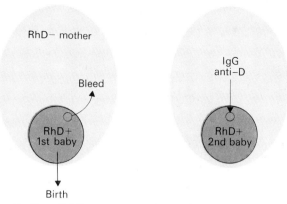

RhD− mother

Bleed

RhD+
1st baby

Birth

IgG
anti−D

RhD+
2nd baby

Sensitization of RhD− mother
by bleed at birth of 1st RhD+
baby leading to synthesis of
anti−D.

D+ erythrocytes in 2nd child
affected by IgG anti−D crossing
the placenta.

Figure 9.11. Haemolytic disease of the
newborn due to rhesus incompatibility.

from a baby carrying RhD antigens (DD or Dd genotype).
This occurs most often at the birth of the first child when a
placental bleed can release a large number of the baby's
erythrocytes into the mother. The antibodies formed are predominantly of the IgG class and are able to cross the placenta
in any subsequent pregnancy. Reaction with the D-antigen
on the fetal red cells leads to their destruction through
opsonic adherence giving haemolytic disease of the newborn
(figure 9.11).

These anti-D antibodies fail to agglutinate RhD + red
cells *in vitro* ('incomplete antibodies') because the low
density of antigenic sites does not allow sufficient antibody
bridges to be formed between the negatively charged erythrocytes to overcome the electrostatic repulsive forces. Erythrocytes coated with anti-D can be made to agglutinate by
addition of albumin or of an anti-immunoglobulin serum
(Coombs' reagent; figure 9.12).

Figure 9.12. The Coombs' test for
antibody-coated red cells used for detecting
rhesus-antibodies and in the diagnosis of
autoimmune haemolytic anaemia (cf. table
11.2, Note 5, p. 315). (Photographs courtesy of Dr. A. Cooke.)

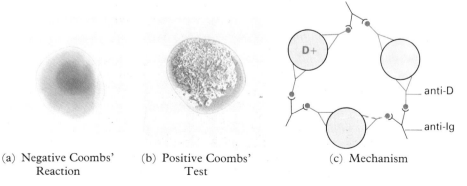

(a) Negative Coombs'
Reaction

(b) Positive Coombs'
Test

(c) Mechanism

If a mother has natural isohaemagglutinins which can react with any fetal erythrocytes reaching her circulation, sensitization to the D antigens is less likely due to 'deviation' of the red cells away from the antigen-sensitive cells. For example, a group O RhD−ve mother with a group A RhD +ve baby would destroy any fetal erythrocytes with her anti-A before they could immunize to produce anti-D. In an extension of this principle, RhD−ve mothers are now treated prophylactically with small amounts of avid IgG anti-D at the time of birth of the first child, and this greatly reduces the risk of sensitization.

Organ transplants

A long-standing homograft which has withstood the first onslaught of the cell-mediated reaction can evoke humoral antibodies in the host directed against surface transplantation antigens on the graft. These may be directly cytotoxic or cause adherence of phagocytic cells or 'non-specific' attack by K-cells (cf. figure 9.2). They may also lead to platelet adherence when they combine with antigens on the surface of the vascular endothelium (figure 10.12, p. 282). Hyperacute rejection is mediated by preformed antibodies in the graft recipient.

AUTOIMMUNE REACTIONS

Autoantibodies to the patient's own red cells are produced in autoimmune haemolytic anaemia. Red cells coated with these antibodies have a shortened half-life largely through their adherence to phagocytic cells. Similar mechanisms account for the anaemia in patients with cold haemagglutinin disease who have monoclonal anti-I after infection with *Mycoplasma pneumoniae,* and in some cases of paroxysmal cold haemoglobinuria associated with the actively lytic Donath–Landsteiner antibodies of specificity anti-blood group P.

The sera of patients with Hashimoto's thyroiditis contain antibodies which in the presence of complement are directly cytotoxic for isolated human thyroid cells in culture. In Goodpasture's syndrome (included here for convenience), antibodies to kidney glomerular basement membrane are present. Biopsies show these antibodies together with complement components bound to the basement membranes where the action of the full complement system leads to serious damage (figure 9.13a). I suppose one could also include the stripping of acetyl choline receptors from the muscle end-plate by autoantibodies in myasthenia gravis as a further example of type II hypersensitivity.

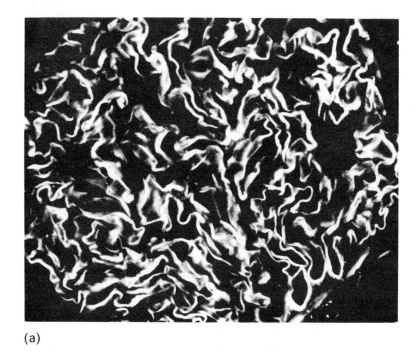

(a)

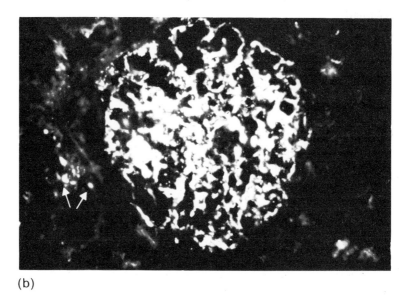

(b)

Figure 9.13. Glomerulonephritis: (a) due to linear deposition of antibody to glomerular basement membrane here visualized by staining the human kidney biopsy with a fluorescent anti-IgG (courtesy of Dr F.J. Dixon) and (b) due to deposition of antigen–antibody complexes which can be seen as discrete masses lining the glomerular basement membrane following immunofluorescent staining with anti-IgG; patches of blue autofluorescence are present in the extraglomerular tissue (arrowed) (courtesy of Dr D. Doniach). Similar patterns to these are obtained with a fluorescent anti-C3.

Very complicated. Drugs may become coupled to body components and thereby undergo conversion from a hapten to a full antigen which will sensitize certain individuals (we don't know which). If IgE antibodies are produced, anaphylactic reactions can result. In some circumstances, particularly with topically applied ointments, cell-mediated hypersensitivity may be induced. In other cases where coupling to serum proteins occurs, the possibility of type III complex-mediated reactions may arise. In the present context we are concerned with those instances where the drug appears to form an antigenic complex with the surface of a formed element of the blood and evokes the production of antibodies which are cytotoxic for the cell–drug complex. When the drug is withdrawn, the sensitivity is no longer evident. Examples of this mechanism have been seen in the *haemolytic anaemia* sometimes associated with continued administration of chlorpromazine or phenacetin, in the *agranulocytosis* associated with the taking of amidopyrine or of quinidine, and the now classic situation of *thrombocytopenic purpura* which may be produced by Sedormid, a sedative of yesteryear. In the latter case, freshly drawn serum from the patient will lyse platelets in the presence, but not in the absence, of Sedormid; inactivation of complement by preheating the serum at 56°C for 30 minutes abrogates this effect.

Type III—complex-mediated hypersensitivity

The body may be exposed to an excess of antigen over a protracted period in a number of circumstances, persistent infection with a microbial organism, autoimmunity to self-components and repeated contact with environmental agents. The union of such antigens and antibodies within the body may well give rise to acute inflammatory reactions (cf. figure 9.3). If complement is fixed, anaphylatoxins will be released as split products of $C3$ and $C5$ and these will cause release of mast cell mediators with vascular permeability changes. The chemotactic factors also produced will lead to an influx of polymorphonuclear leucocytes which begin the phagocytosis of the immune complexes; this in turn results in the extracellular release of the polymorph granule contents, particularly when the complex is deposited on a basement membrane and cannot be phagocytosed (so-called 'frustrated phagocytosis'). The proteolytic enzymes (including neutral proteinases and collagenase), kinin-forming enzymes and polycationic proteins which are released will of course damage local tissues and intensify the inflammatory responses. Further damage may be mediated by reactive lysis

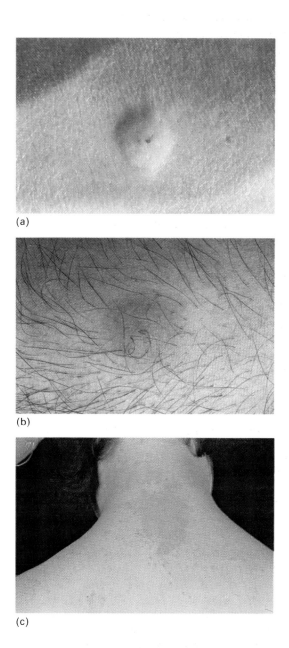

(a)

(b)

(c)

Figure 9.14. Hypersensitivity reactions. (a) Type I anaphylactic intradermal reaction to pollen allergen showing well-developed wheal and a degree of erythema (flare). (b) Type IV cell-mediated hypersensitivity reaction to tuberculin, characterized by induration and erythema. (c) Type IV contact hypersensitivity reaction to nickel caused by the clasp of a necklace. ((a) and (b) kindly provided by Dr J. Brostoff, photographed by Mr B.N. Rice; (c) reproduced from Brit. Soc. Immunol. teaching slides with permission of the Society and Dermatology Department, London Hospital.)

(Chapter 6, p. 169) in which activated C5,6,7 becomes attached to the surface of nearby cells and binds C8,9. Under appropriate conditions, platelets may be aggregated with two consequences: they provide yet a further source of vasoactive amines and may also form microthrombi which can lead to local ischaemia. (The discerning reader will appreciate the need for the complex system of inhibitors present in the body.)

The outcome of the formation of immune complexes *in vivo* depends not only on the absolute amounts of antigen and antibody, which determine the intensity of the reaction, but also on their *relative* proportions which govern the nature of the complexes (cf. precipitin curve, p. 5) and hence their distribution within the body. Between *antibody excess* and *mild antigen excess*, the complexes are rapidly precipitated and tend to be localized to the site of introduction of antigen, whereas in *moderate* to *gross antigen excess*, soluble complexes are formed which circulate and may cause systemic reactions and be widely deposited in the kidneys, joints and skin.

LOCALLY FORMED COMPLEXES

Maurice Arthus found that injection of soluble antigen intradermally into hyperimmunized rabbits with high levels of precipitating antibody produced an erythematous and oedematous reaction reaching a peak at 3–8 hours and then usually resolving. The lesion was characterized by an intense infiltration with polymorphonuclear leucocytes (figure 9.15a). The injected antigen precipitates with antibody often within the venule and the complex binds complement; using fluorescent reagents, antigen, immunoglobulin and complement components can all be demonstrated in this lesion. Anaphylatoxin is soon generated and causes mast cell degranulation. Local intravascular complexes will also cause platelet aggregation and vasoactive amine release and, as a result, erythema and oedema increase. The formation of chemotactic factors leads to the influx of polymorphs. The Arthus reaction can be blocked by depletion of complement or of the neutrophil polymorphs (by nitrogen mustard or specific anti-polymorph sera).

Intrapulmonary Arthus-type reactions to exogenous inhaled antigen appear to be responsible for a number of hypersensitivity disorders in man. The severe respiratory difficulties associated with Farmer's lung occur within 6–8 hours of exposure to the dust from mouldy hay. The patients are found to be sensitized to thermophilic actinomycetes which grow in the mouldy hay, and extracts of these organisms give precipitin reactions with the subject's serum

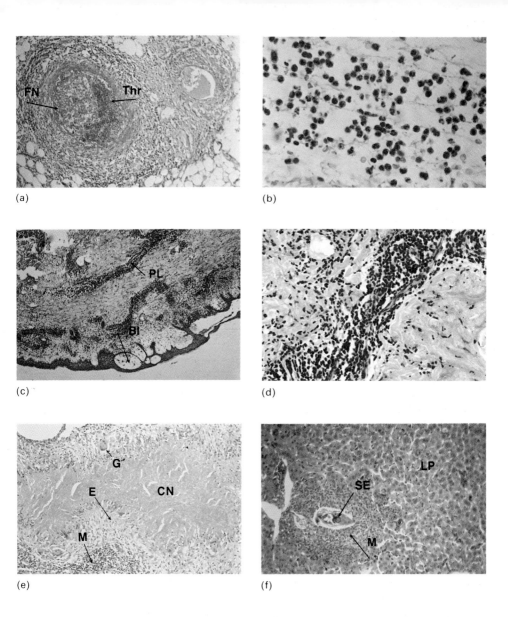

(a)

(b)

(c)

(d)

(e)

(f)

Figure 9.15. Histology of acute and chronic inflammatory reactions. (a) Periarteritis nodosa associated with immune complex formation with hepatitis B surface (HBs) antigen. A vessel showing thrombus (Thr) formation and fibrinoid necrosis (FN) is surrounded by a mixed inflammatory infiltrate, largely polymorphs. (b) High power view of acute inflammatory response in loose connective tissue of patient with periarteritis nodosa—polymorphs (PMN) are prominent. (c) Perivascular lymphocytic infiltrates (PL) and blister (Bl) formation characterize a contact sensitivity reaction of the skin (type IV). (d) High power view to show the lymphocytic nature of the infiltrate in a contact hypersensitivity reaction. (e) Chronic type IV inflammatory lesion in tuberculous lung showing caseous necrosis (CN), epithelioid cells (E), giant cells (G) and mononuclear inflammatory cells (M). (f) Delayed-type hypersensitivity lesion of mononuclear inflammatory cells (M) around schistosome egg (SE) within the liver parenchyma (LP). ((a)–(d) courtesy of Prof. N. Woolf, (e) courtesy of Dr R. Barnetson and (f) courtesy of Dr M. Doenhoff.)

and Arthus reactions on intradermal injection. Inhalation of bacterial spores present in dust from the hay introduces antigen into the lungs and a complex-mediated hypersensitivity reaction occurs. Similar situations arise in pigeon-fancier's disease where the antigen is probably serum protein present in the dust from dried faeces, in rat handlers sensitized to rat serum proteins excreted in the urine (figure 9.16) and in many other quaintly named cases of extrinsic allergic alveolitis resulting from continual inhalation of organic particles, e.g. cheese washer's disease (*Penicillium casei* spores), furrier's lung (fox fur proteins) and maple bark stripper's disease (spores of *Cryptostroma*). Evidence that an immediate anaphylactic type I response may sometimes be of importance for the initiation of an Arthus reaction comes from the study of patients with allergic bronchopulmonary aspergillosis who have high levels of IgE and precipitating IgG antibodies to *Aspergillus* species.

Type III reactions are often provoked by the local release of antigen from infectious organisms within the body, for example, living filarial worms such as *Wuchereria bancrofti* are relatively harmless, but the dead parasite found in lymphatic vessels initiates an inflammatory reaction thought to be responsible for obstruction of lymph flow and the ensuing, rather monstrous, elephantiasis. Chemotherapy may cause an abrupt release of microbial antigens in individuals with high antibody levels, producing quite dramatic immune complex-mediated reactions such as erythema nodosum leprosum in the skin of dapsone-treated lepromatous leprosy patients and the Jarisch–Herxheimer reaction in syphilitics on penicillin.

An interesting variant of the Arthus reaction is seen in rheumatoid arthritis where complexes are formed locally in the joint due to the production of self-associating IgG anti-IgG by synovial plasma cells (cf. p. 339).

It has also been recognized that complexes could be generated at a local site by a quite different mechanism involving non-specific adherence of an antigen to tissue structures followed by the binding of soluble antibody—in other words, the antigens becomes fixed in the tissue *before* not *after* combining with antibody. Although it is not clear to what extent this mechanism operates in patients with immune complex disease, let me describe the experimental observation on which it is based. After injection with bacterial endotoxin, mice release DNA into their circulation which binds specifically to the collagen in the basement membrane of the glomerular capillaries: infusion of anti-DNA now gives rise to antigen–antibody complexes in the kidney.

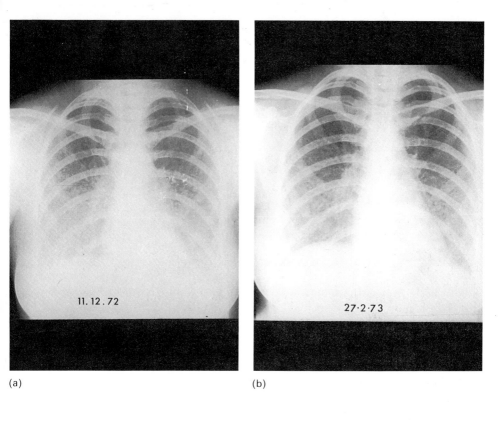

(a)

(b)

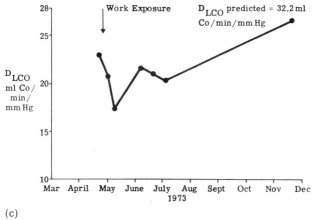

(c)

Figure 9.16. Extrinsic allergic alveolitis due to rat serum proteins in a research assistant handling rats (type III hypersensitivity). Typical systemic and pulmonary reactions on inhalation and positive prick tests were elicited by rat serum proteins; precipitins against serum proteins in rat urine were present in the patient's serum. (a) Bilateral micronodular shadowing during acute episode. (b) Marked clearing within 11 days after cessation of exposure to rats. (c) Temporary fall in pulmonary gas exchange measured by DL_{CO} (gas transfer, single breath) following a 3-day exposure to rats at work (arrowed). (From Carroll K.B., Pepys J., Longbottom J.L., Hughes D.T.D. & Benson H.G. (1975) *Clin. Allergy* **5**, 443; figures by courtesy of Prof. J. Pepys.)

Injection of relatively large doses of foreign serum (e.g. horse anti-diphtheria) used to be employed for various therapeutic purposes. It was not uncommon for a condition known as 'serum sickness' to arise some eight days after the injection. A rise in temperature, swollen lymph nodes, a generalized urticarial rash and painful swollen joints associated with a low serum complement and transient albuminuria could be encountered. These result from the deposition of soluble antigen–antibody complexes formed in antigen excess.

Some individuals begin to synthesize antibodies against the foreign protein—usually horse globulin. Since the antigen is still present in gross excess at that time, circulating soluble complexes of composition Ag_2Ab, Ag_3Ab_2, Ag_4Ab_3, etc. will be formed (cf. precipitin curve, figure 1.3, p. 5). To be pathogenic, the complexes have to be of the right size—too big and they are snapped up smartly by the macrophages of the reticuloendothelial system, too small ($<19S$) and they fail to induce an inflammatory reaction. Even when they are the right size, it seems that they will only localize in

Figure 9.17. Deposition of immune complexes in the kidney glomerulus. (i) Complexes induce release of vasoactive mediators from basophils and platelets which cause (ii) separation of endothelial cells, (iii) attachment of larger complexes to exposed basement membrane, smaller complexes passing through to epithelial side, (iv) complexes induce platelet aggregation, (v) chemotactically attracted neutrophils release granule contents in 'frustrated phagocytosis' to damage basement membrane. Complex deposition is favoured in the glomerular capillary because it is a major filtration site and has a high hydrodynamic pressure. Deposition is greatly reduced in animals depleted of platelets or treated with vasoactive amine antagonists.

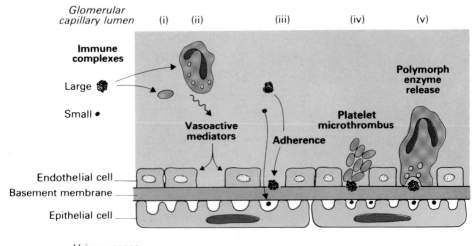

vessel walls if there is a change in vascular permeability. This may come about through release of 5-hydrotryptamine from platelets reacting with larger complexes or through an IgE or complement-mediated degranulation of basophils and mast cells to produce histamine, leukotrienes and platelet activating factor. The effect on the capillaries is to cause separation of the endothelial cells and exposure of the basement membrane to which the appropriately sized complexes attach, the skin, joints, kidneys and heart being particularly affected. As antibody synthesis increases, antigen is cleared and the patient normally recovers.

The deposition of complexes is a dynamic affair and long-lasting disease is only seen when the antigen is persistent as in chronic infections and autoimmune diseases. Experimentally, Dixon produced chronic glomerular lesions by repeated administration of foreign proteins to rabbits. Not all animals showed the lesion and perhaps only those genetically capable of producing low affinity antibody (Soothill & Steward) or antibodies to a restricted number of determinants (Christian) formed soluble complexes in the right size range. The smallest complexes reach the epithelial side but progressively larger complexes are retained in or on the endothelial side of the glomerular basement membrane (figure 9.17). They build up as 'lumpy' granules staining for antigen, immunoglobulin and complement (C3) by immunofluorescence (figure 9.13b) and appear as large amorphous masses in the electron microscope.

It should be said that persistence of circulating complexes does not invariably lead to type III hypersensitivity (e.g. in many cancer patients and in individuals with idiotype–anti-idiotype reactions). Perhaps in these cases the complexes lack the ability to initiate the changes required for complex deposition, but some hold the alternative view that deposited complexes are not preformed in the circulation but are laid down sequentially by the binding to the tissues first of antigen, then of antibody as described in the section on 'locally formed complexes' above. Be that as it may, many cases of glomerulonephritis are associated with circulating complexes and biopsies give a fluorescent staining pattern similar to that of figure 9.13b which depicts DNA/anti-DNA/complement deposits in the kidney of a patient with systemic lupus erythematosus (cf. p. 337). Well known is the disease which can follow infection with certain strains of so-called 'nephritogenic' streptococci and the nephrotic syndrome of Nigerian children associated with quartan malaria where complexes with antigens of the infecting organism have been implicated. Immune complex nephritis can arise in the course of chronic viral infections; for example, mice infected with lymphocytic choriomeningitis virus develop a glomerulonephritis associated with circulating complexes of virus and antibody. This may well represent a model for many cases of glomerulonephritis in man.

The choroid plexus being a major filtration site is also favoured for immune complex deposition and this could account for the frequency of central nervous disorders in systemic lupus. Neurologically affected patients tend to have depressed C_4 in the cerebrospinal fluid and at post-mortem, SLE patients with neurological disturbances and high titre anti-DNA were shown to have scattered deposits of immunoglobulin and DNA in the choroid plexus. Subacute sclerosing panencephalitis is associated with a high c.s.f. to serum ratio of measles antibody, and deposits containing Ig and measles Ag may be found in neural tissue.

The necrotizing arteritis produced in rabbits by experimental serum sickness closely resembles the histology of polyarteritis nodosa and it has recently been reported that in some of these patients, immune complexes containing the HBs antigen of hepatitis B virus are present in the lesions. Another example is the haemorrhagic shock syndrome found with some frequency in South-East Asia during a second infection with a dengue virus. There are four types of virus, and antibodies to one type produced during a first infection may not neutralize a second strain but rather facilitate its entry into, and replication within, human monocytes by attachment of the complex to Fc receptors. The enhanced production of virus leads to immune complex formation and a massive intravascular activation of the classical complement pathway. In some instances drugs such as penicillin become antigenic after conjugation with body proteins and form complexes which mediate hypersensitivity reactions.

DETECTION OF IMMUNE COMPLEX FORMATION

Tissue-bound complexes are usually visualized by the immunofluorescent staining of biopsies with conjugated anti-immunoglobulins and anti-C_3 (cf. figure 9.13b).

Many techniques for detecting circulating complexes have been described and because of variations in the size, complement-fixing ability and Ig class of different complexes, it is useful to apply more than one method. In our laboratory we tend to prefer:

1 precipitation of complexed IgG from serum at concentrations of polyethylene glycol which do not bring down significant amounts of IgG monomer, followed by estimation of IgG in the precipitate by single radial diffusion or laser nephelometry, and

2 binding of serum complexes to plastic tubes coated with Clq and estimation of the amount and class of Ig in the

complex with radio- or enzyme-labelled class-specific anti-Ig (cf. method used for determination of antibody-binding capacity, p. 151).

Other major techniques include (a) estimation of the binding of ^{125}I-Clq to complexes by co-precipitation with polyethylene glycol, (b) inhibition by complexes of rheumatoid factor-induced aggregation of IgG-coated particles and (c) detection with radio-labelled anti-Ig of serum complexes capable of binding to the C3b (and to a lesser extent the Fc) receptors on the Raji cell line. Sera from patients with immune complex disease often form a cryoprecipitate when allowed to stand at 4°. Measurement of serum C3 and its conversion product C3c are sometimes useful.

TREATMENT

The avoidance of exogenous inhaled antigens inducing type III reactions is obvious. Elimination of micro-organisms associated with immune complex disease by chemotherapy may provoke a further reaction due to copious release of antigen. Suppression of the accessory factors thought to be necessary for deposition of complexes would seem logical; for example, the development of serum sickness is prevented by histamine and 5HT antagonists. Disodium cromoglycate, heparin and salicylates are often used, the latter being an effective platelet stabilizer as well as a potent anti-inflammatory agent. Corticosteroids are particularly powerful inhibitors of inflammation and are immunosuppressive. In many cases, particularly those involving autoimmunity, conventional immunosuppressive agents may be justified. Where type III hypersensitivity is thought to arise from an inadequate immune response, the more aggressive approach of immunopotentiation to boost avidity is being advocated, but that is a path that will be trod gently.

Type IV—cell-mediated (delayed type) hypersensitivity

This form of hypersensitivity is encountered in many allergic reactions to bacteria, viruses and fungi, in the contact dermatitis resulting from sensitization to certain simple chemicals and in the rejection of transplanted tissues. Perhaps the best known example is the Mantoux reaction obtained by injection of tuberculin into the skin of an individual in whom previous infection with the mycobacterium had induced a state of cell-mediated immunity (CMI). The reaction is characterized by erythema and induration (figure 9.14b) which appears only after several hours (hence the term 'delayed') and reaches a maximum at 24–48 hours, thereafter subsiding.

Histologically the earliest phase of the reaction is seen as a perivascular cuffing with mononuclear cells followed by a more extensive exudation of mono- and polymorphonuclear cells. The latter soon migrate out of the lesion leaving behind a predominantly mononuclear cell infiltrate consisting of lymphocytes and cells of the monocyte–macrophage series (figure 9.15e and f). This contrasts with the essentially 'polymorph' character of the Arthus reaction (figure 9.15b).

Comparable reactions to soluble proteins are obtained when sensitization is induced by incorporation of the antigen into complete Freund's adjuvant (p. 219). In some but not all cases, if animals are primed with antigen alone or in incomplete Freund's adjuvant (which lacks the mycobacteria), the delayed hypersensitivity state is of shorter duration and the dermal response more transient. This is known as 'Jones–Mote' sensitivity but has recently been termed *cutaneous basophil hypersensitivity* on account of the high proportion of basophils infiltrating the skin lesion.

CELLULAR BASIS

Unlike the other forms of hypersensitivity which we have discussed, delayed-type reactivity cannot be transferred from a sensitized to a non-sensitized individual with serum antibody; lymphoid cells, in particular the T-lymphocytes, are required. Transfer has been achieved in the human using viable white blood cells and interestingly, by a low molecular weight material extracted from them (Lawrence's transfer factor). The nature of this substance is, however, a mystery. The extracts contain a variety of factors which appear capable of stimulating precommitted T-cells mediating delayed hypersensitivity, but whether there is also an informational molecule conferring antigen-specific reactivity is still a highly contentious issue.

It cannot be stressed too often that the hypersensitivity lesion results from an exaggerated interaction between antigen and the *normal* cell-mediated immune mechanisms (cf. p. 75). Following earlier priming, memory T-cells recognize the antigen together with class II MHC molecules on a macrophage and are stimulated into blast cell transformation and proliferation. A proportion of the stimulated T-cells release a number of soluble factors which function as mediators of the ensuing hypersensitivity response particularly by attracting and activating macrophages, while a separate population develops cytotoxic powers.

The cytotoxic drug, cyclophosphamide, enhances cell-mediated hypersensitivity and converts the Jones-Mote reaction to a full tuberculin-type response. This has been attributed to a selective depletion of suppressor B-cells but one should bear in mind also that suppressor T-cells are known to be vulnerable to this drug. CMI is also potentiated by a drug called levamisole whose mechanism of action is unknown, but which might be functioning like transfer factor (possibly not an illuminating comparison at this stage).

IN VITRO TESTS FOR CELL-MEDIATED HYPERSENSITIVITY

Migration inhibition tests

The production of macrophage migration inhibition factor (MIF) by T-cells from sensitized guinea-pigs on incubation with antigen is widely accepted as an *in vitro* correlate of cell-mediated hypersensitivity. The cells are packed into capillary tubes which are placed in small tissue culture chambers. On incubation the macrophages migrate out to form a fan of cells on the bottom of the chamber. If specific antigen is present in the medium, MIF is produced and the migration is inhibited. The degree of inhibition is assessed from the area of the macrophage fan obtained in the presence of antigen and expressed as a percentage of that in the control chambers lacking antigen (figure 9.18), thus correlating with the intensity of the delayed hypersensitivity state.

Greater difficulties have been encountered in attempting migration inhibition tests in the human. One variant is to incubate blood lymphocytes with antigen for several days and then to assay for MIF in the supernatant by addition to guinea-pig macrophages. Another is to mix the lymphocytes directly with the guinea-pig macrophages and to assess the

Figure 9.18. Migration inhibition as an *in vitro* test for cell-mediated hypersensitivity. Migration of peritoneal exudate cells from a sensitized guinea-pig: (a) control in absence of antigen and (b) in the presence of antigen. (Courtesy of Dr J. Brostoff.)

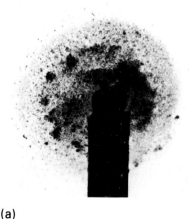

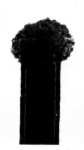

(a)   (b)

effect of antigen on the migratory properties of the macrophages either in a MIF test or in the electric field of a cytopherometer. Inhibitory tests involving migration of buffy coat cells are potentially most useful but the conditions required to define when this represents a direct expression of T-cell reactivity have yet to be rigidly established.

Transformation

The proliferation of sensitized cells on contact with specific antigen and their change in morphology to larger blast-like cells with paler staining nuclei and basophilic cytoplasm (figure 3.7c, p. 55) has frequently been used as an *in vitro* test for cell-mediated hypersensitivity and several studies have shown reasonable correlation with *in vivo* results. The degree of stimulation is assessed either by the percentage of blast-like cells surviving in the culture or by the incorporation of labelled thymidine into newly synthesized DNA.

Comparable changes can be induced in lymphocytes by certain plant mitogens of which the best known are phytohaemagglutinin (PHA) and concanavalin A (conA). These are termed polyclonal T-cell activators because they react with the T-cell surface non-specifically (i.e. not as an antigen) and produce the same series of cellular events as does antigen locking on to its specific surface receptor. Unlike the situation with antigen stimulation where only a small fraction of the cells are sensitive, PHA transforms a major proportion of the T-cells. Additionally, some B-cells are affected although their response appears to be T-cell dependent. The picture is emerging that helper T-cells are preferentially stimulated by PHA and suppressors by conA. Pokeweed activates both T- and B-lymphocytes while lipopolysaccharide (in the mouse at least) is a B-cell mitogen.

TISSUE DAMAGE

Infection

The development of a state of cell-mediated hypersensitivity to bacterial products is probably responsible for the lesions associated with bacterial allergy such as the cavitation, caseation and general toxaemia seen in human tuberculosis and the granulomatous skin lesions found in patients with the borderline form of leprosy. When the battle between the replicating bacteria and the body defences fails to be resolved in favour of the host, persisting antigen provokes a chronic local delayed hypersensitivity reaction. Continual release of lymphokines from sensitized T-lymphocytes leads to the accumulation of large numbers of macrophages, many of which give rise to arrays of epithelioid cells, while others fuse to form giant cells. Macrophages bearing bacterial antigen on their surface may become targets for killer T-cells and be destroyed. Further tissue damage will occur as a result of indiscriminate cytotoxicity by lymphokine-activated macrophages (and NK cells?) and perhaps lymphotoxin itself. Morphologically, this combination of cell types with proliferating lymphocytes and fibroblasts associated with areas of fibrosis and necrosis is termed a *chronic granuloma* and represents an attempt by the body to wall-off a site of persistent infection (figure 9.15e). It should be noted that granulomas can also arise from the persistence of indigestible antigen–antibody complexes or inorganic materials such as talc within macrophages, although non-immunological granulomas may be distinguished by the absence of lymphocytes.

The skin rashes in smallpox and measles and the lesions of herpes simplex may be largely attributed to delayed type allergic reactions with extensive damage to virally infected cells by cytotoxic T-lymphocytes. Cell-mediated hypersensitivity has also been demonstrated in the fungal diseases, candidiasis, dermatomycosis, coccidioidomycosis and histoplasmosis, and in the parasitic diseases, leishmaniasis and schistosomiasis where the pathology has been attributed to a reaction against soluble enzymes derived from the eggs which lodge in the liver capillaries.

Sarcoidosis is a disease of unknown aetiology affecting lymphoid tissue and involving the formation of chronic granulomas. Delayed-type hypersensitivity is depressed and the patients are anergic on skin testing with tuberculin; curiously they give positive responses if cortisone is injected together with the antigen and it has been suggested that cortisone-sensitive T suppressors might be responsible for the anergy. The patients develop a granulomatous reaction a few weeks after intradermal injection of spleen extract from another sarcoid patient—the Kweim reaction.

Contact dermatitis

The epidermal route of inoculation tends to favour the development of a T-cell response through processing by Ia-rich dendritic Langerhans' cells which migrate to the lymph nodes and present antigen to T-lymphocytes (p. 58). Thus, delayed-type reactions in the skin are often produced by foreign materials capable of binding to body constituents, possibly surface molecules of the Langerhans' cell, to form new antigens. The reaction is characterized by a mononuclear cell infiltrate peaking at 12–15 hours, accompanied by oedema of the epidermis with microvesicle formation (figure 9.15c and d). Contact hypersensitivity can occur in people who become sensitized while working with chemicals such as picryl chloride and chromates, or who repeatedly come into contact with the substance urushiol from the poison ivy plant. *p*-Phenylene diamine in certain hair dyes, neomycin in topically applied ointments and nickel salts formed from articles such as nickel jewellery clasps (figure 9.14c) can provoke similar reactions.

Other examples

Delayed hypersensitivity contributes significantly to the prolonged reactions which result from insect bites. The possible implication of homograft rejection by cytotoxic T-cells as a mechanism for the control of cancer cells is discussed in Chapter 10. The contribution made by cell-mediated hypersensitivity reactions to different autoimmune diseases is still rather uncertain (cf. p. 341).

Type V—stimulatory hypersensitivity

Many cells receive instruction by agents such as hormones through surface receptors which specifically bind the external agent presumably through complementarity of structure. This combination may lead to allosteric changes in configuration of the receptor or of adjacent molecules which become activated and transmit a signal to the cell interior. For example, when thyroid stimulating hormone (TSH) of pituitary origin binds to the thyroid cell receptors there appears to be an activation of adenyl cyclase in the membrane which generates cyclic-AMP from ATP and this 'second messenger' acts to stimulate activity in the thyroid cell. The thyroid stimulating antibody present in the sera of thyrotoxic patients (cf. p. 331) is an autoantibody directed against an antigen on the thyroid surface which stimulates the cell and produces the same changes as TSH, similarly utilizing the cyclic-AMP pathway. It is likely that the antibody combines with a site on the TSH receptor or an adjacent molecule to produce the changes required for adenyl cyclase activation. The situation is analogous to lymphocyte stimulation; B-lymphocytes with immunoglobulin surface receptors can be stimulated by changes induced through the receptor molecules either by binding of specific antigen or by an antibody to the immunoglobulin (even anti-Fc) as shown in figure 9.19. Other experimental examples of stimulation by antibodies to cell surface antigens may be cited: the transformation of human T-lymphocytes by monoclonal antibodies to the T3 antigen; the production of cell division in thyroid cells by 'growth' autoantibodies; the induction of pinocytosis by anti-macrophage serum; and the mitogenic effect of anti-

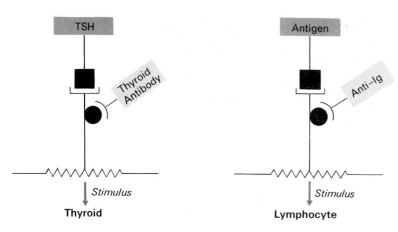

Figure 9.19. Stimulation of thyroid cell and of lymphocyte by physiological agent or by antibody both of which cause compara- ble membrane changes leading to cell acti- vation by reacting with surface receptors.

bodies to sea-urchin eggs. It is worthy of note that although antibodies to enzymes directed against determinants near to the active site can exert a blocking effect, combination with more distant determinants can sometimes bring about allo- steric conformational changes which are associated with a considerable increase in enzymic activity as has been described for certain variants of penicillinase and β- galactosidase.

Summary

The normal effector mechanisms for cell-mediated and humoral immunity are dependent upon the activation of T- and B-cells respectively (figure 9.20). Excessive stimulation of these effector mechanisms by antigen in a sensitized host can lead to tissue damage and we speak of hypersensitivity reactions of which 5 main types can be distinguished.

Type I—anaphylactic hypersensitivity depends upon the reac- tion of antigen with specific IgE antibody bound through its Fc to the mast cell, leading to release from the granules of mediators including histamine, leukotrienes and platelet acti- vating factor, plus eosinophil and neutrophil chemotactic factors. Hay fever and extrinsic asthma represent the most common atopic allergic disorders. The offending antigen is identified by intradermal prick tests giving immediate wheal and erythema reactions or by provocation testing. There is a strong familial disposition; the tendency to produce high levels of IgE is an important contributing factor. Symptom- atic treatment involves the use of mediator antagonists or agents which stabilize the mast cell granules. Courses of

263

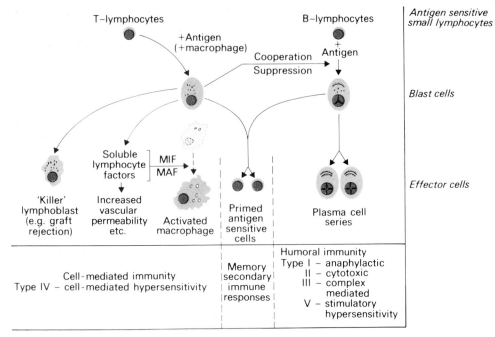

T-lymphocytes

+Antigen
(+macrophage)

Cooperation
Suppression

+
Antigen

B-lymphocytes

Soluble
lymphocyte
factors

MIF
MAF

'Killer'
lymphoblast
(e.g. graft
rejection)

Increased
vascular
permeability
etc.

Activated
macrophage

Primed
antigen
sensitive
cells

Plasma cell
series

Cell-mediated immunity Type IV – cell-mediated hypersensitivity	Memory secondary immune responses	Humoral immunity Type I – anaphylactic II – cytotoxic III – complex mediated V – stimulatory hypersensitivity

Figure 9.20. Relationship of B- and T-cell activity to different forms of hypersensitivity and immunity. Different T-cell functions are mediated by distinct sub-populations.

antigen injection may desensitize by formation of blocking IgG or IgA antibodies or by turning off IgE production.

Type II—antibody-dependent cytotoxic hypersensitivity This involves the death of cells bearing antibody attached to a surface antigen. The cells may be taken up by phagocytic cells to which they adhere through their coating of IgG or C3b or lysed by the operation of the full complement system. Cells bearing IgG may also be killed by myeloid cells (polymorphs and macrophages) or by non-adherent lymphoid K-cells through an extracellular mechanism (antibody-dependent cell-mediated cytotoxicity). Examples are: transfusion reactions, haemolytic disease of the newborn through rhesus incompatibility, antibody mediated graft destruction, autoimmune reactions directed against the formed elements of the blood and kidney glomerular basement membranes, and hypersensitivity resulting from the coating of erythrocytes or platelets by a drug.

Type III—complex-mediated hypersensitivity results from the effects of antigen–antibody complexes through (a) activation of complement and attraction of polymorphonuclear leucocytes which release tissue-damaging enzymes on contact with the complex and (b) aggregation of platelets to cause microthrombi and vasoactive amine release. Where circulating antibody levels are high, the antigen is precipitated near the site of entry into the body. The reaction in the skin is characterized by polymorph infiltration, oedema and erythema maximal at 3–8 hours (Arthus reaction). Examples are Farmer's lung, pigeon fancier's disease and pulmonary aspergillosis where inhaled antigens provoke high antibody levels, reactions to an abrupt increase in antigen caused by microbial cell death during chemotherapy for leprosy or syphilis, and an element of the synovial lesion in rheumatoid arthritis. In relative *antigen excess*, soluble complexes are formed which circulate and are deposited under circumstances of increased vascular permeability at certain preferred sites, the kidney glomerulus, the joints, the skin and the choroid plexus. Complexes can be detected in tissue biopsies by immunofluorescence and in serum by precipitation with polyethylene glycol, reaction with C1q, changes in C3 and C3c, and binding to the C3 receptor on the Raji cell line. Examples are: serum sickness following injection of large quantities of foreign protein, glomerulonephritis associated with systemic lupus or infections with streptococci, malaria and other parasites, neurological disturbances in systemic lupus and subacute sclerosing panencephalitis, polyarteritis nodosa linked to hepatitis B virus, and haemorrhagic shock in dengue viral infection.

Type IV—cell-mediated or delayed-type hypersensitivity is based upon the interaction of antigen with primed T-cells and represents tissue damage resulting from inappropriate cell-mediated immunity reactions. A number of soluble mediators (lymphokines) are released which account for the events which occur in a typical delayed hypersensitivity response such as the Mantoux reaction to tuberculin, namely, the delayed appearance of an indurated and erythematous reaction which reaches a maximum at 24–48 hours and is characterized histologically by infiltration with mononuclear phagocytes and lymphocytes. Another sub-population of T-cells is activated by class I major histocompatibility antigens to become directly cytotoxic to target cells bearing the appropriate antigen. *In vitro* tests for cell-mediated hypersensitivity include macrophage migration inhibition and assessment of blast cell transformation. Examples are: tissue damage occurring in bacterial (tuberculosis, leprosy), viral (smallpox, measles, herpes), fungal (candidiasis, histoplasmosis) and parasitic (leishmaniasis, schistosomiasis) infections, contact dermatitis from exposure to chromates and poison ivy, and insect bites. Continuing provocation of delayed hypersensitivity by persisting antigen leads to formation of chronic granulomata.

Table 9.2. Comparison of different types of hypersensitivity.

	I Anaphylactic	II Cytotoxic	III Complex-mediated	IV Cell-mediated	V Stimulatory
Antibody mediating reaction	Homocytotropic Ab Mast-cell binding	Humoral Ab ±CF*	Humoral Ab ±CF	Receptor on T-lymphocyte	Humoral Ab Non-CF
Antigen	Usually exogenous (e.g. grass pollen)	Cell surface	Extracellular	Associated with MHC antigens on macrophage or target cell	Cell surface
Response to intradermal antigen:					
Max. reaction	30 min.	—	3–8 hours	24–48 hours	—
Appearance	Wheal and flare	—	Erythema and oedema	Erythema and induration	—
Histology	Degranulated mast cells; oedema; eosinophils	—	Acute inflammatory reaction; predominant polymorphs	Perivascular inflammation: polymorphs migrate out leaving predominantly mononuclear cells	—
Transfer sensitivity to normal subject	←———— Serum antibody ————→		←———— Lymphoid cells Transfer factor ————→		Serum antibody
Examples:	Atopic allergy, e.g. hay fever	Haemolytic disease of newborn (Rh)	Complex glomerulonephritis Farmer's lung	Mantoux reaction to TB Granulomatous reaction to schistosome eggs Contact sensitivity	Thyrotoxicosis

* CF = Complement fixation.

266

Type V—stimulatory hypersensitivity where the antibody reacts with a key surface component such as a hormone receptor and 'switches on' the cell. An example is the thyroid hyper-reactivity in Graves' disease due to a thyroid stimulating autoantibody.

Features of the five types of hypersensitivity are compared in table 9.2.

Further reading

Cochrane C.G. & Koffler D. (1973) Immune complex disease in experimental animals and man. *Adv. Immunol.* **16**, 186.

Fudenberg H.H., Stites D.P., Caldwell J.L. & Wells J.V. (1980) *Basic and Clinical Immunology*, 3rd edn. Lange Medical Publications, Los Altos, California.

Lachmann P. & Peters D.K. (eds) (1980) *Clinical Aspects of Immunology*, 4th edn. Blackwell Scientific Publications, Oxford.

Lessof M.H. (ed.) (1981) *Immunology and Clinical Aspects of Allergy*. MTP Press, Lancaster.

Mollison P.L. (1970) Red cell destruction. *Brit.J.Haematol.* **18**, 249.

O'Regan S., Smith M. & Drumond K.N. (1976) Antigens in human immune complex nephritis. *Clin.Nephrol.* **6**, 417.

Pepys J. (1969) *Hypersensitivity Diseases of the Lungs due to Fungi and Organic Dusts*. Karger, Basle.

Rose N.R. & Friedman H. (1976) *Manual of Clinical Immunology*. Amer. Soc. Microbiology, Washington, D.C.

Sachs M.I., Gleich G.J. & Yunginger J.W. (1983) Adverse reactions to foods. *Clin. Immunol. Update.* Franklin, E.C. (ed.). Elsevier Biomedical, New York.

Stanworth D.S. (1973) *Immediate Hypersensitivity*. North Holland, Amsterdam.

Turk J.L. (1975) *Delayed Hypersensitivity*, 2nd edn. North Holland, Amsterdam.

10 Transplantation

The replacement of diseased organs by a transplant of healthy tissue has long been an objective in medicine but has been frustrated to no mean degree by the unco-operative attempts by the body to reject grafts from other individuals. Before discussing the nature and implications of this rejection phenomenon, it would be helpful to define the terms used for transplants between individuals and species:

Autograft—tissue grafted back on to the original donor.

Isograft—graft between syngeneic individuals (i.e. of identical genetic constitution) such as identical twins or mice of the same pure line strain.

Allograft (old term, homograft)—graft between allogeneic individuals (i.e. members of the same species but different genetic constitution), e.g. man to man and one mouse strain to another.

Xenograft (heterograft)—graft between xenogeneic individuals (i.e. of different species), e.g. pig to man.

It is with the allograft reaction that we have been most concerned although it should one day be possible to use grafts from other species. The most common allografting procedure is probably blood transfusion where the unfortunate consequences of mismatching are well known. Considerable attention has been paid to the rejection of solid grafts such as skin and the sequence of events is worth describing. In mice, for example, the skin allograft settles down and becomes vascularized within a few days. Between three and nine days the circulation gradually diminishes and there is increasing infiltration of the graft bed with lymphocytes and monocytes but very few plasma cells. Necrosis begins to be visible macroscopically and within a day or so the graft is sloughed completely (figure 10.1).

Evidence that rejection is immunological

First and second set reactions

It would be expected, if the reaction has an immunological basis, that the second contact with antigen would represent a

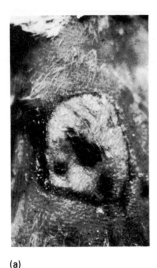

(a)

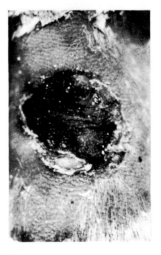

(b)

Figure 10.1. Rejection of CBA skin graft by strain A mouse. (a) 10 days after transplantation; discoloured areas caused by destruction of epithelium and drying of the exposed dermis. (b) 13 days after transplantation; the scabby surface indicates total destruction of the graft. (Courtesy Prof. L. Brent.)

more explosive event than the first and indeed the rejection of a second graft from the same donor is much accelerated. The initial vascularization is poor and may not occur at all. There is a very rapid invasion by polymorphonuclear leucocytes and lymphoid cells including plasma cells. Thrombosis and acute cell destruction can be seen by three to four days.

Specificity

Second set rejection is not the fate of all subsequent allografts but only of those derived from the original donor or a related strain. Grafts from unrelated donors are rejected as first set reactions.

Role of the lymphocyte

Neonatally thymectomized animals have difficulty in rejecting skin grafts but their capacity is restored by injection of lymphocytes from a syngeneic normal donor, suggesting that T-cells are implicated. The recipient of lymphoid cells from a donor which has already rejected a graft will give accelerated rejection of a further graft of the same type (figure 10.2) showing that the lymphoid cells are primed and retain memory of the first contact with graft antigens.

Production of antibodies

After rejection, humoral antibodies with specificity for the graft donor may be recognized. In the mouse where the

270

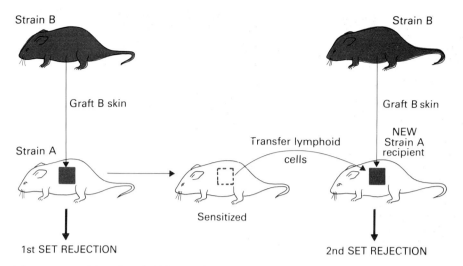

Figure 10.2. Transfer of ability to give accelerated graft rejection with lymphoid cells from a sensitized animal. In fact, successful transfer can be achieved with T-cells. After graft rejection, antibodies to B strain antigens (A anti-B) are detectable.

erythrocytes carry transplantation antigens, haemagglutination tests become positive; in the human, lymphocytotoxins are found. A Jerne plaque test using donor strain thymocytes in place of sheep erythrocytes will often demonstrate the presence of antibody-forming cells in the lymphoid tissues of grafted animals.

Transplantation antigens

GENETICS

The specificity of the antigens involved in graft rejection is under genetic control. Genetically identical individuals such as mice of a pure strain or uniovular twins have identical transplantation antigens and grafts can be freely exchanged between them. The Mendelian segregation of the genes controlling these antigens has been revealed by interbreeding experiments between mice of different pure strains. Since these mice breed true within a given strain and always accept grafts from each other, they must be homozygous for the 'transplantation' genes. Consider two such strains A and B with allelic genes differing at one locus. In each case paternal and maternal genes will be identical and they will have a genetic constitution of, say, A/A and B/B respectively (by convention, the genes are expressed in italics and the antigens they encode in normal type). Crossing strains A and B gives a first familial generation (F1) of constitution A/B. Using an A anti-B serum produced in A strain recipients of B grafts (figure 10.2), and a B anti-A serum obtained in like

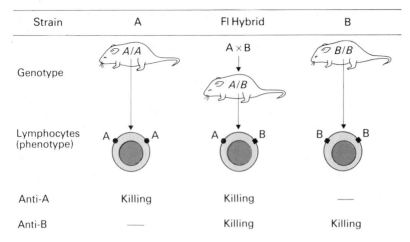

Strain	A	FI Hybrid	B
Genotype	A/A	A × B ↓ A/B	B/B
Lymphocytes (phenotype)	A ● ● A	A ● ● B	B ● ● B
Anti-A	Killing	Killing	—
Anti-B	—	Killing	Killing

Figure 10.3. Co-dominant expression of transplantation antigens. The first familial (FI) generation obtained by crossing the homozygous pure parental strains A and B has the genotype A/B. Since all its lymphocytes are killed in the presence of complement by antibodies to A OR to B (raised as in figure 10.2), antigens encoded by both parental genes must be expressed on each lymphocyte. The same holds for other tissues in the body.

fashion, it can be shown that cells from the FI mice bear both A and B antigens, that is the genes encoding the transplantation antigens are co-dominant (figure 10.3). A consequence of this co-dominant expression is that FI animals will be tolerant to both transplantation antigens and will therefore accept grafts from either parent (figure 10.4). By intercrossing the FI generation, it will be seen from figure 10.4 that three out of four of the F2 generation accept parental strain grafts. Extending the analysis, if instead of one locus with a pair of allelic genes, there were n loci, the fraction of

Figure 10.4. Inheritance of genes controlling transplantation antigens. A represents a gene expressing the A antigen and B the corresponding allelic gene at the same genetic locus. The pure strains are homozygous for A/A and B/B respectively. Since the genes are co-dominant, an animal with an A/B genome will express both antigens, become tolerant to them and therefore accept grafts from either A or B donors. The illustration shows that for each gene controlling a transplantation antigen specificity, three-quarters of the F2 generation will accept a graft of parental skin. For n genes the fraction is $(\frac{3}{4})^n$. If FI A/B animals are back-crossed with an A/A parent, half the progeny will be A/A and half A/B; only the latter will accept B grafts.

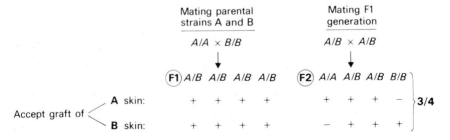

	Mating parental strains A and B				Mating F1 generation			
	$A/A \times B/B$				$A/B \times A/B$			
	↓				↓			
	(F1) A/B	A/B	A/B	A/B	(F2) A/A	A/B	A/B	B/B
A skin:	+	+	+	+	+	+	+	−
Accept graft of **B** skin:	+	+	+	+	−	+	+	+

3/4

272

the F2 generation accepting parental strain grafts would be $(\frac{3}{4})^n$. In this way an estimate of the number of loci controlling transplantation antigens can be made.

In the mouse at least 20 such loci have been established, but of these, one complex locus termed H-2 predominates in the sense that it controls the 'strong' transplantation antigens which provoke intense allograft reactions that are the most difficult to suppress. This H-2 locus constitutes the *major histocompatibility complex* (MHC; cf. figure 3.12), and it is a feature of all the vertebrate species so far studied that each possesses a single MHC which dominates allotransplantation reactivity.

THE MAJOR HISTOCOMPATIBILITY COMPLEX IN MICE

Class I molecules (classical transplantation antigens)

Although the H-2 locus appeared to be a single entity, it is now seen to be far more complicated and may be broken down into regions which are separable by genetic recombination (i.e. by chromosomal crossing over between the subregions). Alloantisera obtained by grafting or immunization between different mouse strains identify two major regions K and D (figure 10.5) each defined by a major genetic locus (with numerous alleles) which encodes a single 'strong' transplantation antigen. Each chromosome therefore controls the synthesis of an H-2K and an H-2D antigenic specificity. Because they are the most potent antigens of the H-2 complex in provoking an antibody response, they were the first to be recognized by sera from allografted animals and the term classical transplantation antigens is appropriate. A third locus codes for H-2L, a minor series of polymorphic antigens structurally similar to H-2D/K. All lymphoid cells are rich in H-2D/K antigens; liver, lung and kidney have moderate amounts whereas brain and skeletal muscle have relatively little. The antigens are on the cell surface since lymphocytes are readily lysed by antibody in the presence of complement. Capping experiments and SDS-polyacrylamide gel analysis of immunoprecipitates of radio-labelled, detergent-solubilized H-2 (cf. figure 6.16) show the K and D specificities to be associated with separate molecules. They are located on peptides of molecular weight 43,000 which are associated non-covalently with β_2-microglobulin. Both β_2-microglobulin and the α_3 domain of the H-2D/K peptides show a high degree of homology with Thy1 and the immunoglobulin constant region domains and appear to adopt a similar tertiary configuration suggesting a common evolutionary origin (figure 10.6). There is evidence that in the

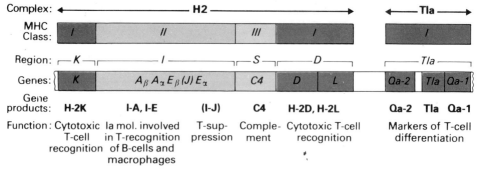

Figure 10.5. The major histocompatibility gene complex in the mouse (H-2). Genes are in italics and their products in normal bold type. I-A and I-E are each composed of α and β chains. Expression of I-J is controlled by a separate gene on chromosome 4. Class I molecules are expressed together with β_2-microglobulin. Other genes within the H-2 complex control: (a) levels of C2, C3 and Factor B, (b) resistance to Gross leukaemia virus (Rgv-1) and mammary tumour virus (RMTV), (c) innate resistance to bone marrow grafts in non-syngeneic irradiated recipients (Hh factors), e.g. parent into F1 (presumably reflecting non-codominant expression of Hh genes), and (d) the level of testosterone and testosterone-binding protein (Hom-1). The *Tla* complex which is downstream from *H-2* (relative to the centromere) encodes class I molecules related to those in the *H-2* complex. Tla appears on the T-cell during intrathymic differentiation and is then lost; it is expressed on activated T-cells and by certain leukaemic T-cells. Qa-1 is associated with the T-helper subset which can induce T-suppressors (cf. figure 4.10, p. 104). There are a large number of relatively quiescent *Qa* loci whose function is unknown, but intriguingly, a recent study suggested that nucleotide changes in the polymorphic region of *H-2K* were effected by a gene conversion mechanism utilizing a particular *Qa* locus sequence. The T-t region (T = normal, t = tailless) affects complex differentiation events in the embryo. Recombination with H-2 is suppressed.

absence of β_2-microglobulin, the classical transplantation antigens fail to be expressed on the cell surface. These antigens are transmembrane glycoproteins and the serological specificity lies in the amino acid sequence rather than the carbohydrate moiety.

Nomenclature If someone says to you in a little-known language, 'I have kicked my commissar', you fail to understand, not because the idea is complicated but because you do not comprehend the language. It is much the same with the shorthand used to describe the H-2 system which looks unnecessarily frightening to the uninitiated. In order to identify and compare allelic genes within the H-2 complex in different strains, it is usual to start with certain pure inbred strains to provide the prototypes. The collection of genes in the H-2 complex is called the haplotype and the haplotype of each prototypic strain will be allotted a given superscript. For example, the DBA strain haplotype is designated $H-2^d$ and the genes constituting the complex are therefore $H-2K^d$, $H-2D^d$ and so on; their products will be H-2K^d and H-2D^d and so forth. When new strains are derived from these by

274

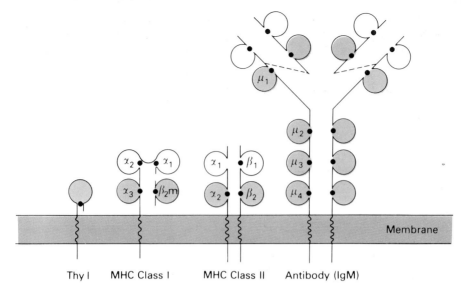

Thy I   MHC Class I   MHC Class II   Antibody (IgM)

Figure 10.6. Comparison of the structures of the thymus differentiation antigen Thy 1, class I and class II major histocompatibility complex molecules and membrane IgM. represents a domain with intrachain disulphide (●). α_1 etc. number the domains of α chains, and β_1 etc. the β chains. β_2 m = β_2-microglobulin. μ_1 etc. number the IgM heavy chain constant region domains (cf. figure 2.17, p. 39). ～～ represents the hydrophobic portion inserted into the membrane. Shaded domains share considerable sequence homology suggesting a common evolutionary ancestry (reproduced, with permission, from *Annual Review of Immunology*, **1**, 529. Copyright 1983 by Annual Reviews Inc).

genetic recombination during breeding, they are assigned new haplotypes but the individual genes are designated by the haplotype of the prototype strain from which they were derived. Thus the A/J strain produced by genetic cross-over during interbreeding between ($H\text{-}2^k \times H\text{-}2^d$) F1 mice is arbitrarily assigned the haplotype $H\text{-}2^a$, but table 10.1 shows that individual genes in the complex are identified by the haplotype symbol of the original parents.

Table 10.1. The haplotypes of the H-2 complex of some commonly used mouse strains and recombinants derived from them.

Strain	Haplotype	K	A	(J)	E	S	D
C57Bl	*b*	*b*	*b*	*b*	*b*	*b*	*b*
CBA	*k*	*k*	*k*	*k*	*k*	*k*	*k*
DBA/2	*d*	*d*	*d*	*d*	*d*	*d*	*d*
A/J	*a*	*k*	*k*	*k*	*k**	*d*	*d*
B.10A(4R)	*h4*	*k*	*k*	*b*	*b*	*b*	*b*

A/J was derived by interbreeding ($k \times d$) F1 mice, recombination occurring between E and S regions(*).

The H-2 complex spans 0.5 centimorgans equivalent to a recombination frequency between the K and D ends of 0.5%. Because the genes are close together, the haplotype appears to segregate as a single Mendelian trait, the complexity only being revealed by recombination events. Each H-2K and D molecule possesses several antigenic specificities corresponding with a number of different epitopes or determinants and these are classed as (i) *private* specificities unique for a given haplotype, (ii) *public* specificities shared between different haplotypes and either restricted to K and D or present on both. Each specificity is assigned a number.

Class II molecules (Ia antigens)

Mixed lymphocyte reaction (MLR)   When lymphocytes from strains of mice which differ at the *I-A* or *I-E* subregion are cultured together, blast cell transformation and mitosis occurs (MLR), each population of lymphocytes reacting against Ia determinants on the surface of the other population. For the 'one-way MLR', the stimulator cells are made unresponsive by treatment with mitomycin C or X-rays and then added to the responder lymphocytes from the other donor. The responding cells belong predominantly to a sub-population of Lyt1 positive T-lymphocytes and they are stimulated by the Ia determinants present mostly on B-cells, macrophages and dendritic antigen-presenting cells. Thus, the MLR is inhibited by anti-Ia sera.

I-A and I-E are transmembrane glycoproteins each consisting of an α- and a β-polypeptide of molecular weights 33K and 28K respectively; both are polymorphic and show sequence homology with class I molecules, antibody and Thy 1 (figure 10.6). It will be recalled that the Ia antigens are concerned in T help and T suppression. Cells bearing I-J evoke suppression and T-lymphocytes which recognize I-A or I-E mediate delayed sensitivity and B-cell help. It now seems clear that they also help in the generation of cytotoxic T-cells.

Cell-mediated lympholysis (CML)   The involvement of Ia antigens in the provocation of transplantation rejection has been brought into some focus by the discovery of the phenomenon of CML which was developed as a possible test for histocompatibility. The principle is illustrated in figure 10.7. In short, responder cells activated by the Ia-induced MLR help in the generation of cytotoxic T-cells directed to the H-2D/K determinants; in essence, the recognition of class II molecules helps to generate effectors against the class I molecules, in some ways reminiscent of the carrier-hapten system

276

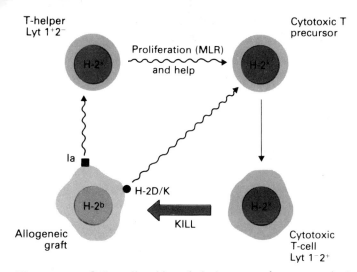

T-helper
Lyt 1⁺2⁻

Proliferation (MLR)
and help

Cytotoxic T
precursor

Ia

H-2D/K

KILL

Allogeneic
graft

Cytotoxic
T-cell
Lyt 1⁻2⁺

Figure 10.7. Cell-mediated lympholysis: generation of *H-2^k* T-cells cytotoxic for *H-2^b* grafts. T-helpers respond to Ia^b on the graft cells by proliferating (mixed lymphocyte reaction) and are then able to help cytotoxic T-cell precursors specific for the H-2D^b or H-2K^b antigens of the graft to become cytotoxic effectors.

in T-B collaboration with class II equivalent to carrier and class I to hapten.

Graft-vs-host (g.v.h.) reaction When competent lymphoid cells are transferred from a donor to a recipient which is incapable of rejecting them, the grafted cells survive and have time to recognize the host antigens and react immunologically against them. Instead of the normal transplantation reaction of host against graft, we have the reverse, the so-called graft-vs-host reaction. In the young rodent there can be inhibition of growth (runting), spleen enlargement and haemolytic anaemia (due to production of red cell antibodies). In the human, fever, anaemia, weight loss, rash, diarrhoea and splenomegaly are observed. The 'stronger' the transplantation antigen difference, the more severe the reaction. Where donor and recipient differ at HLA or H-2 loci, the reaction can be fatal.

Two possible situations leading to g.v.h. reactions are illustrated in figure 10.8. In the human this may arise in immunologically anergic subjects receiving bone marrow grafts, e.g. for combined immunodeficiency (p. 225), for red cell aplasia after radiation accidents or as a possible form of cancer therapy. Competent lymphoid cells in blood or present in grafted organs given to immunosuppressed patients may give g.v.h. reactions; so could maternal cells which adventitiously cross the placenta, although in this case there is as yet no evidence of diseases caused by such a mechanism in the human.

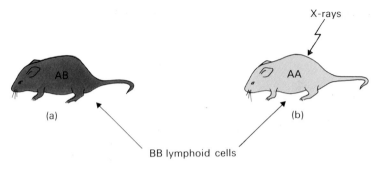

X-rays

AB

(a)

AA

(b)

BB lymphoid cells

Figure 10.8. Graft-vs-host reaction. When competent lymphoid cells are inoculated into a host incapable of reacting against them, the grafted cells are free to react against the antigens on the host's cells which they recognize as foreign. The ensuing reaction may be fatal. Two of many possible situations are illustrated: (a) the hybrid AB receives cells from one parent (BB) which are tolerated but react against the A antigen on host cells (b) an X-irradiated AA recipient restored immunologically with BB cells cannot react against the graft and a g.v.h. reaction will result.

THE MAJOR HISTOCOMPATIBILITY COMPLEX IN MAN

In man, as in the mouse, there is also one dominant group of antigens which provokes strong reactions—the HLA system (figure 10.9). In addition, the ABO group provides strong transplantation antigens.

Of the three class I HLA loci identified, HLA-A and HLA-B probably represent the counterpart of murine H-2K and H-2D in that they most readily evoke the formation of complement-fixing cytotoxic antibodies which can be used for tissue typing. Operationally monospecific sera are selected from patients transfused with whole blood and multigravidas who often become immunized with fetal antigens with specificities defined by paternally derived genes absent from the mother's genome. An individual is typed by setting up his lymphocytes against a panel of such sera in the presence of complement, cell death normally being judged by the inability to exclude trypan blue. Different antigens are arbitrarily assigned numerical specificities (figure 10.10). An individual heterozygous at each locus must express four *major* class I HLA specificities, two from maternally derived and two from the paternally derived chromosomes (figure

Figure 10.9. The major histocompatibility complex loci (HLA) in man. Where the precise order of genes is still uncertain, the loci are separated by commas. The class II molecules each consist of an α- and a β-chain heterodimer.

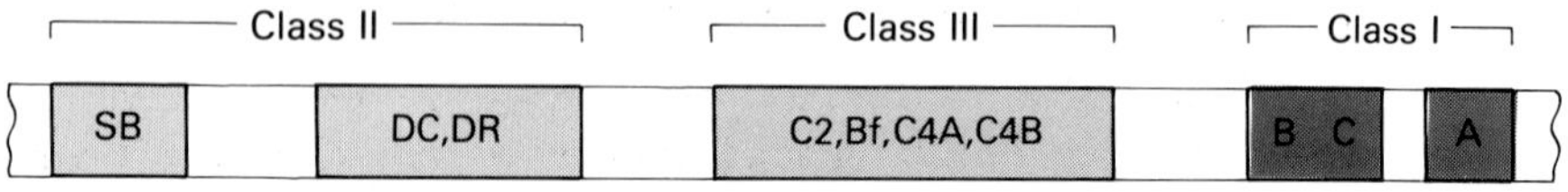

┌─ Class II ─┐	┌─ Class III ─┐	┌─ Class I ─┐
SB	DC,DR	C2,Bf,C4A,C4B	B C	A

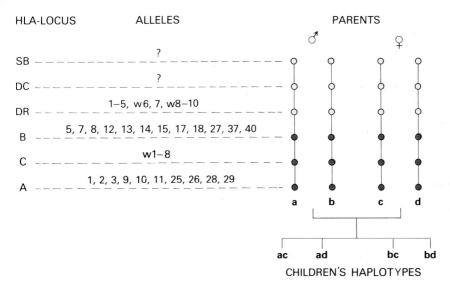

| HLA-LOCUS | ALLELES | PARENTS |
| | | ♂   ♀ |

SB ─ ─ ─ ─ ─ ─ ─ ─ ? ─ ─ ─ ─ ─ ─ ─ ─ ─ ─

DC ─ ─ ─ ─ ─ ─ ─ ─ ? ─ ─ ─ ─ ─ ─ ─ ─ ─ ─

DR ─ ─ ─ ─ ─ 1–5, w6, 7, w8–10 ─ ─ ─ ─ ─ ─ ─

B ─ ─ 5, 7, 8, 12, 13, 14, 15, 17, 18, 27, 37, 40 ─

C ─ ─ ─ ─ ─ ─ ─ ─ w1–8 ─ ─ ─ ─ ─ ─ ─ ─ ─

A ─ ─ ─ 1, 2, 3, 9, 10, 11, 25, 26, 28, 29 ─ ─ ─

                                          a   b   c   d

                 ac   ad   bc   bd

CHILDREN'S HAPLOTYPES

Figure 10.10. HLA specificities and their inheritance. The complex lies on chromosome 6, the SB locus being closest to the centromere. There are several more specificities at the A and B loci but only the most solidly established are given. The numbers at the A and B loci do not overlap. A further locus with just two alleles, HLA-Bw4 and Bw6 (formerly 4a/4b) is intimately linked to HLA-B. The small 'w' before a number stands for 'workshop' and indicates that the specificity concerned has not yet been characterized sufficiently for upgrading to full HLA-status.

Since there are several possible alleles at each locus, the probability of a random pair of subjects from the general population having identical HLA specificities is low. However, there is a 1 : 4 chance that two *siblings* will be identical in this respect because each group of specificities on a single chromosome forms a haplotype which will be inherited *en bloc* giving four possible combinations of paternal and maternal chromosomes. Parent and offspring can only be identical (1 : 2 chance) if the mother and father have one haplotype in common.

10.10). Class I antigens encoded by a third locus, HLA-C induce a somewhat weaker response.

The original class II locus, *HLA-D*, was defined by the MLR using homozygous stimulating cells for typing; if an individual failed to respond to a given typing cell then his own lymphocytes must already have borne that specificity. Subsequently, with serological reagents it transpired that the D locus could be split into *DR* and *DC* each encoding heterodimer class II molecules with homology for murine *I-E* and *I-A* respectively. A further class II locus, SB, has also been identified.

Rejection mechanisms

LYMPHOCYTE-MEDIATED REJECTION

A great deal of the work on allograft rejection has involved transplants of skin or solid tumours because their fate is relatively easy to follow. In these cases there is little support for the view that humoral antibodies are instrumental in destruction of the graft although, as we shall see later, this is not necessarily so with transplants of other organs such as the kidney. Whereas passive transfer of *serum* from an animal which has rejected a skin allograft cannot usually accelerate the rejection of a similar graft on the recipient animal, injection of *lymphoid cells* (particularly recirculating small lymphocytes) is effective in shortening graft survival (cf. figure 10.2).

A primary role of lymphoid cells in first set rejection would be consistent with the histology of the early reaction showing infiltration by mononuclear cells with very few polymorphs or plasma cells (figure 10.11). The dramatic effect of neonatal thymectomy in prolonging skin transplants, as mentioned earlier, and the long survival of grafts on children with thymic deficiencies implicate the T-lymphocytes in these reactions. In the chicken, homograft rejection and g.v.h. reactivity are influenced by neonatal thymectomy but not bursectomy. More direct evidence has come from *in vitro* studies showing that T-cells taken from mice rejecting an allograft could kill target cells bearing the graft antigens *in vitro*. Recent work on the importance of murine Lyt $1^{+}2^{-}$ and human $T4^{+}$ cells as effectors has cast some doubt on the role of cytotoxic cells in graft rejection *in vivo*; although these subsets have sometimes been shown to have cytotoxic potential for class II targets, as a rule they are associated with helper activity and in particular with the production of lymphokines mediating delayed hypersensitivity reactions. Perhaps they act to encourage access of cytotoxic T-cells to their targets?

THE ROLE OF HUMORAL ANTIBODY

It has long been recognized that isolated allogeneic cells such as lymphocytes can be destroyed by cytotoxic (type II) reactions involving humoral antibody. However, although earlier experience with skin and solid tumour-grafts suggested that they were not readily susceptible to the action of cytotoxic antibodies, it is now clear that this does not hold for all types of organ transplants. Consideration of the different ways in which kidney allografts can be rejected illustrates the point:

1 *Hyperacute rejection* within minutes of transplantation, characterized by sludging of red cells and microthrombi in the glomeruli, occurs in individuals with pre-existing humoral antibodies—either due to blood group incompatibility or presensitization through blood transfusion.

2 *Acute early rejection* occurring up to 10 days or so after transplantation is characterized by dense cellular infiltration

280

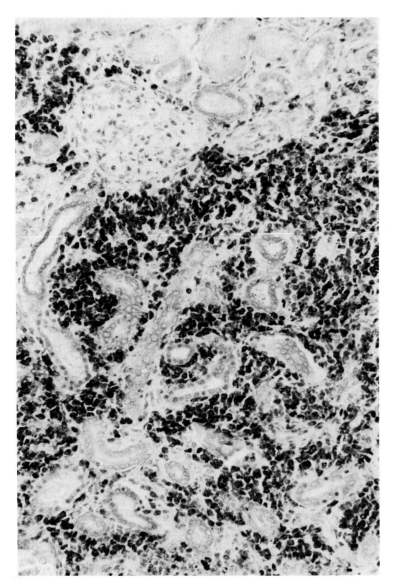

Figure 10.11. Acute early rejection of human renal allograft 10 days after transplantation showing dense cellular infiltration of interstitium by mononuclear cells (pyronin stain). (Courtesy Prof. K. Porter.)

(figure 10.11) and rupture of peritubular capillaries and appears to be a cell-mediated hypersensitivity reaction involving T-lymphocytes.

3 *Acute late rejection*, which occurs from 11 days onwards in patients suppressed with prednisone and azathioprine, is probably caused by the binding of immunoglobulin (presumably antibody) and complement to the arterioles and glomerular capillaries where they can be visualized by immunofluorescent techniques. These immunoglobulin deposits

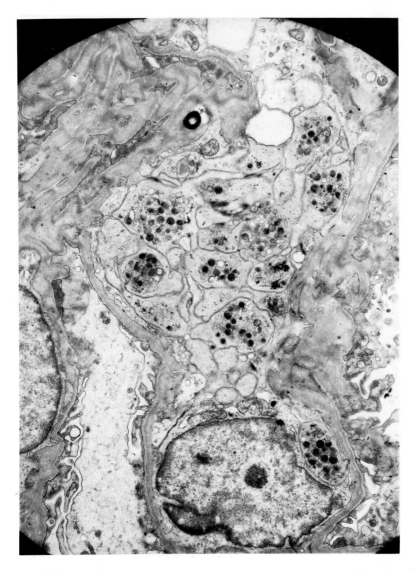

Figure 10.12. Acute late rejection of human renal allograft showing platelet aggregation in a glomerular capillary induced by deposition of antibody on the vessel wall (electron micrograph). (Courtesy Prof. K. Porter.)

on the vessel walls induce platelet aggregation in the glomerular capillaries leading to acute renal shutdown (figure 10.12). The possibility of damage to antibody-coated cells through antibody-dependent cell-mediated cytotoxicity must also be considered.

4 *Insidious and late* rejection associated with subendothelial deposits of immunoglobulin and C3 on the glomerular basement membranes which may sometimes be an expression of an underlying immune complex disorder (originally necessi-

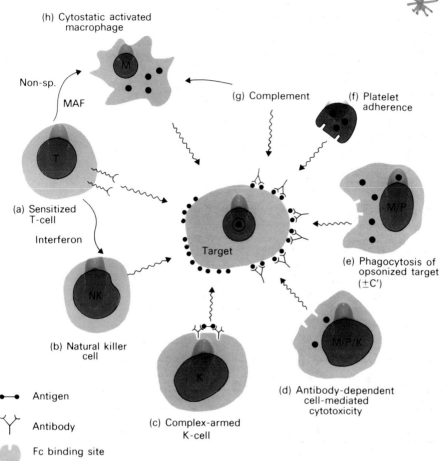

(h) Cytostatic activated macrophage

Non-sp.

MAF

(g) Complement

(f) Platelet adherence

(a) Sensitized T-cell

Interferon

Target

(e) Phagocytosis of opsonized target (±C′)

(b) Natural killer cell

(d) Antibody-dependent cell-mediated cytotoxicity

●—● Antigen

Antibody

Fc binding site

(c) Complex-armed K-cell

Figure 10.13. Mechanisms of target cell destruction. M = macrophage; P = polymorph; K = K cell. (a) Direct killing by cytotoxic T-cells binding through specific surface receptors. Indirect tissue damage through release of lymphokines from delayed-type hypersensitivity T-cells. (b) Killing by NK cells (p. 300) enhanced by interferon. (c) Specific killing by immune-complex-armed K-cell recognizes target through free antibody valencies in the complex. (d) Attack by antibody-dependent cell-mediated cytotoxicity (in a–d the killing is extracellular). (e) Phagocytosis of target coated with antibody (heightened by bound C3). (f) Sticking of platelets to antibody bound to surface of graft vascular endothelium leading to formation of microthrombi. (g) Complement-mediated cytotoxicity. (h) Macrophages activated non-specifically by agents such as BCG, endotoxin, poly-I : C, T-cell macrophage activating factor and possibly C3b are cytostatic and sometimes cytotoxic for dividing tumour cells, perhaps through extracellular action of peroxide and O_2^--derived radicals generated at the cell surface (p. 185). In some situations *in vitro*, sensitized B-cells secrete antibody which coats the target rendering it susceptible to attack by ADCC.

tating the transplant) or possibly of complex formation with soluble antigens derived from the grafted kidney.

The complexity of the action and interaction of cellular and humoral factors in graft rejection is therefore considerable and an attempt to summarize the postulated mechanisms involved is presented in figure 10.13.

There are also circumstances when antibodies may actually *protect* a graft from destruction and this important phenomenon of *enhancement* will be considered further below.

Prevention of graft rejection

TISSUE MATCHING

Based upon experience of matching blood for transfusion and of transplantation between mice of similar specificities it could reasonably be expected that the chances of rejection in the human would be minimized by matching donor and recipient at the HLA loci. Indeed, in the case of human kidney transplantation, the data based upon typing for HLA-A and -B specificities indicate that the closer the match, the better the survival of the graft. This is especially true with matched siblings (figure 10.14) but it would be wrong to conclude that full matching at A and B loci is all that is necessary since grafts between unrelated individuals who fulfil this condition are markedly less successful than those between siblings. Now we have seen that matched siblings have the same haplotypes (figure 10.10) and are therefore identical at all HLA loci, and if we further recall that the

Figure 10.14. Survival of kidney transplants in relation to degree of matching at HLA-A and -B loci. Complete match (siblings) = all antigens identical; partial match (siblings and parent to child) = only antigens on one chromosome (haplotype) identical; mismatch (unrelated) = all antigens different. (Data taken from Dausset J. & Hors J. (1973) *Transpl. Proc.* **V**, 223.)

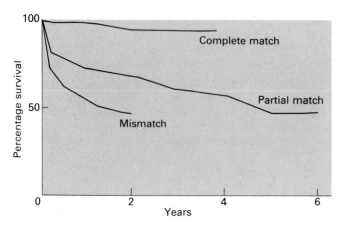

generation of T helpers for cytotoxicity, delayed hypersensitivity and antibody is largely dependent upon class II locus differences (p. 276), it seems likely that matching the D region antigen will prove to be a major factor in improving graft survival.

Because of the many thousands of different HLA phenotypes possible (figure 10.10), it is usual to work with a large pool of potential recipients on a continental basis so that when graft material becomes available the best possible match can be made. The position will be improved when the pool of available organs can be increased through the development of long-term tissue storage banks but techniques are not good enough for this at present except in the case of bone marrow cells which can be kept viable even after freezing and thawing. With a paired organ such as the kidney, living donors may be used; siblings provide the best chance of a good match (cf. figure 10.10). However, the use of living donors poses difficult ethical problems and the objective must be to perfect the use of cadaver material (? or animal organs—or mechanical substitutes—or to prevent the disease in the first place!).

GENERAL IMMUNOSUPPRESSION

Graft rejection can be held at bay by the use of agents which non-specifically interfere with the induction or expression of the immune response. Because these agents are non-specific, patients on immunosuppressive therapy tend to be susceptible to infections; they are also more prone to develop lymphoreticular cancers.

Lymphoid cell ablation

Thymectomy, splenectomy and lymphadenectomy in adult recipients do not appear to help, although extra-corporeal irradiation of blood, injections of anti-lymphocyte globulin (ALG) and thoracic duct cannulation have proved beneficial. Total lymphoid irradiation would appear somewhat Draconian but has been shown to prolong skin grafts in mice when given in divided doses over an extended period, due to the stimulation of powerful non-specific T-suppressors. The most striking feature of this work is that allogeneic bone marrow cells given at the end of this treatment schedule are fully accepted without the development of g.v.h. reactions (Strober & Slavin). Whether the same effects can be produced in man remains to be seen.

Immunosuppressive drugs

The development of an immunological response requires the active proliferation of a relatively small number of antigen-

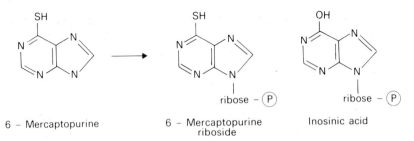

SH

6 – Mercaptopurine

SH

6 – Mercaptopurine
riboside

OH

Inosinic acid

Figure 10.15. Metabolic conversion of aza-thioprine through 6-mercaptopurine to the ribotide: similarity to inosinic acid with which it competes.

sensitive lymphocytes to give a population of sensitized cells large enough to be effective. Many of the immunosuppressive drugs now employed were first used in cancer chemotherapy because of their toxicity to dividing cells. Aside from the complications of blanket immunosuppression mentioned above, these antimitotic drugs are especially toxic for cells of the bone marrow and small intestine and must therefore be used with great care.

One of the most commonly used drugs in this field is *azathioprine* which has a preferential effect on T-cell mediated reactions. It is broken down in the body first to 6-mercaptopurine and then converted to the active agent, the ribotide. Because of the similarity in shape (figure 10.15), this competes with inosinic acid for enzymes concerned in the synthesis of guanylic and adenylic acids; it also inhibits the synthesis of 5-phosphoribosylamine, a precursor of inosinic acid, by a feedback mechanism. The net result is inhibition of nucleic acid synthesis. Another drug, methotrexate, through its action as a folic acid antagonist also inhibits synthesis of nucleic acid. The N-mustard derivative cyclophosphamide probably attacks DNA by alkylation and cross-linking so preventing correct duplication during cell division. These agents appear to exert their damaging effects on cells during mitosis and for this reason are most powerful when administered after presentation of antigen at a time when the antigen-sensitive cells are dividing.

Cyclosporin A represents an exciting and entirely new class of compound which is having a dramatic impact on the human transplantation scene. It is a very insoluble fungal metabolite which is of particular interest since it selectively penetrates antigen-sensitive T-cells in the G_0 to G_1 phase and inhibits their type II RNA polymerase. Resting cells which carry the vital memory for immunity to microbial infections are spared and there is little toxicity for dividing cells in gut and bone marrow. Some studies also point to an 'exquisite' sensitivity of the dendritic antigen-presenting cells to the drug. There are, of course, side-effects. It has to be used at doses below those causing nephrotoxicity so that blood levels have to be monitored regularly by radioimmunoassay. There is also some cause for concern that cyclosporin may make patients susceptible to EB virus-induced lymphomas since the drug inhibits T-cells which control EB virus transformation of B-cells *in vitro*; however, the latest results suggest that the incidence of lymphoma is relatively low in comparison with that reported for allografted patients on conventional immunosuppressive therapy. Whether or not cyclosporin itself proves to be of permanent clinical value, and it seems likely that it will, it does offer an intriguing new pathway towards the development of agents with selective action against dividing lymphocytes.

Steroids such as prednisone intervene at many points in the immune response, affecting lymphocyte recirculation and the generation of cytotoxic effector cells, for example; in addition, their outstanding anti-inflammatory potency rests on features such as inhibition of neutrophil adherence to vascular endothelium in an inflammatory area and suppression of monocyte/macrophage functions such as microbicidal activity and response to lymphokines.

ANTIGEN-SPECIFIC DEPRESSION OF
ALLOGRAFT REACTIVITY

Immunological tolerance

If the disadvantages of blanket immunosuppression are to be avoided, we must aim at knocking out only the reactivity of the host to the antigens of the graft, leaving the remainder of the immunological apparatus intact. One approach is through the induction of tolerance in the patient. Through selective action on antigen-sensitive dividing cells, cyclosporin A may induce clonal abortion. Total lymph node irradiation plus bone marrow (*vide supra*) is thought to induce T-suppression, and grafts of skin and heart from the same donor enjoy prolonged survival. Active suppression is probably also responsible for the long-lasting tolerance to a skin allograft seen in mice given donor liver extract 16 days before the graft and alternating procarbazine hydrochloride and antilymphocyte globulin for a few days afterwards (Brent). As purified histocompatibility antigens become available, it should ultimately not be beyond the wit of *Homo sapiens* to juggle the relative timing and dosages of antigen and various immunosuppressants to produce a specific hyporesponsive state. On rather a different tack, it has been reported that tolerance between rodent strains can be established by autoimmunization with the idiotype of the host receptor for donor transplantation antigens.

The most immunogenic cells in tissue grafts tend to be passenger B-lymphocytes and dendritic accessory cells which are rich in class II, Ia antigens. If these cells are removed, effector T-cells are less likely to differentiate and might even become tolerized by exposure to class I determinants in the absence of a T-helper signal. Thus, the complete reduction in immunogenicity of thyroid, parathyroid and islets of Langerhans after culture for several days in 95% oxygen has been attributed to loss of Ia-positive dendritic cells (Lafferty); such grafts are rapidly rejected if the recipient is injected with as few as 10^3 peritoneal cells of donor origin which present the alloantigen in association with Ia.

Enhancement

There is another possible solution which may be easier to achieve and that is deliberate immunization with these antigens to evoke antibodies which protect rather than destroy the graft. It has long been recognized that such *enhancing* sera are responsible for the prolonged survival of tumour allografts after prior immunization with irradiated tumour cells. The precise mechanism has still to be revealed but explanations usually fall under two headings, masking by antibody and blocking by antigen (figure 10.16).

Masking by antibody The killing of target cells by sensitized lymphocytes from an H-2 incompatible mouse is inhibited by addition of antibodies directed against the H-2K and D antigens of the target. Presumably the antibodies combine with the surface antigens of the target cells which are then no longer accessible to the receptors on the aggressor lymphocytes. The bound antibodies must avoid the activation of complement or indeed of non-specific aggressor K-cells (p. 242). In the case of complement at least, this would occur if the determinants on the surface were too far apart to allow the Fc portions of adjacent antibodies to interact and bind complement (cf. p. 166) and might also be insufficient to allow effective interaction with K-cells; alternatively, if the antigenic determinants were close together, no activation of C1 or of K-cells would be possible if there were a preponderance of antibodies belonging to inappropriate immunoglobulin classes such as IgA. Following the discussion in the last section on the immunological 'silence' of the class I antigens in the absence of Ia, it is clear that block of graft Ia molecules by antibody could achieve a similar effect. Shedding of antigen from the cell surface due to complexing

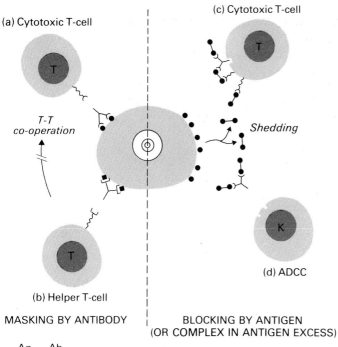

MASKING BY ANTIBODY

BLOCKING BY ANTIGEN
(OR COMPLEX IN ANTIGEN EXCESS)

Ag	Ab	
●	Y	HLA-A and B
■	YY	HLA-D

Figure 10.16. Enhancement: possible mechanisms. *Block by antibody*—(a) Masking the HLA-A or B antigens on the target surface inhibits attack by cytotoxic T-cells. (b) Masking of Ia on the target prevents the induction of T-helpers and hence of cytotoxic T-cells. There is evidence that tolerance may be induced if classical transplantation antigens are presented in the absence of Ia-induced T-helpers (cf. the idea that 1 signal tolerizes and 2 signals trigger a B-cell, p. 72). *Block by antigen*— Sufficient antigen shed from the surface of the target, either free or as a complex in antigen excess, can (c) block the receptors on cytotoxic T-cells and possibly tolerize their precursors or (d) block the antibody involved in antibody-dependent cell-mediated cytotoxicity.

It has also been suggested that antibody could opsonize antigen-sensitive cells which had bound antigen to their surface, so causing their elimination.

with antibody (p. 159) would also leave the cell resistant to attack.

Blocking by antigen   If graft or tumour antigen is shed from the surface as a result of stripping by antibody, it will be released as a complex, but it may also occur spontaneously. The shed antigen might block the receptors on specific cytotoxic T-cells, the complex possibly being more effective in this than free antigen to the extent that it can establish multivalent linking to both antigen and Fc receptors. Alternatively, the antigen may pre-emptively neutralize antibody which would otherwise render the graft vulnerable to ADCC.

Successful enhancement of kidney and bone-marrow grafts has been reported in isolated instances and one supposes this will inevitably be extended. There are indications that serum-enhancing factors may inhibit tumour destruction by cell-mediated mechanisms in some cancer patients as will be discussed later.

Clinical experience in grafting

Privileged sites

Corneal grafts survive without the need for immunosuppression. Because they are avascular they do not sensitize the recipient although they become cloudy if the individual has been pre-sensitized. Grafts of cartilage are successful in the same way but an additional factor is the protection afforded the chondrocytes by the matrix. With bone and artery it doesn't really matter if the grafts die because they can still provide a framework for host cells to colonize.

Kidney

Thousands of kidneys have been transplanted and with improvement in patient management there is a high survival rate (figure 10.14). Patients are partially immunosuppressed at the time of transplantation because uraemia causes a degree of immunological anergy. Recipients sharing three or four of the A and B locus antigens with the donor show improved results if they have previously been transfused with blood; will this prove to be a case of serendipitous enhancement through production of Ia antibodies? Unquestionably the importance of D-locus matching is widely recognized. The combination of azathioprine and prednisone is commonly employed in the long-term management of kidney grafts but replacement of the azathioprine with cyclosporin A looks very promising. If kidney function is poor during a rejection crisis renal dialysis can be used. When transplantation is performed because of immune complex induced glomerulonephritis, the immunosuppressive treatment used may help to prevent a similar lesion developing in the grafted kidney. Patients with glomerular basement membrane antibodies (e.g. Goodpasture's syndrome) are likely to destroy their renal transplants unless first treated with plasmapheresis and immunosuppressive drugs.

290

Heart

Something like 40–50% of transplant patients survive by one year but this figure is improving with the introduction of cyclosporin A therapy. The results have not been as good as with kidney grafting but special factors should be taken into account. The recipient patients were in irreversible cardiac failure with wasting and advanced secondary changes of passive congestion, and the clinical urgency made it difficult to find well-matched donor organs. Aside from the rejection problem it is likely that the number of patients who would benefit from cardiac replacement is much greater than the number dying with adequately healthy hearts. More attention will have to be given to the possibility of xenogeneic grafts and mechanical substitutes.

Liver

Survival rates for orthotopic liver grafts are broadly in line with those receiving heart transplants. Three-quarters of the patients transplanted for hepatic cancer have had recurrence of their tumour within one year.

Experience with liver grafting between pigs revealed an unexpected finding. Many of the animals retained the grafted organs in a healthy state for many months without any form of immunosuppression. The transplanted liver represented a large antigen pool which induced a state of unresponsiveness to grafts of skin or kidney from the same donor. The mechanism is not clear but may involve true tolerance or enhancement. There is as yet no evidence that this highly desirable state can be established by a hepatic transplant in man.

Bone marrow

Patients with certain immunodeficiency disorders and aplastic anaemia are obvious candidates for treatment with bone marrow stem cells as are acute leukaemia patients treated radically with intensive chemotherapy and possibly whole body irradiation in attempts to eradicate the neoplastic cells. Successful results with bone marrow transfers require highly compatible donors if fatal graft-vs-host reactions are to be avoided, and here siblings offer the best chance of finding a matched donor (figure 10.10). Matching for antigens quite distinct from those controlled by the major HLA loci may prove to be essential (cf. the murine Hh locus, figure 10.5 legend). The incidence of chronic graft-vs-host disease is reduced if T-cells in the grafted marrow are first removed by a cytotoxic cocktail of anti-T-cell monoclonals and significant improvements have also been reported both for success of primary engraftment and the prevention of g.v.h. disease when patients are treated with cyclosporin A. A curious effect that requires further exploration is the observation that leukaemia patients with g.v.h. disease have a lower incidence of relapse.

Other organs

It is to be expected that improvement in techniques of control of the rejection process will encourage transplantation in several other areas—not, of course, in most cases of endocrine disorders where exogeneous replacement therapy is available, but one looks forward to the successful transplantation of lungs, and of skin for lethal burns.

Biological significance of the major histocompatibility complex

RECOGNITION SYSTEMS

It is becoming increasingly clear that the major transplantation antigens subserve an intercellular recognition function. We do not know whether they are involved in phenomena like the reassortment of dispersed kidney cells in culture which preferentially reaggregate with each other despite admixture with hepatocytes but they do undoubtedly play a central role in directing T-cell interactions.

Haplotype restriction

Of dramatic significance has been the revelation that the MHC is intimately involved in the T-cell recognition of macrophage-processed antigens (cf. p. 99), collaboration with B-cells (p. 99) and killing of virally infected cells (cf. p. 201). In essence, T-cells recognize antigen in association with one of the products of the MHC complex. Memory T-cells are most effectively triggered by exposure to antigen in association with the MHC haplotype used for priming.

Let us look at an example of this phenomenon of so-called 'haplotype restriction' in more detail. If I may be permitted to refresh your mind, dear reader, cytotoxic T-cells provoked by a virus infection will only kill target cells infected with that virus *in vitro* if they share the same classical transplantation antigens as the original host. Thus cytotoxic T-cells arising in a mouse of H-2^d haplotype infected with lymphocytic choriomeningitis virus (LCM) will kill LCM-infected cells of H-2^d but not H-2^k haplotype (figure 10.17). By using target cells from strains derived by genetic recombination within the H-2 complex, the relevant MHC molecule recog-

HLA -A
-B

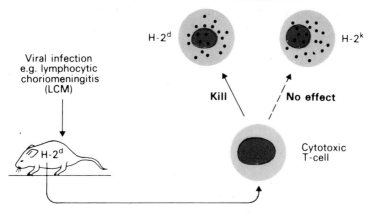

(a) MHC RESTRICTED CYTOTOXICITY OF T-CELLS FOR VIRALLY INFECTED TARGETS *IN VITRO*

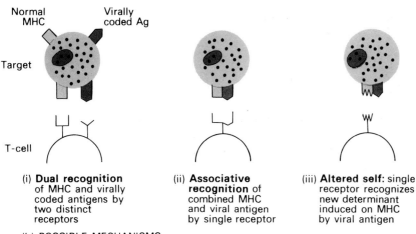

(i) **Dual recognition** of MHC and virally coded antigens by two distinct receptors

(ii) **Associative recognition** of combined MHC and viral antigen by single receptor

(iii) **Altered self**: single receptor recognizes new determinant induced on MHC by viral antigen

(b) POSSIBLE MECHANISMS

Figure 10.17. The Doherty and Zinkernagel phenomenon of haplotype restriction in recognition of virally infected targets by cytotoxic T-cells. On recovery from infection, cytotoxic T-cells can be demonstrated which kill virus-infected cells of the same H-2 haplotype but not cells bearing a different haplotype, even though both targets express the same viral antigen as shown by the cytotoxic effect of antiviral antibody plus complement. The same mechanisms apply to the recognition of H-2 linked minor transplantation antigens such as the male (Y) antigen and to the response to Ia associated antigen on the macrophage surface.

A consequence of the altered self model is that there must be as many new determinants inducible on the MHC molecule as there are distinct cytotoxic T cell specificities. Furthermore, if the individual H-2 polymorphic specificity becomes changed due to this alteration in self this would not explain how specific anti-H-2 sera block T-cell recognition unless they cause dissociation of the antigen–MHC complex. Both dual and associative models involve recognition of self MHC + viral antigen; whether it is stereochemically likely that determinants on MHC and a separate surface antigen, even in a fluid membrane, can become sufficiently closely apposed to fit into a single receptor has not been established. However, if a T-cell hybridoma which recognizes antigen A in the context of H-2^d is fused with one recognizing antigen B in association with haplotype H-2^k, the resulting cell retains the original haplotype restriction for the recognition of each antigen and cannot respond to antigen A/H-2^k or antigen B/H-2^d; this is not the result to be expected if there are separate receptors for antigen and H-2 unless there is some restriction in their association with each other.

nized by the T-cell has been pinpointed as H-2D. With certain other viruses such as vaccinia, the target cell shows H-2K restriction. Various models have been proposed for these recognition processes: (i) two distinct receptors combine with self H-2D (or H-2K) and virally coded antigen respectively, (ii) a single receptor recognizes a determinant formed by association of H-2D/K and viral antigen, or (iii) the virus modifies the synthesis or configuration of the H-2D/K molecule to produce a new 'altered self' determinant. These are discussed further in the legend to figure 10.17.

Based upon the inhibition of T-cell reactions by antibodies to various human T-cell markers and to unique, presumably idiotypic, molecules on individual clones (Ti), a model for recognition by T-lymphocytes has been proposed in which the foreign antigen in association with the polymorphic part of the MHC molecule is bound by a receptor consisting of Ti and T3 while the non-polymorphic part is bound by either T4 or T8 (figure 10.18). Although the T4 and T8 subsets correspond rather loosely with helper/inducer and cytotoxic/suppressor functions respectively (cf. p. 62), a small proportion of T4 clones have been found to be cytotoxic and the relationship is more precisely with the type of MHC molecule involved, T4 lymphocytes interacting with class II and T8 with class I molecules. The Ti molecule, like the idiotypic component identified in murine T-cell clones (p. 138), is a heterodimer composed of 43K and 49K polypeptide chains and presumably has a type of variable region binding site for the antigen-MHC complex. T3 is present on all immunocompetent T-cells and can be modulated by anti T3 which induces shedding of the molecule together with the Ti component. Since anti-T3 is mitogenic and can also induce IL-2 receptors, it is speculated that T3 transduces a signal generated on target cell recognition, to activate the lymphocyte.

Figure 10.18. Model for T-cell structures. T4 and T8 recognize monomorphic class II and class I MHC determinants respectively. Antigen (▬) in the context of the polymorphic MHC specificity (◣ and ◥) is bound by the receptor Ti, unique to each T-cell, in association with the transducing protein T3. Antibodies to T3, Ti and to T4 or T8 inhibit the T-cell response (after Reinherz E.L., Meuer S.C. & Schlossman S.F. (1983) *Immunol. Today* **4**, 5, courtesy of the authors and publishers).

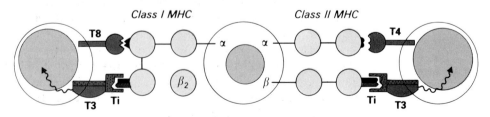

Class I MHC   Class II MHC

T8 lymphocyte   Target cell   T4 lymphocyte

There is evidence that the T-cells are programmed to recognize the appropriate self MHC antigens during their differentiation in the thymus and they learn the haplotype of the cells they meet in the thymus gland. This is shown by experiments in which thymectomized irradiated F1 offspring of two parental strains, A and B, injected with F1 bone marrow, are reconstituted with different thymuses and then tested in the LCM haplotype restriction system. Cytotoxic cells generated by LCM infection of mice given an F1 thymus could kill both A and B targets infected with virus; A strain thymus restricted killing to A targets and B thymus to B targets. However, similar results were not obtained when thymus-grafted nude mice were used as bone marrow recipients and the situation awaits some clarification.

Facilitation of the appropriate immune response

When a cell is first infected with virus, there is an eclipse phase during which the machinery of the cell is being switched for viral replication and the only marker of the complete microbe is the viral antigen on the cell surface. At this stage, killing of the cell by a cytotoxic T-cell will prevent viral replication.

How does the killer T-cell know when it has reached its target? It has to recognize two features before striking: one is the presence of viral antigen and the other is its location on the surface of a body cell. The microbial antigen is recognized by the specific T-receptor and the cell through its marker, the class I antigens which are present on nearly every cell in the body. Thus the killer cell, in the mouse for example, operates on the basis that:

$$\text{viral antigen} + \text{H-2D/K} = \text{virally infected cell}$$

In other words, viral antigen is the code for 'viral infection' and class I molecules are the code for 'cell', and that is why its receptors have to see both antigens. The human utilizes the HLA-A and B (and probably C) loci in the same way.

The situation is quite different with intracellular bacteria and protozoa which do not go through an eclipse phase after phagocytosis by macrophages but are held as infectious entities; lysis by cytotoxic T-cells will merely release the organisms, not kill them. A separate strategy utilizing the delayed-type hypersensitivity T-cell population is required and in this case, the effector T-lymphocyte recognizes the infected macrophage by the presence of microbial antigen on the surface in association with an I-region molecule which is now a code for 'macrophage'. This interaction triggers the release of lymphokines which enable the macrophage to kill the intracellular parasites (p. 196). Similarly, in T-B cooperation, the B-cell is recognized through its Ia molecule associated with the foreign antigen while I-J is used as a marker for T-cells mediating suppression. In summary, each

Function	Cell interaction	MHC marker on target cell
T-help	T-B	I-A/E
T-proliferation	T-macrophage	I-A/E
T-delayed sensitivity	T-macrophage	I-A/E
T-suppression	T-T	I(-J)
T-cytotoxic	T-infected cell	D/K

Table 10.2.
Guidance of
T sub-populations
to appropriate
target cell by MHC
molecules in the
mouse.

T-lymphocyte subset has to communicate with a particular cell type in order to make the *appropriate* immune response and it does so by recognizing not only foreign antigen (or idiotype, cf. p. 106) but also the particular MHC molecule used as a marker of that cell (table 10.2).

In addition to the I region on chromosome 17, the quite separate M locus on chromosome 1 in the mouse provokes a strong mixed lymphocyte reaction and, following the theme of a link with recognition systems, it is exciting to note that a gene controlling susceptibility to leishmania infection maps in the close vicinity.

POLYMORPHISM

With loci for at least seven peptides on each of two chromosomes and several alleles at each locus, there are literally millions of different possible phenotypes, in other words the MHC is an extraordinarily polymorphic system. That this holds for widely divergent species like man, mouse and chicken implies that the maintenance of such polymorphism confers a survival advantage in evolutionary terms. One suggestion is that a polymorphic system provides a defence against microbial molecular mimicry in which a whole species might be put at risk by its inability to recognize as foreign an organism which displays determinants similar in structure to those of the host. It is also possible that in some way the existence of a high degree of polymorphism helps to maintain the diversity of antigenic recognition within the lymphoid system of a given species.

One consequence of this multi-allelic complex is that it ensures *heterozygosity*, with its connotation of 'hybrid vigour' (yet another phenomenon whose mechanisms remain obscure but could involve almost anything from fertilization onwards).

IMMUNOLOGICAL RELATIONSHIP
OF MOTHER AND FETUS

A further consequence of polymorphism in an outbred population is that mother and fetus will almost certainly have different MHCs. Some examples of selection for heterozygotes (where maternally and paternally derived haplotypes are different) over homozygotes (both fetal haplotypes identical with the mother's) in viviparious animals suggest that this is beneficial. Likewise, the placentae of FI offspring are larger than normal when mothers are preimmunized to the paternal H-2 haplotype and smaller when mothers are tolerant to these antigens.

The threat posed to the fetus as a potential graft due to the possession of paternal transplantation antigens so intrigued Lewis Thomas that he was moved to suggest that rejection of the fetus might initiate parturition, although it would be difficult to account for the normal birth of female offspring to pure strain mating pairs where fetus and mother would have identical histocompatibility antigens without further postulating a placenta-specific surface antigen.

Nonetheless, in the human haemochorial placenta, maternal blood with immunocompetent lymphocytes does circulate in contact with the fetal trophoblast and we have to explain how the fetus avoids allograft rejection, despite the development of an immunological response in a proportion of mothers as evidenced by the appearance of anti-HLA antibodies and cytotoxic lymphocytes. In fact, prior sensitization with a skin graft fails to affect a pregnancy, showing that trophoblast cells are immunologically protected. Some of the many speculations which have been aired on this subject are summarized in figure 10.19. The low density or absence of

Figure 10.19. Mechanisms postulated to account for the survival of the fetus as an allograft in the mother. (After L. Brent.)

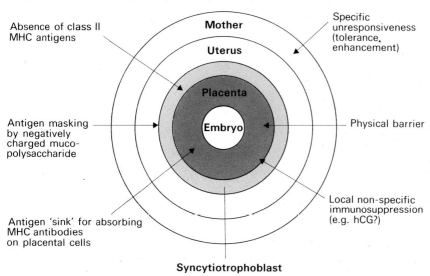

class II antigens on the syncytiotrophoblast cells which are in front-line contact with the maternal circulation makes it more likely that paternal class I antigens will induce tolerance rather than a cytotoxic T-cell response. This alone might be sufficient to explain the invulnerability of the placenta to immunological attack, but in addition, trophoblast cells may be protected against cytotoxic lymphocytes by a surrounding barrier (admittedly incomplete) of sialic acid-rich mucopolysaccharide.

THE CANCER CELL AND THE
ALLOGRAFT REACTION

The ability to reject transplants of tissue may be traced back a long way down the evolutionary tree—back even as far as the annelid worms. Long before the studies on the involvement of self-MHC in immunological responses, Lewis Thomas suggested that the allograft rejection mechanism represented a means by which the body's cells could be kept under *immunological surveillance* so that altered cells with a neoplastic potential could be identified and summarily eliminated. For this to operate, cancer cells must display a new surface antigen which can be recognized by the lymphoid cells and examples have been discovered although the phenomenon is not universal.

Tumour surface antigens (figure 10.20)

(a) *Virally controlled* Cells infected with oncogenic viruses usually display two new antigens on their surface, one (V)

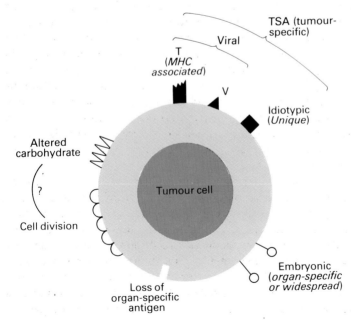

Figure 10.20. Tumour-associated antigens. Even virally induced tumours may possess idiotypic specificities.

298

identical with an antigen on the isolated virion and the other (T), also a product of the viral genome, present only on infected cells; the latter represents a strong transplantation antigen and generates haplotype-restricted cytotoxic T-cells. All syngeneic tumours induced by a given virus carry the same surface antigen, irrespective of their cellular origin, so that immunization with any one of these tumours confers resistance to subsequent challenge with the others.

(b) *Embryonic* If the uncontrollable cell division of a cancer cell is attributable to the abnormal expression of one of a number of normal differentiation genes (so-called cellular oncogenes), their products or the products encoded by other genes which secondarily might become derepressed could be differentiation antigens normally associated with an earlier fetal stage. Thus tumours derived from the same cell type are often found to express such oncofetal antigens which are also present on embryonic cells. Examples would be α-fetoprotein in hepatic carcinoma and carcinoembryonic antigen (CEA) in cancer of the intestine. Certain monoclonal antibodies raised against human melanoma cells also react with tumours of neural crest origin and fetal melanocytes. Another monoclonal antibody defines the SSEA-1 antigen found on a variety of human tumours and early mouse embryos but absent from adult cells with the exception of human granulocytes and monocytes.

(c) *Division* The carbohydrate moiety of surface membrane glycoproteins may change during cell division. For example, Thomas found that the density of surface sugar determinants cross-reacting with blood group H fell as murine mastocytoma cells moved into the G_1 phase of the division cycle while, reciprocally, group B determinants increased. We have found that surface components binding the lectin, wheatgerm agglutinin, are abundant on myeloid cells (polys and macrophages) but poorly represented on resting T- and B-cells; however, within 24 hours of stimulation by lymphocyte polyclonal activators and before DNA synthesis begins, high concentrations of lectin binding sites appear on the surface. Transferrin receptors are also abundant on dividing cells which presumably are keen to take more iron on board.

(d) *Idiotypic* Tumours induced by chemical agents, benzopyrene for example, also possess specific transplantation antigens, but each tumour produced by a given chemical carcinogen has its own individual idiotypic antigen; even when a carcinogen produces two different primary tumours in the same animal, they do not exhibit the same antigenic specificities and do not confer cross-resistance by immunization. In the light of the potentially exciting observation that a retroviral gp 70 molecule on the surface of a methylcholanthrene-induced tumour behaved as a tumour-specific transplantation antigen, it is conceivable that this tumour individuality could be based on diversity in gp 70 produced by some form of random recombination events. Perhaps the nearest one can get to a really tumour-specific antigen is the Ig idiotype on the surface of chronic lymphocytic leukaemic cells.

Immune response to tumours

When present, these antigens can provoke immune responses in experimental animals which lead to resistance against tumour growth but they vary tremendously in their efficiency. Powerful antigens associated with tumours induced by oncogenic viruses or ultraviolet-light generate strong resistance while chemically induced tumours are weaker and somewhat variable; disappointingly, tumours which arise spontaneously in animals produce little or no response. This would seem to reason against the immune surveillance theory, although it might be argued that most tumours were silenced at their inception by immunological control and that only the very few which lacked a provocative surface component were 'successful'. However, athymic nude mice have a normal incidence of spontaneous tumours and this makes a single, exclusively T-cell surveillance system most unlikely. Furthermore, the only increase in cancer reported in immunosuppressed patients was related to the lympho-reticular system which could have been the direct target for the drugs employed; one exception was the considerable increase in skin cancer in immunosuppressed patients living in high sunshine regions north of Brisbane and we have already noted the 'antigen strength' of such tumours provoked in experimental animals.

Perhaps in speaking of immunity to tumours, one too readily thinks in terms of acquired responses whereas it is possible that innate mechanisms will prove to be of greater significance. Macrophages taken from BCG-infected animals, or activated by a diversity of factors, bacterial lipopolysaccharide, double-stranded RNA, T-cell lymphokine and so forth, destroy tumour cells in tissue culture through the copious production of hydrogen peroxide and a cytolytic protease. There is an uncommon flurry of interest in the natural killer (NK) cell which is probably the same as the K cell of ADDC fame (p. 242) except that it works in the absence of antibody. NK cells are spontaneously cytolytic for certain, but by no means all, tumour lines in culture as well as for cells infected with herpes and mumps viruses or *Listeria monocytogenes*. The target molecule might be a surface membrane glycoprotein with altered carbohydrate and the blocking of cytotoxicity by anti-Ly5 sera tentatively suggests that this differentiation antigen could be the NK receptor. Interferon markedly enhances the activity of NK cells and, at the same time, increases the resistance of *normal* cells to lysis. Agents such as BCG and *Corynebacterium parvum* which stimulate macrophages also increase NK activity. A recently described mouse strain with a mutant gene (*beige*) which leads to complete and selective impairment of NK activity should help to define the role of these cells in resistance to spontaneous tumours much the same as the nude mouse allowed more precise delineation of thymus function.

Immunotherapy

On one point all are agreed, if immunotherapy is to succeed, it is essential that the tumour load should first be reduced by surgery, irradiation or chemotherapy, since not only is it unreasonable to expect the immune system to cope with a large tumour mass, but considerable amounts of antigen released by shedding would tend to prevent the generation of any significant response in some cases due to the stimulation of T-suppressors. This leaves the small secondary deposits as the proper target for immunotherapy.

For active immunization we need antigen. Based on the not unreasonable belief that certain forms of cancer (e.g. lymphoma) are caused by oncogenic viruses, attempts are being made to isolate the virus and prepare a suitable vaccine from it. In fact, large-scale protection of chickens against the development of Marek's disease lymphoma has been successfully achieved by vaccination with another herpes virus native to turkeys. In the human, patients with Burkitt's lymphoma develop antibodies which react with antigens on cells of their own and other Burkitt tumours which are controlled by a herpes group organism, the Epstein–Barr (EB) virus. The unique idiotype on monoclonal B-cell tumours with surface Ig also offers a potentially feasible target for immunotherapy and successful treatment of one patient has had wide publicity. Immunologists have for long been bemused by the idea of eliminating tumour cells by specific antibody linked to a killer molecule. Not surprisingly, the 'magic bullet' devotees were greatly encouraged by experiments in which guinea-pig B lymphoma cells were killed *in vitro* by anti-idiotype conjugated with ricin, a toxin of such devastating potency that one molecule entering the cell is lethal (those readers who still maintain contact with the outside world will recollect that minute amounts of ricin on the end of a pointed walking stick provide a favourite weapon for the liquidation of unwanted intelligence agents). There is optimism that by using monoclonal antibodies, it may be

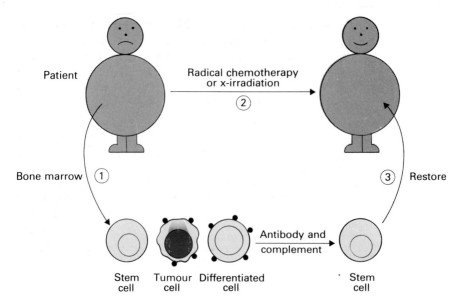

Figure 10.21. Treatment of leukaemias by autologous bone marrow rescue. By using cytotoxic antibodies to a differentiation antigen (●) present on leukaemic cells and even on other normal differentiated cells, but absent from stem cells, it should be possible to obtain a tumour-free population of the latter which can be used to restore haematopoietic function in patients subsequently treated radically to destroy the leukaemic cells. However, techniques to clean up the marrow effectively still leave room for improvement.

feasible to apply this approach to the human. It should be mentioned that differentiation antigens present on leukaemic cells but absent on bone-marrow stem cells, even though not tumour-specific, can be used to prepare tumour-free autologous stem cells to restore function in patients treated with chemotherapy or x-irradiation which destroys both their tumour cells and their haematopoietic tissue (figure 10.21).

Despite reports of cytotoxic antibodies in a proportion of patients with malignant melanoma and cytotoxic leukocytes from patients with neuroblastoma or bladder cancer, which indicate that some form of immunological response to tumour antigens is possible, it must be said that attempts to control human cancer by immunization with tumours plus adjuvants have had very mixed and in many ways somewhat disappointing results. Presumably we can only expect results from this approach with those tumours which possess some potential antigen such as the oncofetal proteins. Many attempts are being made to boost the inherently weak autoantigenicity of these cells by infection with viruses, membrane insertion of chemical haptens or fusion with highly immunogenic allogeneic or xenogeneic normal cells. Another interesting attack is suggested by the finding of two different groups that a proportion of tumour cells after treatment with mutagenic drugs and cloning can be shown to have acquired new antigens which induce an immunological response conferring resistance to the parent tumour.

With respect to putatively non-antigenic tumours, there have been numerous, not very successful, attempts to boost 'non-specific' effector mechanisms mediated by macrophages and NK cells through the injection of BCG or *C. parvum*. Intimate contact of the adjuvant with the tumour itself can produce dramatic results and one hopeful study records the beneficial effects of intrathoracic BCG in lung cancer. The status of interferon therapy is not yet clear. Interferon can be anti-mitotic; it augments NK activity and it can increase the expression of MHC products which might have an effect on immunogenicity. γ-Interferon is now becoming available through gene cloning and since it might have considerably higher anti-cancer potency than IFNα or -β, the results of clinical trials will be eagerly awaited.

Immunodiagnosis

Analysis of blood for the oncofetal antigens, α-fetoprotein in hepatoma and carcinoembryonic antigen in tumours, of the colon has provided valuable diagnostic information, but enthusiasm has been slightly curtailed by the knowledge that there is a high incidence of so-called 'false positives'. Reappearance of these proteins after surgical removal of the primary is strongly indicative of fresh tumour growth. The GM1 monosialoganglioside has been demonstrated in the blood of 96% of patients with pancreatic carcinoma and 64% of colorectal carcinomas as against 2% in normal subjects. Identification of the cell type by surface markers is of increasing value for the diagnosis and treatment of childhood leukaemias such as non-T, non-B ALL (p. 122).

Preliminary results on the localization of tumours *in vivo* by scanning after injection of radio-labelled monoclonal antibodies to oncofetal antigens holds promise that this will provide a useful adjunct to existing imaging techniques.

RELATION OF MHC TO THE COMPLEMENT SYSTEM

Class III genes controlling levels of C4, C2 and Factor B are all located within the major histocompatibility complex. Two C4 isotypes, C4A and C4B are present in each individual and were previously thought to be the red cell antigens, Rodgers and Chido respectively, because of their adsorption to the surface of erythrocytes. Both are highly polymorphic but C4A alleles seem to be less active than C4B and individuals may differ greatly in their ability to generate classical ($\overline{C4,2}$) C3 convertase activity even though possessing comparable molecular concentrations of plasma C4. C2 deficiency in man has been linked to the HLA-A10/Bw18 haplotype.

These genes therefore are concerned with C3 and the factors which react with it, viz. the classical (C4,2) and the alternative pathway (Factor B,C3b) enzymes which split C3, and their clustering in this region is provocative. Since a function of the MHC relates to the interaction between cells in the immune response, it is tempting to consider that complement-related signals might be concerned in some of these intercellular events.

ASSOCIATION WITH DISEASE

An impressive body of data is accumulating which links specific HLA antigens with particular disease states in the human (table 10.3) and even more striking relationships may be uncovered as the complexity of the HLA-D region is unravelled. The relationships are influenced by *linkage disequilibrium*, a state where closely linked genes on a chromosome tend to remain associated rather than undergo genetic randomization in a given population, so that the frequency of a pair of alleles occurring together is greater than the product of the individual gene frequencies (figure 10.22a). This could result from natural selection favouring a particular haplotype or from insufficient time elapsing since the first appearance of closely located alleles to allow them to become randomly distributed throughout the population. Be that as it may, a significant association between a disease and a given HLA-specificity does not imply that we have identified the disease susceptibility gene because we might find an even better correlation with another HLA gene in linkage disequilibrium with the first. To take an example: in multiple sclerosis, an association with the B7 allele was first established but when patients were typed for the D locus, a much stronger correlation with DR2 emerged (figure 10.22b). The initial correlation with B7 resulted from linkage disequilibrium between B7 and DR2. We still cannot be sure that DR2 itself is the disease susceptibility gene since, carrying the argument a stage further, one cannot exclude the possibility of finding an even greater association with another closely linked gene.

With the odd exception such as idiopathic haemochromatosis and congenital adrenal hyperplasia resulting from a 21-hydroxylase deficiency, HLA-linked diseases are intimately bound up with immunological processes. By and large, the HLA-D related disorders are autoimmune with a tendency for DR3 to be associated with organ-specific diseases involving cell-surface receptors. The question of some link between DR3 and these receptors has been mooted, though not with much confidence. It has also been suggested

Table 10.3.
Association
of HLA with
disease.

Disease	HLA allele	Relative risk
(a) Class II associated:		
Hashimoto's disease	DR5	3.2
Rheumatoid arthritis	DR4	5.8
Dermatitis herpetiformis	DR3	56.4
Chronic active hepatitis (autoimmune)	DR3	13.9
Coeliac disease	DR3	10.8
Sjögren's syndrome	DR3	9.7
Addison's disease (adrenal)	DR3	6.3
Insulin-dependent diabetes	DR3	5.0
	DR4	6.8
	DR3/4	14.3
	DR2	0.2
Thyrotoxicosis (Graves')	DR3	3.7
Primary myxoedema	DR3	5.7
Goodpasture's syndrome	DR2	13.1
Tuberculoid leprosy	DR2	8.1
Multiple sclerosis	DR2	4.8
(b) Class I, HLA-B27 associated:		
Ankylosing spondylitis	B27	87.4
Reiter's disease	B27	37.0
Post-salmonella arthritis	B27	29.7
Post-shigella arthritis	B27	20.7
Post-yersinia arthritis	B27	17.6
Post-gonococcal arthritis	B27	14.0
Uveitis	B27	14.6
Amyloidosis in rheumatoid arthritis	B27	8.2
(c) Other class I associations:		
Subacute thyroiditis	Bw35	13.7
Psoriasis vulgaris	Cw6	13.3
Idiopathic haemochromatosis	A3	8.2
Myasthenia gravis	B8	4.4

(Data mainly from Ryder *et al.*: see legend to figure 10.22b.)

that HLA antigens might also affect the susceptibility of a cell to viral attachment or infection, thereby influencing the development of autoimmunity to associated surface components.

Inevitably, because class II genes are dominant in these relationships (for the time-being), the temptation is to think in terms of immune response genes controlling the nature of the reaction to the relevant autoantigen or to whatever might be a causative agent. On this basis, DR3 and DR4 must influence separate but synergistic immune responses which mediate the onset of insulin-dependent diabetes. In both that disease and in rheumatoid arthritis, the DR2 allele is under-represented and DR2 positive patients have less severe disease, implying that DR2 might be considered a poor-

HLA Genes	Gene frequency %		
	Single gene	Paired genes Expected	Paired genes Observed
A1 B8	16 10	1.6	8.8
A3 B7	13 10	1.3	2.8

Figure 10.22. Linkage disequilibrium and the association between HLA and disease.

(a) Two examples of linkage disequilibrium. The expected frequency for a pair of genes is the product of each individual gene frequency. B8 and DR3 are in linkage disequilibrium as are B7 and DR2; thus the haplotypes A1, B8, DR3 and A3, B7, DR2 are *relatively* common.

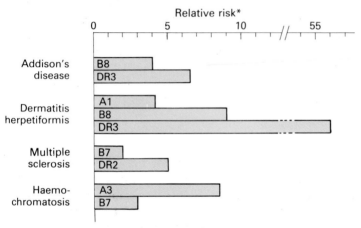

(b) Influence of linkage disequilibrium on disease association. *Relative risk: the increased chance of contracting the disease for individuals bearing the antigen relative to those lacking it. (Data from Ryder L.P., Andersen E. & Svejgaard A. (1979) HLA and disease Registry 1979. *Tissue Antigens*, Supplement.)

responder gene. In the case of multiple sclerosis where DR2 is a major risk factor, it is conceivable that these individuals are poor T-cell responders to measles since defective cell-mediated immunity to this virus is to date the only major immunological abnormality recognized. However, the B7 allele also correlates positively with an increased incidence of paralytic polio and with relatively poor T-cell activity *in vitro* for heterologous target cells. This raises another interpretation of this phenomenon, which does not necessarily exclude some contribution from immune response genes, in which it is postulated that individual DR alleles control overall cellular interactions and reactivity rather than individual antigenic specificities.

The association with HLA in ankylosing spondylitis is quite extraordinary; up to 95% of patients are of B27 phenotype as compared with around 5% in controls. The incidence of B27 is also markedly raised in other conditions when accompanied by sacroiliitis, e.g. Reiter's disease, acute anterior uveitis, psoriasis and other forms of infective sacro-iliitis such as yersinia, gonococcal and salmonella arthritis. The very close association with B27 makes it unlikely that as good a correlation with any other gene will be found. The involvement of infective agents may provide a clue: does molecular similarity to B27 imply a tolerance to certain microbial antigens, or is there some more subtle interaction with microbial products? Reports by Ebringer and colleagues of a cross-reaction of B27 with *Klebsiella pneumoniae* and a higher faecal carriage rate for these organisms in patients with active disease are certainly provocative in this respect.

Deficiencies in C4 and C2, which are MHC class III molecules, clearly predispose to the development of immune complex disease (p. 173) and so it would be expected that the inheritance of null genes or alleles coding for the less active complement allotypes would increase the risk of rheumatological disorders and add yet further complexity to the correlations between HLA types and disease.

Summary

Graft rejection is an immunological reaction: it shows specificity, the second set response is brisk, it is mediated by lymphocytes, and antibodies specific for the graft are formed. In each vertebrate species there is a major histocompatibility complex (MHC) which is responsible for provoking the most intense graft reactions. MHC antigens inherited from mother and father are co-dominantly expressed on the cell surface. The MHC in the mouse (H-2) is a complex region with two loci encoding the class I major classical transplantation antigens, H-2K and H-2D each with many polymorphic specificities defined by the antibodies they so readily evoke. The molecules contain two peptides, one of H-2 specificity and the other β_2-microglobulin. Another major region, I, codes for class II Ia molecules which provoke a mixed lymphocyte reaction of proliferation and blast transformation when genetically dissimilar lymphocytes interact; this reaction stimulates the formation of helper T-cells required for the generation of cytotoxic T-cells directed against H-2D/K class I determinants (cf. T-B co-operation with carrier-hapten), the process being termed cell-mediated lympholysis. Ia differences are largely responsible for the reaction of tolerated grafted lymphocytes against host antigens (g.v.h.). The genes in the whole MHC being closely linked tend to be inherited *en bloc* and are referred to as a haplotype. The MHC in man (HLA) consists of three loci (HLA-A, B and C) for class I antigens and three (HLA-DR, DC and SB) for the class II. Individuals are typed by cytotoxic antisera and by the mixed lymphocyte reaction for the original D locus. Siblings have a 1 : 4 chance of identity with respect to MHC.

Grafts are rejected either by sensitized T-cells or by antibody inducing platelet aggregation or type II hypersensitivity reactions (e.g. antibody-dependent cell-mediated cytotoxicity). Rejection may be prevented by: (a) tissue matching including the D-locus, (b) anti-mitotic drugs (e.g. azathioprine), anti-inflammatory steroids and anti-lymphocyte globulin which produce general immunosuppression, and a new drug cyclosporin A which is more selective, (c) antigen-specific depression through tolerance induction or enhancement by deliberate immunization.

Cornea and cartilage grafts are avascular and comparatively well tolerated. Kidney grafting has been the most widespread although immunosuppression must normally be continuous. Bone marrow grafts for immunodeficiency and aplastic anaemia are accepted from matched siblings but it is difficult to avoid g.v.h. disease with allogeneic marrow although this can be kept more under control with cyclosporin A.

The very high degree of polymorphism of the MHC may protect a species from molecular mimicry by parasites, maintain diversity of antigenic recognition and ensure heterozygosity ('hybrid vigour'). Differences between MHC of mother and fetus may be beneficial to the fetus but as a potential graft it must be protected against transplantation attack by the mother; suggested defence mechanisms are (i) lack of class II antigens on syncytiotrophoblast, (ii) mucopolysaccharide coat around trophoblast, and (iii) local production of immunosuppressant.

The MHC subserves recognition functions. The immune response (Ir) genes code for molecules (Ia) which in association with carrier determinants optimally regulate priming of T-cells by macrophage-processed antigen and interactions between T- and B-cells. Other MHC antigens are involved in the generation of cytotoxic T-cells in response to viral infection. Thus *the MHC would appear to be part of a system for signalling changes in 'self'* which enables the T-cells to make the appropriate immune response. Each cell in the body bears H-2D/K determinants so the cytotoxic T-cells use these to recognize a virally infected cell. The antigens of organisms such as TB, *Leishmania* and *Toxoplasma* which live within macrophages are processed to form an association with Ia on the macrophage surface which can stimulate 'delayed hypersensitivity' T-cells; these release factors enabling the macrophages to kill their intracellular parasites.

The immune surveillance theory of cancer postulates that changes in the surface of the neoplastic cell are recognized by the immune system and eliminated. However, although virally coded, idiotypic and oncofetal antigens may be detected on experimentally induced tumour cells together with components linked to cell division, the incidence of spontaneous cancers in immunosuppressed individuals is not generally higher than normal. Examples of immune responses to tumours in human cancer are known but attempts at control by immunization with tumour plus adjuvant have not been encouraging. Other strategies involve non-specific activation of macrophages and NK cells by adjuvants such as BCG, *C. parvum* and by interferon. Oncofetal antigens may be useful in diagnosis (e.g. α-fetoprotein in primary hepatoma) while monoclonal antibodies directed against them are being developed for tumour imaging *in vivo*.

Genes controlling C2, C4A, C4B and Factor B map in the MHC. HLA specificities are often associated with particular diseases, e.g. HLA-B27 with ankylosing spondylitis, B8 with myasthenia gravis, DR3 with autoimmune chronic active hepatitis, DR4 with rheumatoid arthritis and DR2 with multiple sclerosis.

Further reading

Batchelor J.R. & Welsh K.I. (1982) Association of HLA antigens with disease. In *Clinical Aspects of Immunology*, 4th edn. Lachmann P.J. & Peters D.K. (eds). Blackwell Scientific Publications, Oxford.

Billingham R. & Silvers W. (1971) *The Immunology of Transplantation*. Foundations of Immunology Series. Prentice-Hall, New Jersey.

Bodmer W.F. (ed.) (1978) The HLA system. *Brit. Med. Bull.* **34**, No. 3.

Castro J.E. (ed.) (1978) *Immunological Aspects of Cancer*. MTP Press, Lancaster.

Dausset J. & Hors J. (1973) Statistics of 416 consecutive kidney transplants in the France-Transplant organization. *Transpl. Proc.* **5**, 223.

Festenstein H. & Demant P. (1978) *Immunogenetics of the Major Histocompatibility System*. Edward Arnold, London.

Fudenberg H.H., Stites D.P., Caldwell J.L. & Wells J.V. (eds) (1980) *Basic & Clinical Immunology*, 3rd edn. Lange Medical Publications, Los Altos, California.

Hogarth P.J. (1982) *Immunological Aspects of Mammalian Reproduction*. Praeger, New York.

Lance E.M., Medawar P.B. & Taub R.N. (1973) Antilymphocyte serum. *Adv. Immunol.* **17**, 2.

McConnell I., Munro A. & Waldmann H. (1981) *The Immune System. A Course on the Molecular and Cellular Basis of Immunology*, 2nd edn. Blackwell Scientific Publications, Oxford.

Mitchinson N.A. (1982) Protective immunity (to tumours) *in vivo*. In *Clinical Aspects of Immunology*, 4th edn. Lachmann P. & Peters D.K. (eds). Blackwell Scientific Publications, Oxford.

Möller G. (ed.) (1979) Natural killer cells. *Immunol. Rev.* **44**.

Rose N.R., Bigazzi P.E. & Warner N.L. (eds) (1978) *Genetic Control of Autoimmune Disease*. Elsevier North-Holland, New York.

Smith, R.T. & Landy M. (1975) *Immunobiology of the Tumour—Host Relationship*. Academic Press, New York.

Yamamura T. & Tada T. (eds) (1984) *Progress in Immunology V*. Academic Press, Tokyo.

Zinkernagel R.M. & Doherty P.C. (1979) MHC-restricted cytotoxic T cells: studies on the biological role of polymorphic major transplantation antigens determining T-cell restriction—specificity, function and responsiveness. *Adv. Immunol.* **27**, 51.

11 Autoimmunity

The monumental repertoire of the adaptive immune system has evolved to allow it to recognize and ensnare virtually any shaped microbial molecules either at present in existence or yet to come, and in so doing, has been unable to avoid the generation of lymphocytes which react with the body's own constituents. We have already discussed the mechanisms which exist to prevent these self-components from provoking an immune response but, as with all machinery, there is always a chance that these systems might break down, and the older the individual, the greater the chance of a breakdown. When this happens *autoantibodies* (i.e. antibodies capable of reacting with 'self' components) are produced. Grabar is of the opinion that autoantibodies have a biological function to act as 'transporting' agents for cellular breakdown products thereby aiding their disposal. While antibodies can act in this way, we are here concerned more with autoimmune phenomena which appear in relation to certain defined human diseases. Ideally we wish to apply the term 'autoimmune disease' to those cases where it can be shown that the autoimmune process contributes to the pathogenesis of the disease rather than situations where apparently harmless autoantibodies are formed following tissue damage, e.g. heart antibodies appearing after a myocardial infarction. Yet the role of autoimmunity in many disorders is still not clearly defined, and it is as a matter of convenience that we will refer to all maladies firmly associated with autoantibody formation as 'autoimmune diseases', except where it can be shown that the immunological phenomena are purely secondary findings.

The spectrum of autoimmune diseases

These disorders may be looked upon as forming a spectrum. At one end we have '*organ-specific diseases*' with organ-specific autoantibodies. Hashimoto's disease of the thyroid is an example: there is a specific lesion in the thyroid involving infiltration by mononuclear cells (lymphocytes, histiocytes and plasma cells), destruction of follicular cells and germinal

Table 11.1. Spectrum of autoimmune diseases.

Organ specific◄──►Non-organ specific				
Hashimoto's thyroiditis	Myasthenia gravis	Autoimmune haemolytic	Primary biliary cirrhosis	Systemic lupus erythematosus
Primary myxoedema	Juvenile diabetes	anaemia	Active chronic hepatitis	(SLE)
Thyrotoxicosis	Goodpasture's syndrome	Idiopathic thrombocytopenic	HB_s-ve	Discoid LE
Pernicious anaemia	Pemphigus	purpura	Cryptogenic	Dermatomyositis
Autoimmune atrophic gastritis	vulgaris	Idiopathic leucopenia	cirrhosis (some cases)	Scleroderma
Addison's disease	Pemphigoid		Ulcerative	Rheumatoid arthritis
Premature meno-	Sympathetic ophthalmia		colitis	
pause (few cases)	Phacogenic		Sjögren's	
Male infertility (few cases)	uveitis		syndrome	
	(?? Multiple sclerosis ??)			

centre formation, accompanied, as we showed originally, by the production of circulating antibodies with absolute specificity for certain thyroid constituents (Roitt, Doniach & Campbell).

Moving towards the centre of the spectrum are those disorders where the lesion tends to be localized to a single organ but the antibodies are non-organ specific. A typical example would be primary biliary cirrhosis where the small bile ductule is the main target of inflammatory cell infiltration but the serum antibodies present—mainly mitochondrial—are not liver specific.

At the other end of the spectrum are the '*non-organ-specific diseases*' exemplified by systemic lupus erythematosus (SLE) where both lesions and autoantibodies are not confined to any one organ. Pathological changes are widespread and are primarily lesions of connective tissue with fibrinoid necrosis. They are seen in the skin (the 'lupus' butterfly rash on the face is characteristic), kidney glomeruli, joints, serous membranes and blood vessels. In addition the formed elements of the blood are often affected. A bizarre collection of autoantibodies are found some of which react with the DNA and other nuclear constituents of all cells in the body.

An attempt to fit the major diseases considered to be associated with autoimmunity into this spectrum is shown in table 11.1.

Autoantibodies in human disease

At this stage in the discussion it may be of value to have a more precise account of the major autoantibodies detected in the different diseases to provide a framework for reference. Table 11.2 documents a list of these antibodies and the methods employed in their detection. The notes following

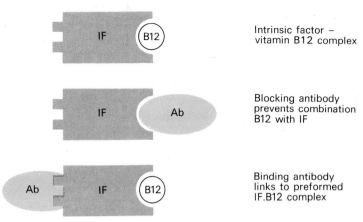

Intrinsic factor –
vitamin B12 complex

Blocking antibody
prevents combination
B12 with IF

Binding antibody
links to preformed
IF.B12 complex

Figure 11.1. Intrinsic factor autoantibodies: sites of determinants for binding and blocking. (Roitt I.M., Doniach D. & Shapland C. (1964) *Lancet* **II**, 469.)

the table amplify specific points while some of the tests are illustrated in figures 11.1, 11.2, 6.17 and 6.18.

Overlap of autoimmune disorders

There is a tendency for more than one autoimmune disorder to occur in the same individual and when this happens the association is often between diseases within the same region of the autoimmune spectrum (cf. table 11.1). Thus patients with autoimmune thyroiditis (Hashimoto's disease or primary myxoedema) have a much higher incidence of pernicious anaemia than would be expected in a random population matched for age and sex (10% as against 0.2%). Conversely both thyroiditis and thyrotoxicosis are diagnosed in pernicious anaemia patients with an unexpectedly high frequency. Other associations are seen between Addison's disease and autoimmune thyroid disease and in the rare cases of juveniles with pernicious anaemia and polyendocrinopathy which includes Addison's disease, hypoparathyroidism, diabetes and thyroiditis.

There is an even greater overlap in serological findings. 30% of patients with autoimmune thyroid disease have concomitant parietal cell antibodies in their serum. Conversely, thyroid antibodies have been demonstrated in up to 50% of pernicious anaemia patients. It should be stressed that these are not cross-reacting antibodies. The thyroid-specific antibodies will not react with stomach and *vice versa*. When a serum reacts with both organs it means that two populations of antibodies are present, one with specificity for thyroid and the other for stomach.

At the non-organic-specific end of the spectrum, SLE is clinically associated with rheumatoid arthritis and several

Table 11.2. Autoantibodies in human disease. (IFT = immunofluorescent test; CFT = complement fixation test.)

Disease	Antigen	Detection of antibody
Hashimoto's thyroiditis Primary myxoedema	Thyroglobulin	Precipitins; passive haemaggln.
	2nd colloid Ag (CA2)	IFT on fixed thyroid
	Cytoplasmic microsomes	IFT on unfixed thyroid; passive haemaggln.
	Cell surface	IFT on viable thyroid cells; C′-mediated cytotoxicity
Thyrotoxicosis	Cell surface TSH receptors	Bioassay—stimulation of mouse thyroid *in vivo*; blocking combination TSH with receptors; stimulation adenyl cyclase
	'Growth' receptors	Induction of cell division in thyroid fragments
Pernicious anaemia[1]	Intrinsic factor	Neutralization; blocking combination with vit-B_{12}; binding to Int.Fact-B_{12} by copptn.
	Parietal cell microsomes	IFT on unfixed gastric mucosa
Addison's disease	Cytoplasm adrenal cells	IFT on unfixed adrenal cortex
Premature onset of menopause[2]	Cytoplasm steroid-producing cells	IFT on adrenal and interstitial cells of ovary and testis
Male infertility (some)[3]	Spermatozoa	Sperm agglutination in ejaculate
Insulin-dependent (juvenile) diabetes[4]	Cytoplasm of islet cells	IFT on unfixed human pancreas
	Cell surface	IFT on isolated cells
Type B insulin resistance c̄ acanthosis nigricans	Insulin receptor	Block hormone binding to receptor Radioimmunoassay with purified receptor
Atopic allergy (some)	β-Adrenergic receptor	Blocking radioassay with hydroxybenzylpindolol
Myasthenia gravis	Skeletal and heart muscle	IFT on skeletal muscle
	Acetyl choline receptor	Blocking or binding radioassay with α-bungarotoxin
(Multiple sclerosis)	Brain	Cytotoxic effects on cerebellar cultures by serum and lymphocytes (? secondary to disease)
Goodpasture's syndrome	Glomerular and lung basement membrane	Linear staining by IFT of kidney biopsy with fluorescent anti-IgG Radioimmunoassay with purified Ag
Pemphigus vulgaris	Desmosomes between prickle cells in epidermis	IFT on skin
Pemphigoid	Basement membrane	IFT on skin
Phacogenic uveitis	Lens	Passive haemagglutination
Sympathetic ophthalmia	Uvea	(Delayed skin reaction to uveal extract)
Autoimmune haemolytic anaemia[5]	Erythrocytes	Coombs' antiglobulin test
Idiopathic thrombocytopenic purpura	Platelets	Shortened platelet survival *in vivo*
Primary biliary cirrhosis	Mitochondria (mainly)	IFT on mitochondria-rich cells (e.g. distal tubules of kidney)
Active chronic hepatitis (HB$_s$-ve)	Smooth muscle, nuclei	IFT (e.g. on gastric mucosa)
	Cell surface lipoprotein	Leucocyte cytotoxicity
Ulcerative colitis	Colon 'lipopoly-saccharide'	IFT; passive haemaggln. (cytotoxic action of lymphocytes on colon cells)
Sjögren's syndrome[6]	Ducts, mitochondria, nuclei, thyroid	IFT
	IgG	Antiglobulin (rheumatoid factor) tests

Table 11.2. (*contd.*)

Disease	Antigen	Detection of antibody
Rheumatoid arthritis[7]	IgG	Antiglobulin tests: latex aggln., sheep red cell aggln. test (SCAT; commercial product, RAHA test) and radioassay
	RANA[8]	IFT on EB-transformed cell line
	Collagen	Passive haemaggln.
Discoid lupus erythematosus ⎱	Nuclear	IFT
Dermatomyositis	IgG	Antiglobulin tests
Scleroderma[9] ⎰		
Mixed connective tissue disease[10]	Extractable nuclear	IFT; countercurrent electro-phoresis
Systemic lupus erythematosus	DNA	Radioassay[11]; pptn; CFT
	Nucleoprotein	IFT; latex aggln. L.E. cells[12]
	Cytoplasmic sol.Ag	'Non-organ sp.CFT'
	Array of other Ag incl. formed elements of blood, clotting factors, IgG and Wasserman antigen	'Biological false positive' CFT

Notes:

1 Two major types of antibody to intrinsic factor are detected, viz. blocking and binding (figure 11.1). Binding antibody combines with preformed Int.Fact.—radioactive B_{12} ($*B_{12}$) complex which can then be precipitated at 50% ammonium sulphate (cf. Farr test—salt copptn., p. 151) and the radioactivity in the precipitate counted. Blocking antibody prevents binding of $*B_{12}$ to Int.Fact. and the uncombined $*B_{12}$ can then be adsorbed to charcoal and counted.

2 Antibodies occur in the minority of patients with associated Addison's disease.

3 Only small percentage show agglutinins. Spermatozoa may be agglutinated head to head, tail to tail or joined through their mid-piece. Seen also in small percentage of infertile women.

4 Most if not all insulin-dependent diabetics have islet cell antibodies at some stage during the first year of onset. In contrast, islet cell antibodies in diabetic patients with an associated autoimmune polyendocrinopathy persist for many years.

5 The Coombs' test involves the demonstration of bound antibody on the washed red cell by agglutination with an antiglobulin. Erythrocyte autoantibodies, which bind well over the temperature range $0–37°C$ ('warm' Ab), are mostly IgG; approximately 60 per cent of cases are primary, the remainder being associated with other autoimmune disorders, e.g. SLE, ulcerative colitis. 'Cold' Ab, which react best over the range $0–20°C$, are mostly IgM and red cells coated with this Ab can often be agglutinated by anti-complement sera; approximately half are primary, the others being associated with *Mycoplasma pneumoniae* infection or generalized neoplastic disease of the lymphoreticular tissues.

6 Antibodies specifically reacting with the epithelium of salivary gland excretory ducts are demonstrable by immunofluorescence in up to half the cases.

7 The main antiglobulin factors react with the Fc portion of IgG which is usually adsorbed on to latex particles (human IgG) or present in an antigen–antibody complex (sheep red cells coated with sub-agglutinating dose of rabbit antibody). In the radioassay test, rabbit IgG is bound to a plastic tube, patient's serum added and the antiglobulin bound assessed by subsequent binding of labelled anti-human IgG or IgM (cf. p. 152). Rheumatoid factors specific for human IgG can be detected by this test using human Fcγ to coat the tubes and labelled anti-human Fdγ or IgM for the final stage.

8 The rheumatoid arthritis nuclear antigen (RANA) is revealed as speckled staining by IFT using cells transformed by EB virus; normal cells are negative.

9 In scleroderma (progressive systemic sclerosis) antinucleolar antibodies are frequently found.

10 This syndrome combines features of scleroderma, rheumatoid arthritis, SLE and dermatomyositis. The antigen is an extractable nuclear antigen which gives speckled fluorescence and RNase-sensitive precipitation by countercurrent electrophoresis.

11 Antibodies to single or double-stranded DNA are assayed by the Farr test (cf. p. 151) using labelled Ag, or by a DNA-coated tube test similar to the radioassay for antiglobulins (note 7 above).

12 When blood from an SLE patient is incubated at $37°C$, some white cells are damaged and allow the entry of antibodies. Certain of the antibodies combining with the nuclear surface bind complement and attract polymorphs which strip away the cytoplasm and engulf the nucleus. The polymorph containing the engulfed homogenized nucleus is called an LE-cell.

other diseases which are themselves uncommon: haemolytic anaemia, idiopathic leucopenia and thrombocytopenic purpura, dermatomyositis and Sjögren's syndrome. Anti-nuclear antibodies, non-organic-specific complement fixation reactions, and anti-globulin (rheumatoid) factors are a general feature of these disorders.

Sjögren's syndrome occupies an interesting position (table 11.3); aside from the clinical and serological features associated with non-organ-specific disease mentioned above, characteristics of an organ-specific disorder are evident. Antibodies reacting with salivary ducts are demonstrable and there is an abnormally high incidence of thyroid autoantibodies; histologically the affected lacrimal and salivary glands reveal changes of a similar nature to those seen in Hashimoto's disease, namely a replacement of the glandular elements by patchy lymphocytic and plasma cell granulomatous tissue. Associations between diseases at the two ends of the spectrum have been reported, but, as might be predicted from the serological data (table 11.3), they are not common.

There is still no entirely satisfactory explanation to account for the rare tendency to develop hypo-gammaglobulinaemia and the increased incidence of certain cancers occurring in autoimmune disease. Patients with organ-specific disorders are slightly more prone to develop cancer in the affected organ whereas generalized lympho-reticular neoplasia shows up with uncommon frequency in non-organ-specific disease.

Genetic factors in autoimmune disease

Autoimmune phenomena tend to aggregate in certain families. For example, the first degree relatives (sibs, parents and children) of patients with Hashimoto's disease show a high incidence of thyroid autoantibodies (figure 11.3) and of overt

Figure 11.2. (a) Thyroid microsomal antibodies staining cytoplasm of acinar cells. (b) PHA-stimulated thyroid cell in culture showing surface staining for the microsomal antigen (orange rhodamine conjugate) and HLA-DR (green fluorescein conjugate). (c) Fluorescence of cells in the pancreatic islets of Langerhans after treatment with serum from insulin-dependent diabetic. (d) The same showing cells stained simultaneously for somatostatin (the yellow cells are stained with rhodamine anti-somatostatin and fluorescein anti-human IgG which localizes the bound patient's autoantibody). (e) Serum of patient with Addison's disease staining cytoplasm of monkey adrenal granulosa cells. (f) Fluorescence of distal tubular cells of the kidney after reaction with mitochondrial autoantibodies. (g) Diffuse nuclear staining on a thyroid section obtained with nucleoprotein antibodies from an SLE patient. (h) Serum of a scleroderma patient staining the nucleoli of SV-40-transformed human keratinocytes (K14) in monolayer culture. ((a)–(g) courtesy of Dr G.F. Bottazzo; (b) taken from Pujol-Borrell R., Hanafusa T., Chiovata L. & Bottazzo G.F. (1983) *Nature* **303**, 5921; (h) courtesy of Dr F.T. Woj-narowska.)

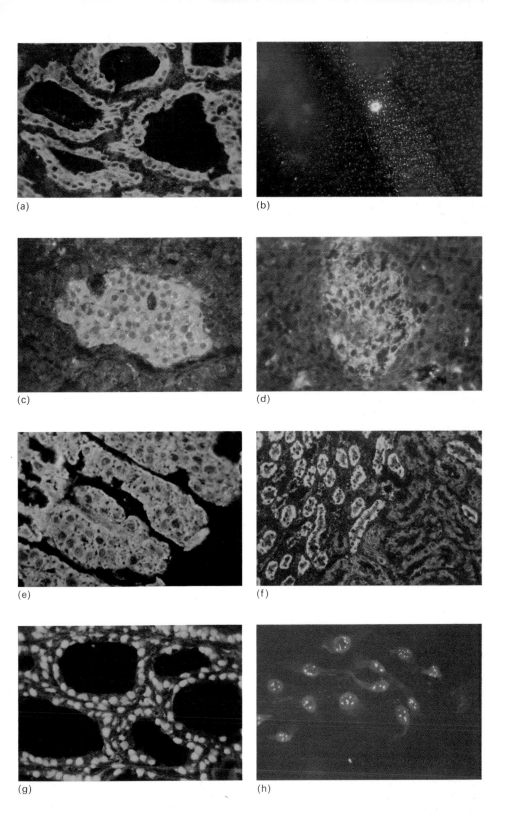

Table 11.3. Organ-specific and non-organ-specific serological interrelationships in human disease.

Disease	% Positive reactions for antibodies to:				
	Thyroid*	Stomach*	Nuclei*	Non-organ-specific antigen**	IgG†
Hashimoto's thyroiditis	99.9	32	8	5	2
Pernicious anaemia	55	89	11	7	
Sjögren's syndrome	45	14	56	19	75
Rheumatoid arthritis	11	16	50	10	75
SLE	2	2	99	66	35
Controls‡	0–15	0–16	0–19	0–10	2–5

* Immunofluorescence test   ** CFT with kidney   † Rheumatoid factor classical tests
‡ Incidence increases with age and females > males

and subclinical thyroiditis. Interestingly there is also an increased frequency of 'non-immunological' thyroid disorders, such as non-toxic nodular goitre. The proportion with autoantibodies is higher in those families where more than one member is clinically affected. Parallel studies have disclosed similar relationships in the families of pernicious anaemia patients in that gastric parietal cell antibodies are prevalent in the relatives who are wont to develop achlorhydria and atrophic gastritis. Familial aggregation of mito-

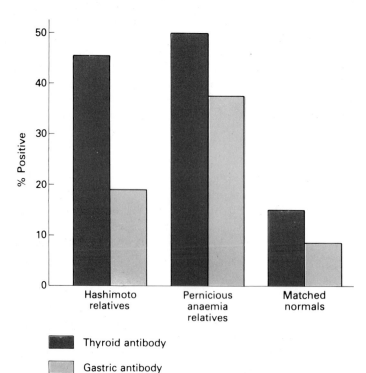

Figure 11.3. The high incidence of thyroid and gastric autoantibodies in the first degree relatives of patients with Hashimoto's disease or pernicious anaemia. Note the overlap of gastric and thyroid autoimmunity and the higher incidence of gastric autoantibodies in pernicious anaemia relatives. (Data from Doniach D. & Roitt I.M. (1964) *Semin. Haematol.* **I**, 313.)

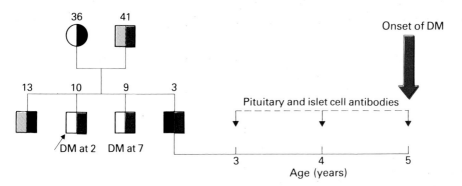

Figure 11.4. HLA-haplotype linkage and onset of insulin-dependent diabetes (DM). Haplotypes: ▨ A3, B14, DR6; ■ A3, B7, DR4; ▦ A28, B51, DR4; and ▨ A2, B62, C3, DR4. Disease is linked to possession of the A2, B62, C3, DR4 haplotype. The 3-year-old sister had complement-fixing antibodies to the islet cell surface for 2 years before developing frank diabetes. (From Gorsuch A.N. *et al.* (1981) *Lancet* **II**, 1363.)

chondrial antibodies has been observed, albeit to a lesser extent, in primary biliary cirrhosis. Turning to SLE, disturbances of immunoglobulin synthesis and a susceptibility to develop 'connective tissue diseases' have been reported but there are some conflicting accounts still not resolved.

These familial relationships could be ascribed to environmental factors such as an infective micro-organism, but there is evidence that one or more genetic components must be given serious consideration. In the first place, when thyrotoxicosis occurs in twins there is a greater concordance rate (i.e. both twins affected) in identical than in non-identical twins. Secondly, thyroid autoantibodies are more prevalent in individuals with ovarian dysgenesis having X-chromosome aberrations such as XO and particularly the iso-chromosome X abnormality. Furthermore, there are strong associations between several autoimmune diseases and particular HLA specificities, e.g. DR3 in Addison's disease and DR4 in rheumatoid arthritis (Table 10.3, p. 305). Figure 11.4 shows a multiplex family, with insulin-dependent diabetes in which the disease is linked to a particular HLA-haplotype. Since only very restricted determinants on the autoantigenic molecules evoke autoantibodies (e.g. thyroglobulin of molecular weight 650,000, has a valency of only 4), one is tempted to think in terms of Ir genes, it being precisely under such conditions that Ir genes can be recognized.

It is also worthy of note that lines of animals have been bred which spontaneously develop autoimmune disease. In other words, the autoimmunity is genetically programmed. There is an Obese line of chickens with autoimmune thyroiditis and the New Zealand Black (NZB) mouse with autoimmune haemolytic anaemia. The hybrid of NZB with another strain, the New Zealand White (B × W hybrid), actually develops LE-cells, antinuclear antibodies and a fatal immune complex induced glomerulonephritis. Suitable intercross and backcross breeding of these mice has established that a *minimum* of three genes determines the expression of autoimmunity and that the production of both red cell and nuclear antibodies may be under separate genetic control, i.e. there may be different factors predisposing to autoimmunity on the one hand, and to the selection of antigen on the other. This view finds support in the genetic analysis of Obese chickens which has delineated an influence of the MHC, abnormalities in T-cell control and a defect in the thyroid gland.

The facts presented by human autoimmune disease also attest to multifactorial control. The overlaps in autoantibodies and disease discussed above point to a general tendency to develop autoimmunity in these individuals and further, the factors which predispose to organ-specific disease must be different from those in non-organ-specific disorders (as judged by the minimal overlap between them). There must be additional factors which are organ-related in that relatives of patients with pernicious anaemia are more prone to gastric autoimmunity than members of Hashimoto families (figure 11.3).

Autoantibodies are demonstrable in comparatively low titre in the general population and the incidence of positive results increases steadily with age (figure 11.5) up to around

Figure 11.5. Incidence of autoantibodies in the general population. A serum was considered positive for thyroid antibodies if it reacted at a dilution of 1/10 in the tanned red cell test or neat in the immunofluorescent test and positive for antinuclear antibodies if it reacted at a dilution of 1/4 by immunofluorescence.

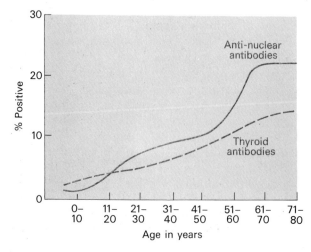

60–70 years. In the case of the thyroid and stomach at least, biopsy has indicated that the presence of antibody is almost invariably associated with minor thyroiditis or gastritis lesions (as the case may be), and it is of interest that post-mortem examination has identified 10% of middle-aged women with significant degrees of lymphadenoid change in the thyroid similar in essence to that characteristic of Hashimoto's disease.

The point should also be made here that, in general, autoantibodies and autoimmune diseases are found more frequently in women than in men.

Aetiology of autoimmune response

How do autoantibodies arise? Our earliest view, with respect to organ-specific antibodies at least, was that the antigens were sequestered within the organ, and through lack of contact with the lymphoreticular system failed to establish immunological tolerance. Any mishap which caused a release of the antigen would then provide an opportunity for auto-antibody formation. For a few body constituents this holds true and in the case of sperm, lens and heart for example, release of certain components directly into the circulation can provoke autoantibodies. But in general, the experience has been that injection of *unmodified* extracts of those tissues concerned in the organ-specific autoimmune disorders does not readily elicit antibody formation. Indeed detailed investigation of the thyroid autoantigen, thyroglobulin, has disclosed that it is not completely sequestered within the gland but gains access to the extracellular fluid around the follicles and leaves via the thyroid lymphatics (figure 11.6) reaching the serum in normal human subjects at concentrations of approximately 0.01–0.05 μg/ml. In fact, in the majority of cases—e.g. red cells in autoimmune haemolytic anaemia, DNA released from dying cells in SLE and surface receptors in many cases of organ-specific autoimmunity—the autoantigens are accessible to circulating lymphocytes.

There is also mounting evidence that auto-reactive B- and T-cells are present normally. A small proportion of the B-cells in normal individuals bind autoantigens such · as human thyroglobulin, myelin basic protein and DNA, through their surface receptors. Furthermore, the B-cells in a wide range of vertebrate hosts can be persuaded by various means to synthesize autoantibodies which react with these antigens. Almost certainly the lymphocytes which bind the autoantigens include the population which produces the autoantibodies, a view sustained by 'antigen suicide' experiments in which lymphocytes from thyroglobulin-primed animals fail to make antibodies when challenged in a second-

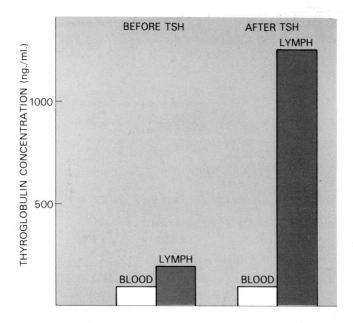

Figure 11.6. Thyroglobulin in the cervical lymph draining the thyroid in the rat. The concentration of thyroglobulin is increased after injection of pituitary thyroid stimulating hormone (TSH) suggesting that the release from thyroid follicles is linked to the physiological activity of the acinar cells. (From Daniel P.N., Pratt O.E., Roitt I.M. & Torrigiani G. (1967) *Quart.J.Exp.Physiol.* **52**, 184.)

ary host if they are allowed to bind thyroglobulin of very high specific radioactivity *in vitro* before transfer; the implication is that cells binding the 'hot' antigen through surface receptors are inactivated by irradiation.

Auto-reactive T-cells can also be demonstrated—witness the establishment of T-cell lines *in vitro* which react specifically with myelin basic protein, thyroglobulin and other autoantigens such as collagen. In addition, self-reactive effector T-cells have been generated when lymphocytes have been cultured with a variety of autologous tissues in the presence of an agent such as a mitogenic lectin or fetal calf serum. The message then is that we are all sitting on a minefield of potentially self-reactive cells, with access to their respective autoantigens, but since autoimmune disease is more the exception than the rule, the body must have homeostatic mechanisms to prevent them being triggered under normal circumstances. Accepting its limitations, figure 11.7 provides a framework for us to examine ways in which these mechanisms may be circumvented to allow autoimmunity to develop. It is assumed that the key to the system is control of the auto-reactive T-inducer/helper cell. Presumably these cells are unresponsive because of clonal deletion, T-suppression or failure of autoantigen presentation.

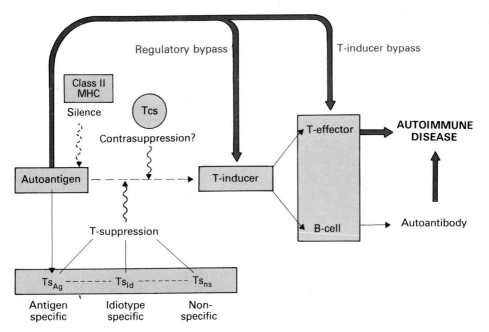

Figure 11.7. The control of auto-reactivity. The constraints on the stimulation of autoantigen with self-reactive inducer/helper T-cell can be circumvented either through bypassing the inducer cell or by disturbance of the regulatory mechanisms.

T-INDUCER BYPASS MECHANISMS

Provision of new carrier determinant

Allison and Weigle argued independently that if auto-reactive T-cells are tolerized and thereby unable to collaborate with B-cells to generate autoantibodies, provision of new carrier determinants to which no self-tolerance had been established would bypass this mechanism and lead to auto-antibody production (figure 11.8).

(i) *Modification of the autoantigen* A new carrier could arise through some modification to the molecule, for example, by defects in synthesis or by an abnormality in lysosomal breakdown yielding a split product exposing some new groupings. Experimentally it has been found that large proteolytic fragments of thyroglobulin are autoantigenic when injected alone but no evidence for such a mechanism has yet been uncovered in man. In fact studies on spontaneous autoimmune disease have never revealed any abnormality in the antigen. Consider the following as an illustration. Neonatal thyroidectomy prevents the spontaneous development of thyroglobulin autoantibodies in Obese strain chickens; however, these animals will now make autoantibodies if injected with thyroglobulin prepared from *normal* chickens suggesting that

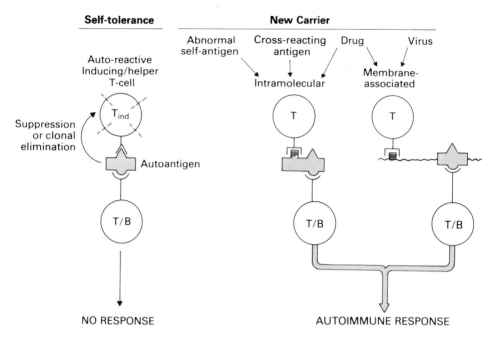

Figure 11.8. T-inducer bypass through new carrier determinant generates auto-immunity.

the immunological response rather than the antigen is abnormal.

Incorporation into Freund's complete adjuvant frequently endows many autologous proteins with the power to induce autoallergic disease in laboratory animals. It is conceivable that the physical constraints on the proteins at the water–oil interface of the emulsion provide the required alteration in configuration of the 'carrier portions' of the molecules.

Modification can also be achieved through combination with a drug. The autoimmune haemolytic anaemia associated with administration of α-methyl dopa might be attributable to modification of the red-cell surface in such a way as to provide a carrier for stimulating B-cells which recognize the rhesus *e* antigen. This is normally regarded as a 'weak' antigen and would be less likely to induce B-cell tolerance than the 'stronger' antigens present on the erythrocyte. Isoniazid may produce arthritis associated with nuclear antibodies and unlike most other cases of drug-induced autoimmunity, synthesis of these antibodies is said to continue after cessation of drug therapy. A high proportion of patients on continued treatment with procainamide develop nuclear antibodies and 40% present with clinical signs of SLE. Myasthenia gravis and symptoms of pemphigus have been described in some patients on penicillamine. It is not clear in every case whether the drug provides carrier help through direct modification of the autoantigen or of some independent molecule concerned in associative recognition.

(ii) *Cross-reactions* Many examples are known in which potential autoantigenic determinants are present on an exogenous cross-reacting antigen which provides the new carrier that provokes autoantibody formation. Post-rabies vaccine encephalitis is thought to result from an autoimmune reaction to brain initiated by heterologous brain tissue in the vaccine (cf. experimental allergic encephalomyelitis below). Some micro-organisms carry determinants which cross react with the human and this may prove to be an important way of inducing autoimmunity. In rheumatic fever antibodies produced to the streptococcus also react with heart, and the sera of 50% of children with the disease who develop Sydenham's chorea give neuronal immunofluorescent staining which can be absorbed out with streptococcal membranes. Colon antibodies present in ulcerative colitis have been found to cross-react with *Escherichia coli* 014. There is also some evidence for the view that antigens common to *Trypanosoma cruzi* and cardiac muscle provoke some of the immunopathological lesions seen in Chagas' disease.

(iii) *Associative recognition* This term applies to the phenomenon in which one membrane component may provide help for the immune response to another. In the context of autoimmunity, a new helper determinant may arise through drug modification as mentioned above, or through the insertion of viral antigen into the membrane of an infected cell. That this can promote a reaction to a pre-existing cell component is clear from the studies in which infection of a tumour with influenza virus elicited resistance to uninfected tumour cells. The appearance of cold agglutinins often with blood group I specificity after *Mycoplasma pneumonia* infection could have a similar explanation.

Idiotype bypass

Knowing that T-helpers with specificity for the idiotype on a lymphocyte receptor can be instrumental in the stimulation of that cell (figure 4.15, p. 109), it is conceivable that an environmental agent such as a parasite or virus which triggered antibody carrying a public idiotype (CRI) which happened to be shared with the receptor of an auto-reactive T- or B-cell, could provoke an autoimmune response (Cooke & Lydyard). The same thing could happen if the CRI was similar in shape to a determinant on the environmental antigen (figure 11.9). The occurrence of major cross-reactive idiotypes associated with the DNA autoantibodies in

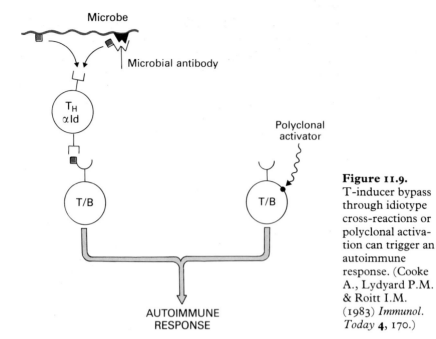

Microbe

Microbial antibody

T_H
αId

T/B

Polyclonal
activator

T/B

AUTOIMMUNE
RESPONSE

Figure 11.9.
T-inducer bypass
through idiotype
cross-reactions or
polyclonal activa-
tion can trigger an
autoimmune
response. (Cooke
A., Lydyard P.M.
& Roitt I.M.
(1983) *Immunol.
Today* **4**, 170.)

(NZB × NZW)F1 and MRL mice and the autoantibodies in
rheumatoid arthritis, SLE and Hashimoto's disease, lend
some credence to this view.

Polyclonal activation

Microbes often display adjuvant properties through their
possession of polyclonal lymphocyte activators such as bacterial endotoxins which may act by providing the second
(non-specific) inductive signal for B-cell stimulation (p. 72),
so bypassing the need for specific T-cell help (figure 11.9).
This can occur by direct interaction with the B-lymphocyte
or indirectly through stimulating the secretion of non-
specific factors from T-cells or macrophages. A good
example is the thymus-dependent production of autoantibodies by injection of mice with thyroglobulin and endotoxin
(LPS). The variety of autoantibodies detected in cases with
infectious mononucleosis must surely be attributable to the
polyclonal activation of B-cells by EB virus. They are seen
also in lepromatous leprosy where the abundance of mycobacteria reproduces some of the features of Freund's adjuvant. However, unlike the usual situation in human
autoimmune disease, these autoantibodies tend to be IgM
and, in addition, do not persist when the microbial components are cleared from the body. Curiously, lymphocytes
from mice with spontaneous autoimmunity (e.g. NZB)
produce abnormally large amounts of IgM when cultured *in*

vitro as if they were under polyclonal activation; so do lymphocytes from many patients with SLE. On the other hand, the failure of neonatally thyroidectomized Obese strain chickens to make thyroglobulin autoantibodies (p. 323) implies that autoantigen itself is needed for the induction of autoimmunity, in organ-specific disease at least, although the possible need for spontaneous production of accessory signals as in the thyroglobulin/LPS experiment just cited, cannot be excluded.

REGULATORY BYPASS MECHANISMS

Failure of suppressor circuits

It should be emphasized that these T-inducer bypass mechanisms for the induction of autoimmunity do not by themselves ensure the continuation of the response, since normal animals have been shown to be capable of damping down autoantibody production through T-suppressor interactions as, for example, in the case of red cell autoantibodies induced in mice by injection of rat erythrocytes (figure 11.10). When T-suppressor activity is impaired by low doses of cyclophosphamide or if strains like the SJL which have prematurely ageing suppressors are used, autoimmunity is prolonged and more severe.

In general, manipulations which reduce T-suppressors encourage the development of autoantibodies. Thus, irradiated mice reconstituted with spleen cells deprived of Lyt 2

Figure 11.10. Regulation of self-reactivity. When CBA mice are injected with rat red cells, autoantibodies are produced by this cross-reacting antigen (p. 325) which coat the host erythrocytes and are detected by the Coombs' test (p. 315). The SJL strain, in which suppressor activity declines rapidly with age, is unable to regulate the autoimmune response and develops particularly severe disease. The response is also prolonged in the autoimmune NZB strain (after A. Cooke & P. Hutchings).

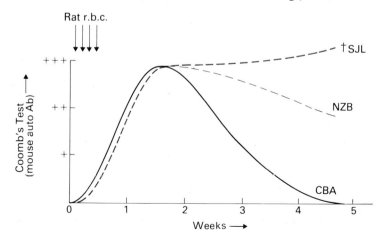

positive T-cells produce antibodies to thyroglobulin, nuclei and lymphocytes. When rats were thymectomized at a few weeks of age and given divided doses of X-rays, they developed thyroglobulin autoantibodies and thyroiditis. Neonatal thymectomy which greatly depletes the T-suppressor population, induces or exacerbates spontaneous autoimmune states in susceptible animals—autoimmune haemolytic anaemia in NZB mice and thyroiditis in Obese strain chickens and Buffalo rats. Coombs' positivity (i.e. the state in which circulating red cells are coated with antibody) can be transferred with the spleen cells of a Coombs' positive NZB to a young negative mouse of the same strain, but the continued production of red cell antibodies is short-lived unless the recipient's T-cells are first depleted by pretreatment with anti-lymphocyte serum. Other changes seen with age in the NZB are an increasing resistance to the induction of tolerance to soluble proteins and a sudden fall in the plasma concentration of the thymic peptide thymulin (p. 118) before the onset of disease (note: thymulin is said to inhibit the auto-reactive response of spleen cells to syngeneic fibroblasts in culture). Thus, there is a widely held view that one defect in the NZB is a progressive loss of T-suppressors with age and it is relevant that Lyt 1,2 cells which are needed for the induction of suppressors are low in diseased mice. Defects are possible at various other control points in the regulatory mechanism: for example, another mutant mouse strain with a spontaneous SLE-like syndrome, the MRL/l, has ample numbers of effective Lyt 1,2 cells but Lyt 1 helpers are resistant to their suppressor action.

This raises another possibility. A sub-population of Lyt 1^+2^- cells with binding sites for the lectin *Vicia villosa* are said to have *contrasuppressor* activity in so far as they protect T-helpers from the influence of suppressor cells. While this area is still relatively unexplored, it requires no gigantic leap of imagination to realize that undue activity by such cells will lower the threshold for autoimmunity (figure 11.11).

Less is known of regulatory circuits in man although there is increasing evidence that non-specific T-suppressor function in SLE may be poorly regulated. B-lymphocytes from patients with active disease secrete larger amounts of Ig when cultured *in vitro* than normal B-cells. Concanavalin A-induced non-specific suppressors are reduced or absent and T_G cells which suppress pokeweed mitogen-stimulated lymphocytes (p. 104) are low, the defect being greater the more active the disease. The production of thymulin and of interleukin-2 is also depressed in these patients. A significant proportion of clinically unaffected close relatives also demonstrate abnormally low levels of non-specific suppressors indicating that the deficit in SLE patients is not a consequence of

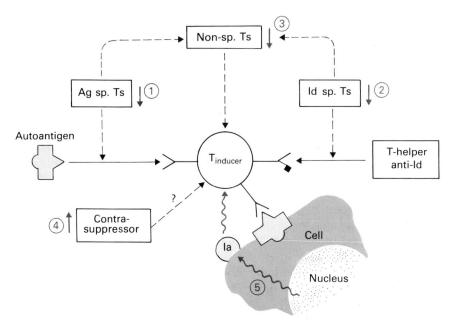

Figure 11.11. Bypass of regulatory mechanisms leads to triggering of auto-reactive T-inducer cell through defects in (1) antigen-specific, (2) idiotype-specific or (3) non-specific suppressors, through (4) stimulation of contrasuppressors or (5) derepression of class II genes with inappropriate cellular expression of Ia.

the illness or its treatment and that additional factors must be implicated in the causation of disease.

In any case, it is difficult to account for the antigenic specificity of different autoimmune disorders on the basis of a generalized depression of non-specific suppressors alone, without invoking defects in either antigen- or idiotype-specific suppressor T-cells (figure 11.11). There is, however, a further possibility which is both novel and exciting.

Inappropriate Ia expression

The majority of organ-specific autoantigens normally appear on the surface of the cells of the target organ in the context of class I but not class II MHC molecules. As such they cannot communicate with T-inducers and are therefore immunologically silent (Mitchison; p. 114). Bottazzo and colleagues reasoned that if the class II genes were somehow derepressed and Ia molecules were now synthesized, they would endow the surface molecules with potential autoantigenicity (figure 11.11). Indeed, they have been able to show that human thyroid cells in tissue culture can be persuaded to express HLA-DR (Ia) molecules on their surface after stimulation with the plant lectin, phytohaemagglutinin (figure 11.2b, p. 316), and further, that the cytoplasm of epithelial cells from the glands of patients with Graves' disease (thyrotoxicosis) stains strongly with anti-HLA-DR reagents, indicating active synthesis of class II polypeptides.

The autoimmune diseases have a multifactorial aetiology. Perhaps most, if not all, the defects we have discussed may contribute in different combinations to different disorders. Although these defects individually may be not uncommon, their origin remains obscure. They might be the consequence of some subtle virus infection, perhaps of the target organ in the case of organ-specific disease and of the lymphoid system at the non-organ-specific pole; the shedding of tremendous amounts of a C type oncornavirus from NZB T-cell lines may be of relevance to this. Or one may be dealing with some ageing process affecting the thymus or the lymphoid stem cells. Sex hormones may also contribute to the increased frequency of autoimmunity in females. Thus, oopherectomy and testosterone treatment alleviate the disease in female (NZB × NZW)F1 hybrids.

Pathogenic mechanisms in autoimmune disease

We have mentioned that despite certain exceptions as, for instance, myocardial infarction or damage to the testis, traumatic release of organ constituents does not in general elicit antibody formation. Destruction of thyroid tissue by therapeutic doses of radio-iodine does not initiate thyroid autoimmunity, nor does damage to the liver in alcoholic cirrhosis result in the synthesis of mitochondrial antibodies, to give but two examples. We should now look at the evidence which bears directly on the issue of whether autoimmunity, however it arises, plays a *primary* pathogenic role in the production of tissue lesions in the group of diseases labelled as 'autoimmune'.

EFFECTS OF HUMORAL ANTIBODY

Blood

The erythrocyte antibodies play a role in the destruction of red cells in autoimmune haemolytic anaemia. Normal red cells coated with autoantibody eluted from Coombs' positive erythrocytes have a shortened half-life after reinjection into the normal subject. Platelet antibodies are apparently responsible for idiopathic thrombocytopenic purpura (ITP). IgG from a patient's serum when given to a normal individual causes a depression of platelet counts and the active principle can be absorbed out with platelets. The transient neonatal thrombocytopenia which may be seen in infants of mothers with ITP is explicable in terms of transplacental passage of IgG antibodies to the child.

Some children with immunodeficiency associated with very low white cell counts have a serum lymphocytotoxic factor which requires complement for its activity. Lymphopenia occurring in patients with SLE and rheumatoid arthritis may also be a direct result of antibody since non-agglutinating antibodies coating the white cells have been reported.

Thyroid

Cytotoxic antibodies The serum of patients with Hashimoto's disease is cytotoxic for human thyroid cells growing in monolayer culture after dispersal by trypsin. This is a typical complement-mediated antibody reaction directed against a cell surface antigen which is identical with the microsomal antigen revealed by intracytoplasmic staining of thyroid sections with sera from Hashimoto patients. Curiously, this antigen is expressed only on the apical portion of the follicular cells in contact with the colloid so that it is not normally accessible to circulating antibody. This explains why simple fragments of thyroid which have intact follicles are unaffected by incubation in the presence of medium containing cytotoxic antibody and complement, and also why there is no evidence that infants born to Hashimoto mothers have defective thyroid function despite the presence of the antibody in their serum. Nonetheless, antibody can be detected on the inner surface of thyroid follicles in tissue removed from patients with autoimmune thyroiditis, and it seems necessary to postulate that thyroid damage only occurs when there is collaboration with other factors such as immune complex deposition or mechanisms mediated by sensitized T-cell effectors.

Thyroid-stimulating antibodies Under certain circumstances antibodies to the surface of a cell may stimulate rather than destroy (cf. type V sensitivity; Chapter 9). This would seem to be the case in thyrotoxicosis (Graves' or Basedow's disease). There has long been indirect evidence suggesting a link between autoimmune processes and this disease: thyroid antibodies are detectable in up to 85% of thyrotoxic patients and histologically the majority of the glands removed at operation show varying degrees of thyroiditis and local antibody formation in addition to the characteristic acinar cell hyperplasia; thyrotoxicosis is found with undue frequency in the families of Hashimoto patients; there is an association with gastric autoimmunity in that 30% have gastric antibodies and up to 10% pernicious anaemia. The direct link came with the discovery by Adams and Purves of thyroid stimulating activity in the serum of thyrotoxic patients. Using a new bioassay they found that the serum caused a stimulation of the thyroid gland of the recipient animal which was considerably prolonged relative to the time course of action of the physiological thyroid stimulating hormone (TSH) from the pituitary; it was ultimately shown that this was due to the presence of thyroid stimulating antibodies (TSAb). These antibodies can block the binding of TSH to thyroid membranes and seem to act in the same manner as TSH, probably by stimulating the identical receptors (cf. figure 9.19). Both operate through the adenyl cyclase system as indicated by the potentiating effect of theophylline, and both produce similar changes in ultrastructural morphology in the thyroid cell, but it is one of Nature's 'passive transfer experiments' which links TSAb most directly with the pathogenesis of Graves' disease. When TSAb from a thyrotoxic mother crosses the placenta it is associated with the production of neonatal hyperthyroidism (figure 11.12), which resolves after a few weeks as the maternal IgG is catabolized.

There is a good correlation between the titre of TSAb and the severity of hyperthyroidism. Because TSAb act independently of the pituitary–thyroid axis, iodine uptake by the gland is unaffected by administration of thyroxine or triiodothyronine, whereas normally this would cause feedback inhibition and suppression of uptake; this forms the basis of an important diagnostic test for thyrotoxicosis.

Figure 11.12. Neonatal thyrotoxicosis. (a) The autoantibodies which stimulate the thyroid through the TSH-receptors are IgG and cross the placenta. (b) The thyrotoxic mother therefore gives birth to a baby with thyroid hyperactivity which spontaneously resolves as the mother's IgG is catabolized. (Photograph courtesy of Dr A. MacGregor.)

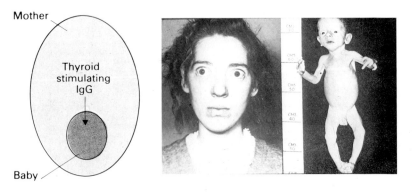

Mother

Thyroid stimulating IgG

Baby

(a)

(b)

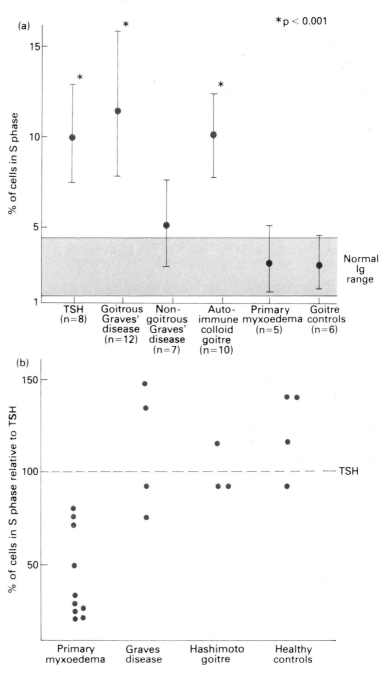

Figure 11.13. Autoantibodies affecting thyroid growth. (a) Stimulating antibodies in goitrous Graves' disease and auto-immune colloid goitre shown by the increase of cells entering the DNA synthetic (S) phase of the cell cycle in thyroid fragments treated with IgG from the patient's serum. n = number of patients studied. p values relate to differences from results with normal Ig. (b) Blocking antibodies in primary myxoedema revealed by the ability of patient's IgG to inhibit the growth stimulation caused by TSH. (Data from Drexhage H.A., Bottazzo G.F., Doniach D., Bitensky I. & Chayen J. (1980) *Lancet* **II**, 287 and from (1981) *Nature* **289**, 594.)

There is reason to believe that enlargement of the thyroid in this disorder is due to the action of antibodies which react with a 'growth' receptor and directly stimulate cell division as distinct from metabolic hyperactivity (figure 11.13a). In contrast, sera from patients with primary myxoedema contain antibodies capable of blocking the mitogenic action of TSH (figure 11.13b) thereby preventing the regeneration of follicles which is a feature of the enlarged Hashimoto goitre. We see now that there is considerable diversity in the autoimmune response to the thyroid leading to tissue destruction, metabolic stimulation, growth promotion or mitotic inhibition which in different combinations account for the variety of forms in which autoimmune thyroid disease presents (figure 11.14).

Intrinsic factor

Autoantibodies to this product of gastric mucosal secretion were first demonstrated in pernicious anaemia patients by oral administration of intrinsic factor, vitamin B_{12} and the serum from a patient with this disease. The serum was found to prevent intrinsic factor from mediating the absorption of B_{12} into the body, and further studies showed the active principle to be an antibody. Circulating antibody does not seem to be capable of neutralizing the physiological activity of intrinsic factor; a patient immunized parenterally with hog intrinsic factor in complete Freund's adjuvant had high serum antibody levels and good cell-mediated skin responses but still absorbed B_{12} well when fed with hog intrinsic factor. These data imply that the antibodies have to be present within the lumen of the gastrointestinal tract to be biologically effective, and indeed they can be identified in the gastric juice of these patients, synthesized by plasma cells in the gastritic lesion.

Sperm

In some infertile males, agglutinating antibodies cause aggregation of the spermatozoa and interfere with their penetration into the cervical mucus.

Glomerular basement membrane (gbm)

With immunological kidney disease the experimental models preceded the finding of parallel lesions in the human. Injection of cross-reacting heterologous gbm preparations in complete Freund's adjuvant produces glomerulonephritis in sheep and other experimental animals. Antibodies to gbm can be picked up by immunofluorescent staining of biopsies

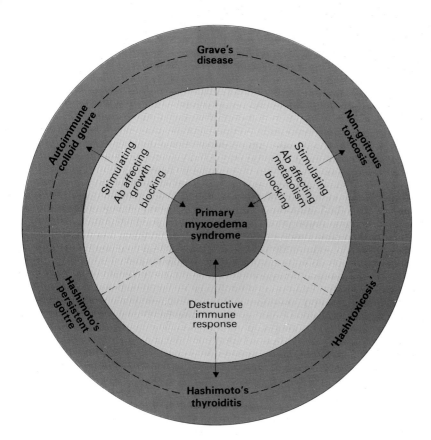

Figure 11.14. Relationship of different autoallergic responses to the circular spectrum of autoimmune thyroid diseases. Responses involving thyroglobulin and the microsomal/surface microvillous antigen lead to tissue destruction whereas other autoantibodies can stimulate or block metabolic activity or thyroid cell division. 'Hashitoxicosis' is the down-to-earth term used by our Scots' colleagues to describe a gland showing Hashimoto's thyroiditis and thyrotoxicosis simultaneously (courtesy of Prof. D. Doniach and Dr G.F. Bottazzo).

from nephritic animals with anti-IgG. The antibodies are largely if not completely absorbed out by the kidney *in vivo* but they appear in the serum on nephrectomy and can passively transfer the disease to another animal of the same species.

An entirely analogous situation occurs in man in certain cases of glomerulonephritis, particularly those associated with lung haemorrhage (Goodpasture's syndrome). Kidney biopsy from the patient shows *linear* deposition of IgG and C3 along the basement membrane of the glomerular capillaries (figure 9.13a). After nephrectomy, gbm antibodies can be detected in the serum. Dixon and his colleagues eluted the gbm antibody from a diseased kidney and injected it into a squirrel monkey. The antibody rapidly fixed to the gbm of the recipient animal and produced a fatal nephritis (figure

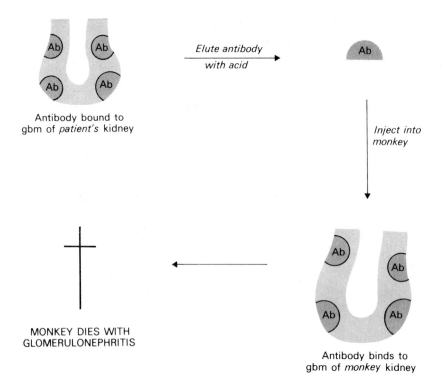

Antibody bound to
gbm of *patient's* kidney

Elute antibody
with acid

Ab

Inject into
monkey

MONKEY DIES WITH
GLOMERULONEPHRITIS

Antibody binds to
gbm of *monkey* kidney

Figure 11.15. Passive transfer of glomerulonephritis to a squirrel monkey by injection of antiglomerular basement membrane
(anti-gbm) antibodies isolated by acid elution from the kidney of a patient with
Goodpasture's syndrome (after Lerner
R.A., Glassock R.J. & Dixon F.J. (1967)
J.Exp.Med. **126**, 989).

11.15). It is hard to escape the conclusion that the lesion in
the human was the direct result of attack on the gbm by these
complement-fixing antibodies. The lung changes in Goodpasture's syndrome may be attributable to cross-reaction
with some of the gbm antibodies.

Muscle

The transient muscle weakness seen in babies born to
mothers with myasthenia gravis calls to mind neonatal
thrombocytopenia and hyperthyroidism and would certainly
be compatible with the transplacental passage of an IgG
capable of inhibiting neuromuscular transmission. Strong
support for this view is afforded by the consistent finding of
antibodies to muscle acetyl choline receptors in myasthenics
and the depletion of these receptors within the motor end
plates.

Table 11.4 summarizes these direct pathogenic effects of
humoral autoantibodies.

Table 11.4. Direct pathogenic effects of humoral antibodies.

Disease	Autoantigen	Lesion
Autoimmune haemolytic anaemia	Red cell	Erythrocyte destruction
Lymphopenia (some cases)	Lymphocyte	Lymphocyte destruction
Idiopathic thrombocytopenic purpura	Platelet	Platelet destruction
Male infertility (some cases)	Sperm	Agglutination of spermatozoa
Pernicious anaemia	Intrinsic factor	Neutralization of ability to mediate B_{12} absorption
Hashimoto's disease	Thyroid surface antigen	Cytotoxic effect on thyroid cells in culture
Thyrotoxicosis	TSH receptors	Stimulation of thyroid cells
	'Growth' receptors	Induction of thyroid cell division
Goodpasture's syndrome	Glomerular basement membrane	Complement-mediated damage to basement membrane
Myasthenia gravis	Acetyl choline receptor	Blocking and destruction of receptors
Acanthosis nigricans (type B) and ataxia telangiectasia with insulin resistance	Insulin receptor	Blocking of receptors
Atopic allergy (some cases)	β-Adrenergic receptors	Blocking of receptors

EFFECTS OF COMPLEXES

Systemic lupus erythematosus (SLE)

Where autoantibodies are formed against soluble components to which they have continual access, complexes may be formed which can give rise to lesions similar to those occurring in serum sickness (cf. p. 254). In SLE, complexes of DNA and other nuclear antigens, and possibly C-type viral components, together with immunoglobulin and complement can be detected by immunofluorescent staining of kidney biopsies from patients with evidence of renal dysfunction. The staining pattern with a fluorescent anti-IgG or anti-C3 is punctate or 'lumpy-bumpy' as some would describe it (figure 9.13b) in marked contrast with the linear pattern caused by the gbm antibodies in Goodpasture's syndrome (figure 9.13a; p. 247). The complexes grow in size to become large aggregates visible in the electron microscope as amorphous humps on the epithelial side of the glomerular basement membrane. During the active phase of the disease, serum complement levels fall as components are affected by immune aggregates in the kidney and circulation. Attempts to detect autoantigens in the circulating complexes have not been conspicuously successful; immunoglobulins and complement components make up the usual tally of constituents which can be identified. Although in a way negative evidence, this is consistent with the possibility that anti-idiotype may perpetuate an autoimmune state once it is initiated (i.e. acts as a surrogate autoantigen) and generate circulating idiotype—anti-idiotype complexes.

Immunofluorescent studies on skin biopsies from patients with the related disease discoid lupus erythematosus also reveal the presence of immune complexes.

Rheumatoid arthritis

A strong case can be made for the fairly straightforward proposition that an autoimmune response to the Fc portion of IgG gives rise to complexes which are ultimately responsible for the pathological changes characteristic of the rheumatoid joint. Virtually all patients with rheumatoid arthritis have demonstrable antibodies to IgG—the so-called rheumatoid or anti-globulin factors. The majority have IgM anti-globulins which react in the classical latex and sheep cell agglutination tests (table 11.2; note 7) and both they and the 'sero-negative' patients who fail to react in these tests can be shown to have elevated levels of IgG antiglobulins detectable by solid phase techniques (cf. p. 152) (figure 11.16). Sensiti-

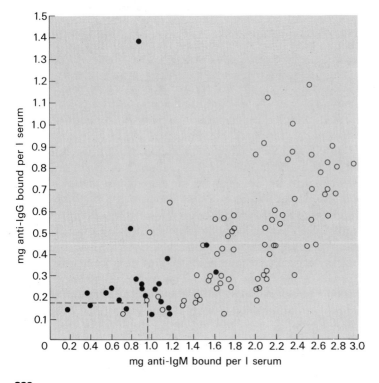

Figure 11.16. IgM and IgG antiglobulins determined by tube radioassay in patients with sero-positive (◉) and seronegative (●) rheumatoid arthritis. The dotted lines indicate the 95% confidence limits (mean + 2 S.D.) of the normal group. (From Nineham L., Hay F.C. & Roitt I.M. (1976) *J. Clin. Path.* **29**, 1121.)

zation to self IgG is therefore an almost universal feature of the disease.

The synovium typically is very heavily infiltrated with mononuclear cells often aggregated in the form of lymphoid follicles; there are many plasma cells and it has been estimated that the synthesis of IgG can be as high as that of a stimulated lymph node. If IgG is the main antigen responsible for evoking this response, most of the plasma cells should be synthesizing antiglobulins, yet only a minority (say 10–20%) bind fluoresceinated IgG, either in the form of heat-aggregated material or immune complexes (rheumatoid factor is a low affinity antibody and good binding is only seen when multivalent IgG is used as antigen). However, we must take into account a strange and unique feature of IgG antiglobulins; because they are both antigen and antibody at the same time, they are capable of self-association (figure 11.17b) and this hides the majority of free antiglobulin valencies. Cleverly realizing that destruction of the Fc regions by pepsin would liberate these hidden binding sites (figure 11.17c), Munthe & Natvig observed that as many as 40–70% of the plasma cells in the synovium

Figure 11.17. Self-associated complexes of IgG antiglobulins and the exposure of 'hidden' binding sites by pepsin. Such complexes in the joint may be stabilized by IgM antiglobulin and C1q which have polyvalent binding sites for IgG.

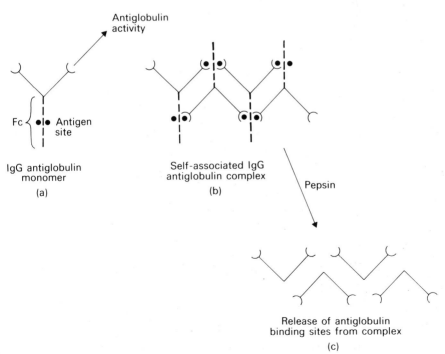

Antiglobulin activity

Fc — Antigen site

IgG antiglobulin monomer

(a)

Self-associated IgG antiglobulin complex

(b)

Pepsin

Release of antiglobulin binding sites from complex

(c)

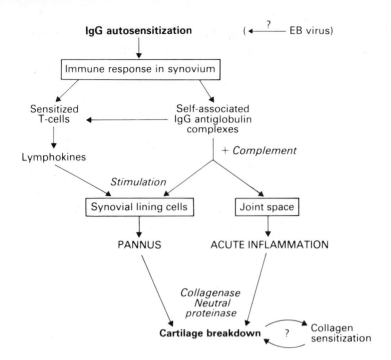

Figure 11.18. Hypothetical scheme showing how initial autosensitization to IgG can lead to the pathogenetic changes characteristic of rheumatoid arthritis.

displayed an anti-IgG specificity following treatment with this enzyme.

IgG aggregates, presumably products of these plasma cells, can be regularly detected in the synovial tissues and fluid. Analysis shows them to consist almost exclusively of immunoglobulins and complement while a major proportion of the IgG is present as self-associated antiglobulin as shown by binding to an Fcγ immunosorbent after treatment with pepsin. The complexes can mediate cartilage breakdown through different pathways (figure 11.18). In the joint space itself they initiate an Arthus reaction leading to an influx of polymorphs with which they react to release lysosomal enzymes. These include neutral proteinases and collagenase which can damage the articular cartilage by breaking down proteoglycans and collagen fibrils. More damage results if the complexes are adherent to the cartilage since the polymorph binds but is unable to internalize them ('frustrated phagocytosis'); as a result the lysosomal hydrolases are released extracellularly into the space between the cell and the cartilage where they are protected from enzyme inhibitors such as α_2-macroglobulin.

The aggregates may also stimulate the macrophage-like cells of the synovial lining, either directly through their surface receptors or indirectly through the release of lympho-kines from sensitized T-cells. The activated synovial cells grow out as a malign pannus (cover) over the cartilage and at the margin of this advancing granulation tissue, breakdown can be seen, almost certainly as a result of enzyme release. Activated macrophages also secrete plasminogen activator and the plasmin formed as a consequence activates a latent collagenase produced by synovial cells. Sensitization to partially degraded collagen may occur and this could lead secondarily to amplification of the lesion. Prostaglandin E_2, another product of the stimulated macrophage, can bring about bone resorption which is a further complication of severe disease. Subcutaneous nodules are granulomata possibly formed through local production of insolubilized self-associating antiglobulins.

The rheumatological pulse has quickened perceptibly with the discovery that a high proportion of patients with rheumatoid arthritis have elevated titres of circulating antibodies to a nuclear antigen present in EB virus transformed but absent from normal lymphocytes. This has led to the finding that the T-cells in these patients are deficient in the γ-interferon-mediated control of EB virus transformation of B-lymphocytes. Whether this betokens a primary aetiological role for EB virus infection or represents a basic regulatory abnormality which results in defective handling of virus is not yet resolved.

CELLULAR HYPERSENSITIVITY

The inflammatory infiltrate in organ-specific autoimmune disease is usually essentially mononuclear in character and, although not an infallible guide, this has been taken as an expression of cell-mediated hypersensitivity. Direct evidence is still thin. At the time of writing, skin reactions to autoantigens have proved difficult to assess and *in vitro* leucocyte inhibition tests have not been unequivocally accepted although, for example in autoimmune thyroiditis and thyrotoxicosis, there is a consistent finding of inhibition of leucocyte migration by thyroid microsomes. The killing of colon cells in culture by lymphocytes from patients with ulcerative colitis is encouraging and it has been reported that long-term culture of thyroid target cells with Hashimoto leucocytes leads to significant failure in the metabolic handling of iodine. Firm evidence for a direct participation of T-lymphocytes in any of these reactions has yet to be provided. There is more inclination to think in terms of ADCC, either by pre-armed cells or of targets coated with antibody secreted into the cultures by the effector cell population.

Thus the destruction of isolated liver cells by leucocytes from patients with HB_s-negative active chronic hepatitis can be blocked by antigen (hepatic lipoprotein) or by aggregated normal IgG (which would bind to K-cell Fc receptors), but is not affected by removal of T-cells.

Indirect evidence for a destructive role of the inflammatory cells comes from the observation that high doses of steroids may restore gastric function in certain patients with pernicious anaemia. In one such case studied, biopsy after intensive treatment with prednisone showed a diminution in the cellular infiltrate and new formation of parietal and chief cells in the gastric mucosa; acid and intrinsic factor were now produced after histamine stimulation and the ability to absorb vitamin B_{12} assessed by the Schilling test was restored to near normal values. The most likely explanation is that attack by the inflammatory cells and attempts to regenerate by mucosal cells were more or less in balance in the atrophic mucosa. Elimination of inflammatory cells by the prednisone allowed the regeneration of gastric mucosal cells to become dominant.

Our views on the pathogenesis of pernicious anaemia may be stated as follows. Autoimmune attack based on the parietal cell antigen gives rise to an atrophic gastritis which in many cases settles down to a dynamic equilibrium where the rate of destruction roughly balances the rate of regeneration; the loss of capacity to make intrinsic factor is evident in tests showing defective B_{12} absorption but sufficient vitamin is absorbed to keep the body in balance. These patients often have parietal cell antibodies and go on for 15 years or so without developing megaloblastic anaemia. However, if they should produce antibodies to intrinsic factor in the lumen of the gastrointestinal tract, these will neutralize the small amount of intrinsic factor still available and the body will move into negative balance for B_{12}. The symptoms of B_{12} deficiency will then appear some considerable time later as the liver stores become exhausted (figure 11.19). A similar long latent period before the onset of clinical disease is evident in the prospective study of a family with insulin-dependent diabetes documented in figure 11.4 (p. 319) where complement-fixing islet cell antibodies were detected two years before overt signs of pancreatic deficiency were apparent. Note also that the disease occurs after the autoimmunity pointing yet again to a primary pathogenetic role for the immune process.

The nature of the cellular attack in organ-specific disorders is still not resolved but it is not improbable that cell-mediated hypersensitivity, antibody-mediated cytotoxicity and inflammatory reactions due to immune complexes may operate alone or in concert.

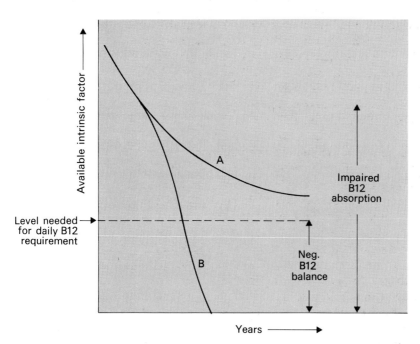

Figure 11.19. Pathogenesis of pernicious anaemia. Group A: Patients with long standing atrophic gastritis having parietal cell but no intrinsic factor antibodies. Group B: Pernicious anaemia patients with intrinsic factor antibodies superimposed upon the atrophic gastritis. (After Doniach D. & Roitt I.M. (1964) *Semin. Hematol.* **1**, 313.)

EXPERIMENTAL MODELS OF AUTOIMMUNE DISEASE

If autoimmune processes are pathogenic in human diseases we would expect that the production of autoimmunity should lead to comparable lesions in experimental animals.

Experimental autoallergic disease

When animals are injected with extracts of certain organs emulsified in oil containing killed tubercle bacilli (i.e. in complete Freund's adjuvant), autoantibodies and destructive inflammatory lesions specific to the organ used for immunization result. Thus, Rose and Witebsky found that rabbits receiving rabbit thyroglobulin in Freund's adjuvant developed antibodies to thyroglobulin and thyroiditis involving invasion of the gland by mononuclear cells of lymphocytic and histiocytic types with destruction of the normal follicular architecture. Histologically there are many points of similarity between this experimental autoallergic lesion and human autoimmune thyroiditis (figure 11.20).

In some of the earliest work in this field it was shown that injection of central nervous tissue produced encephalomyelitis and paralysis in monkeys and guinea-pigs; the parallel

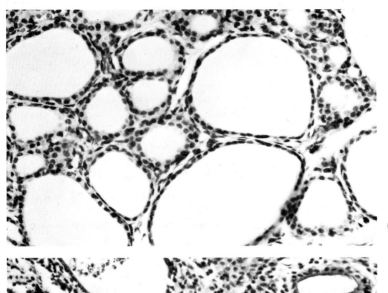

(a) Normal
rat thyroid

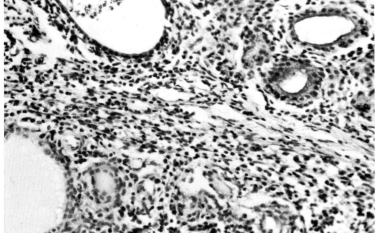

(b) Thyroiditis
in the rat

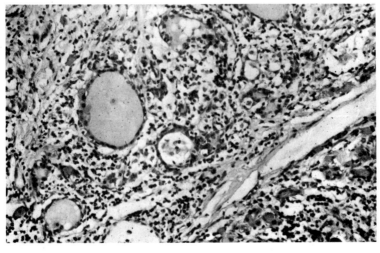

(c) Spontaneous
human autoimmune

with post rabies vaccine encephalitis is clear since the vaccine contains brain extracts, and optimistic comparisons with multiple sclerosis have been made. Just as with the thyroid, the most convenient model for the production of allergic encephalomyelitis involves immunization with the antigen, in this case myelin basic protein, incorporated in complete Freund's adjuvant. Similar lesions can be induced in the adrenal (cf. Addisonian idiopathic adrenal atrophy) and the testis (? model for granulomatous orchitis), while experimental myasthenia gravis can be induced by immunization with acetyl choline receptor. Heterologous glomeruli stimulate the formation of glomerular basement membrane autoantibodies which localize in the kidney of the host to cause severe glomerulonephritis (Steblay model) resembling closely that seen in Goodpasture's syndrome.

The experimental disease can usually be transmitted to syngeneic animals by lymphoid cells from immunized donors and occasionally by serum. In the case of experimental autoallergic orchitis, a synergism between cell-mediated hypersensitivity and antibody was recognized in the transfer studied. Allergic encephalomyelitis can be induced in syngeneic animals by injection of purified T-cells from sensitized donors and in particular by T-cell lines which respond *in vitro* to myelin basic protein. On the other hand, transfer of monoclonal autoantibodies raised to acetyl choline receptors produces the muscle weakness characteristic of myasthenia.

The pre-eminent ability of Freund's complete adjuvant to enhance the production of experimental autoallergic disease may depend upon several factors acting concomitantly: modification of antigen, stimulation of T-helpers and (more controversially) disruption of normal T-suppressor feedback perhaps through priming of contrasuppressor cells. Although the precise nature of the events leading to tissue damage has yet to be resolved, it is abundantly clear that the deliberate provocation of an autoallergic state can produce lesions which closely mimic those seen in human organ-specific autoimmune disease and add weight to the notion that the immunological events are directly concerned in the pathogenesis of these disorders.

Figure 11.20. Similarity of lesions in spontaneous human autoimmune thyroiditis and the experimental disease produced by injection of rats with homologous thyroid in complete Freund's adjuvant. Other features of Hashimoto's disease such as the eosinophilic metaplasia of acinar cells (Askenazy cells) and local lymphoid follicles are not seen in this experimental model although the latter occur in the spontaneous thyroiditis of Obese strain chickens.

The message from animal models in which autoimmune disease develops spontaneously is the same. Neonatal bursectomy largely prevents the appearance of thyroglobulin antibodies and thyroiditis in Obese strain chickens, so pointing to a primary involvement of thyroid antibodies in the tissue lesions. Immunological control is also implicated by the exacerbation of disease caused by neonatal thymectomy.

The now famous strain of mouse, the New Zealand Black (NZB), consistently develops an autoimmune haemolytic anaemia with positive Coombs' tests (agglutination of antibody-coated erythrocytes by an antiglobulin serum). As discussed earlier, the disease can be provoked in young unaffected NZB's by transfer of spleen cells from a Coombs' positive donor suggesting that it is the production of red cell antibodies which leads to shortened erythrocyte survival and consequent anaemia. A high proportion of these mice, and especially their hybrids with the partially related New Zealand White (B × W F1), have circulating antinuclear antibodies and an immune complex induced glomerulonephritis. Several other mutant mouse strains which have SLE-like symptoms are also positive for anti-DNA and die with type III hypersensitivity kidney lesions.

Diagnostic value of autoantibody tests

Serum autoantibodies frequently provide valuable diagnostic markers. The most useful routine test is screening of the serum by immunofluorescence on a frozen section prepared from a composite block of unfixed human thyroid and stomach, and rat kidney and liver. This is supplemented by agglutination tests for rheumatoid factors and for thyroglobulin, thyroid microsome and red cell antibodies and by radioassay for antibodies to intrinsic factor, DNA and IgG (see table 11.2). The salient information is summarized in table 11.5.

The tests will also prove of value in screening for people at risk, e.g. relatives of patients with autoimmune disease, thyroiditis patients (for gastric autoimmunity and *vice versa*) and ultimately the general population.

Treatment of autoimmune disorders

The majority of approaches to treatment, not unnaturally, involve manipulation of immunological responses (figure 11.21). However, in many organ-specific diseases, metabolic control is usually sufficient, e.g. thyroxine replacement in primary myoedema, insulin in juvenile diabetes, vitamin B_{12}

Table 11.5. Autoantibody tests and diagnosis.

Disease	Antibody	Comment
Hashimoto's thyroiditis	Thyroid	Distinction from colloid goitre, thyroid cancer and subacute thyroiditis. Thyroidectomy usually unnecessary in Hashimoto goitre
Primary myxoedema	Thyroid	Tests +ve in 99% of cases. If suspected hypothyroidism assess 'thyroid reserve' by TRH stimulation test
Thyrotoxicosis	Thyroid	High titres of cytoplasmic Ab indicate active thyroiditis and tendency to post-operative myxoedema: anti-thyroid drugs are the treatment of choice although HLA-B8 patients have high chance of relapse
Pernicious anaemia	Stomach	Help in diagnosis of latent PA, in differential diagnosis of non-auto-immune megaloblastic anaemia and in suspected subacute combined degeneration of the cord
Idiopathic adrenal atrophy	Adrenal	Distinction from tuberculous form
Myasthenia gravis	Muscle	When positive suggests associated thymoma (more likely if HLA-B12)
	ACh receptor	Positive in >80%
Pemphigus vulgaris and pemphigoid	Skin	Different fluorescent patterns in the two diseases
Autoimmune haemolytic anaemia	Erythrocyte (Coombs' test)	Distinction from other forms of anaemia
Sjögren's syndrome	Salivary duct cells	
Primary biliary cirrhosis (PBC)	Mitochondrial	Distinction from other forms of obstructive jaundice where test rarely +ve. Recognize subgroup within cryptogenic cirrhosis related to PBC with +ve mitochondrial Ab
Active chronic hepatitis	Smooth muscle anti-nuclear and 20% mitochondrial	Smooth muscle Ab distinguish from SLE
Rheumatoid arthritis	Antiglobulin, e.g. SCAT and latex fixation	High titre indicative of bad prognosis
SLE	High titre antinuclear, DNA; LE-cells	DNA antibodies present in active phase. Ab to double-stranded DNA characteristic
Scleroderma	Nucleolar	
Other 'collagenoses'	Nuclear	

in pernicious anaemia, anti-thyroid drugs for Graves' disease and so forth. Anticholinesterase drugs are commonly used for long-term therapy in myasthenia gravis; thymectomy is of benefit in most cases and it is conceivable that the gland contains ACh receptors in a particularly antigenic form (? associated with HLA-D expression).

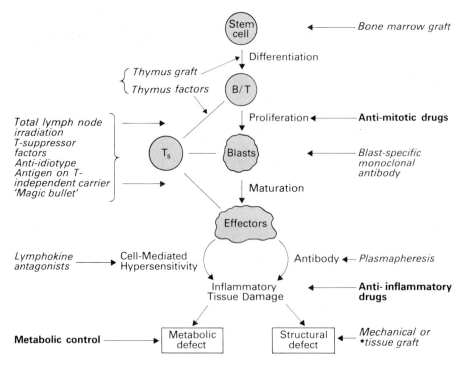

Figure 11.21. The treatment of autoimmune disease. Current conventional treat-
ments are in bold type; some feasible
approaches are given in italics. (*In the case
of a live graft, the immunosuppressive
therapy used may protect the tissue from
the autoimmune damage which affected the
organ being replaced.)

Patients with severe myasthenic symptoms respond well to
high doses of steroids and the same is true for serious cases
of other autoimmune disorders such as SLE and immune
complex nephritis where the drug helps to suppress the
inflammatory lesions.

In rheumatoid arthritis, apart from steroids, anti-
inflammatory drugs such as salicylates, indomethacin,
phenylbutazone and newer preparations such as fenoprofen
and ibuprofen are widely used. Penicillamine, gold salts and
antimalarials such as chloroquine all find an important place
in therapy but their mode of action is unknown.

Therapeutic blocking of other mediators directly concerned in immunological tissue damage will be feasible if
lymphokine and complement antagonists become available.
Plasma exchange to lower the rate of immune complex deposition in SLE provides only temporary benefit although it
may be of value in life-threatening cases of arteritis. Successful results have been obtained in Goodpasture's syndrome when the treatment has been applied in combination
with anti-mitotic drugs (figure 11.22), the rationale being an
increased tendency for antigen-reactive cells to divide as the

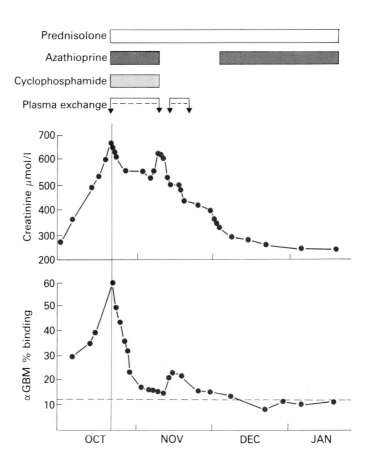

Figure 11.22.
Treatment of a patient with anti-glomerular basement membrane (α-GBM) nephritis with plasma exchange, steroids and immunosuppressive drugs. Kidney function is here monitored by the serum creatinine level. The treatment leads to loss of autoantibody (the dotted line represents the amount of GBM antigen bound in the assay by normal serum) and restoration of kidney function (courtesy of Dr C.M. Lockwood).

negative feedback effect of IgG is lowered following removal of plasma proteins.

Cyclosporin A which preferentially influences dividing lymphocytes (p. 286) should similarly discriminate against the antigen-sensitive cells responding during autoimmune disease, and although a pilot study in SLE has not been encouraging it would be expected that this drug would find a place in the treatment of some of these disorders. If these cells carry a characteristic blast specific antigen, they should be vulnerable to attack by an appropriate anti-lymphocyte globulin. Several groups are trying to evolve a strategy based upon the 'magic bullet' (cf. p. 301), the essence of which is to fashion different types of cytotoxic weaponry by coupling bacterial toxins or lots of radioactivity to the antigen which selectively homes on to the lymphocytes bearing specific surface receptors.

While awaiting more selective therapy, conventional non-specific anti-mitotic agents such as azathioprine, cyclophosphamide and methotrexate have been used effectively in SLE, chronic active hepatitis and autoimmune haemolytic anaemia for example. It should one day be practical to correct any relevant defects in stem cells or in thymus processing by bone marrow or thymus grafting or perhaps, in the latter case, by thymic hormones.

We have already discussed the possible role of thymic factors in maintaining T-suppressor control of autoimmunity and one anticipates some interesting advances now that purified materials are available. Hybridoma technology or even gene cloning should ultimately provide the clinician with antigen-specific suppressor factors. Other features of regulatory bypass mechanisms such as excessive contrasuppressor activity or inappropriate HLA-DR expression may also become feasible targets for therapy one day. The powerful immunosuppressive action of anti-idiotype antibodies has led to much rumination on the feasibility of controlling autoantibody production by provoking appropriate interactions within the immune network (cf. p. 105). Another potentially valuable approach for the future involves 'switching off' primed B-cells by presenting hapten linked to a thymus-independent carrier like the copolymer of D-glutamic and D-lysine (D-GL) or isologous IgG particularly when given with high cortisone doses. This has certainly worked well in NZB hybrid mice where anti-DNA levels have been reduced using nucleosides as the haptens: we shall have to see whether man and mouse really are that different.

Summary: comparison of organ-specific and non-organ-specific diseases

Organ-specific (e.g. thyroiditis, gastritis, adrenalitis)	Non-organ specific (e.g. systemic lupus erythematosus)
Differences	
1 Antigens only available to lymphoid system in low concentration	Antigens accessible at higher concentrations
2 Antibodies and lesions organ-specific	Antibodies and lesions non-organ-specific
3 Clinical and serologic overlap—thyroiditis, gastritis and adrenalitis	Overlap SLE, rheumatoid arthritis, and other connective tissue disorders
4 Familial tendency to organ-specific autoimmunity	Familial connective tissue disease ? Abnormalities in immunoglobulin synthesis in relatives
5 Lymphoid invasion, parenchymal destruction by ? ± cell-mediated hypersensitivity ? ± antibodies	Lesions due to deposition of antigen–antibody complexes
6 Therapy aimed at controlling metabolic deficit	Therapy aimed at inhibiting inflammation and antibody synthesis
7 Tendency to cancer in organ	Tendency to lymphoreticular neoplasia

8 Antigens evoke organ-specific antibodies in normal animals with complete Freund's adjuvant	No antibodies produced in animals with comparable stimulation
9 Experimental lesions produced with antigen in Freund adjuvant	Diseases and autoantibodies arise spontaneously in certain animals (e.g. NZB mice and hybrids and some dogs) or after injection of parental lymphoid tissue into F1 hybrids

Similarities

1 Circulating autoantibodies react with normal body constituents
2 Patients often have increased immunoglobulins in serum
3 Antibodies may appear in each of the main immunoglobulin classes
4 Greater incidence in women
5 Disease process not always progressive; exacerbations and remissions
6 Association with HLA
7 Spontaneous diseases in animals genetically programmed
8 Autoantibody tests of diagnostic value

Further reading

Bottazzo G.F., Pujol-Borrell R., Hanufusa T. & Feldman M. (1983) Hypothesis: role of aberrant HLA-DR expression and antigen presentation in the induction of endocrine autoimmunity. *Lancet* **II**, 1115.

Davies T.F. (ed.) (1983) *Autoimmune Endocrine Disease*. John Wiley & Sons, New York.

Doniach D. & Bottazzo G.F. (1977) Autoimmunity and the endocrine pancreas. In *Pathobiology Annual*, Iochim H.L. (ed.). Appleton–Century–Crofts, New York.

Fudenberg H.H., Stites D.P., Caldwell J.L. & Wells J.V. (1980) *Basic and Clinical Immunology*, 3rd edn. Lange Medical Publications, Los Altos, California.

Glynn L.E. & Holborow E.J. (1964) *Autoimmunity and Disease*. Blackwell Scientific Publications, Oxford.

Lachmann P.J. & Peters D.K. (eds) (1982) *Clinical Aspects of Immunology*, 4th edn. Blackwell Scientific Publications, Oxford.

Maini R.N. (1977) *Immunology of the Rheumatic Diseases*. Edward Arnold, London.

Marchalonis J.J. & Cohen N. (eds) (1980) *Self/Non-self Discrimination*. Contemporary Topics in Immunobiology, Vol. 9. Plenum Press, New York.

Miescher P.A. *et al.* (1978) Menarini Symposium on *Organ Specific Autoimmunity*. Schwabe & Co., Basle.

Rose N.R., Bigazzi P.E. & Warner N.L. (eds) (1978) *Genetic Control of Autoimmune Disease*. Elsevier-North Holland, New York.

Talal N. (ed.) (1977) *Autoimmunity*. Academic Press, New York.

Turk J.L. (1978) *Immunology in Clinical Medicine*, 3rd edn. Heinemann, London.

Yamamura T. & Tada T. (eds) (1984) *Progress in Immunology V.* Academic Press, Tokyo.

World Health Organisation Technical Report Series (1973) No. 496, *Clinical Immunology*.

Appendix

Table 1. Recommended schedule for active routine immunization of normal individuals in the UK[1].

Age	Vaccine	Interval	Notes
During the first year of life	Dip/tet/pert and oral polio vaccine (first dose)		The earliest age at which the first dose should be given is 3 months, but a better general immunological response can be expected if the first dose is delayed until 6 months of age
	Dip/tet/pert and oral polio vaccine (second dose)	Preferably after an interval of 6–8 weeks	
	Dip/tet/pert and oral polio vaccine (third dose)	Preferably after an interval of 4–6 months	
During the second year of life	Measles vaccine	After an interval of not less than 3 weeks	Although measles vaccination can be given in the second year of life, delay until 3 years of age or more will reduce the risk of occasional severe reactions to the vaccine which occur mainly in children under the age 3 years
At 5 years of age or school entry	Dip/tet and oral polio vaccine or dip/tet/polio vaccine		These may be given, if desired, at 3 years of age to children entering nursery schools, attending day nurseries or living in children's homes
Between 10 and 13 years of age	BCG vaccine	There should be an interval of not less than 3 weeks between BCG and rubella vaccination	
All girls aged 11–13 years	Rubella vaccine		All girls of this age should be offered rubella vaccine whether or not there is a past history of an attack of rubella
At 15–19 years of age or on leaving school	Polio vaccine (oral or inactivated) and tetanus toxoid		

[1] Data from *Immunisation Against Infectious Diseases* (1972), DHSS, London. (Reproduced from *Immunisation*, by G. Dick (1978) Update Books, London, with permission of author and publisher.)

Table 2. Recommended schedule for active routine immunization of normal individuals in the USA[1].

Age	Vaccine	Notes
2 months	Dip/tet/pert and oral polio vaccine	Suitable for breast-fed as well as bottle-fed babies
4 months	Dip/tet/pert and oral polio vaccine	
6 months	Dip/tet/pert and oral polio vaccine	
1 year	Measles, rubella, mumps, tuberculin test	May be given at 1 year as combined measles–rubella or measles–mumps–rubella vaccines
		Measles vaccine may be given at 6 months in places where measles frequent in first year of life. In such circumstances a repeat dose should be given at 1 year
		Frequency of repeated tuberculin tests depends on risk of exposure and prevalence of tuberculosis
		Initial test shoould be at time of, or preceding, measles immunization
$1\frac{1}{2}$ years	Dip/tet/pert and oral polio vaccine	
4–6 years˙	Dip/tet/pert and oral polio vaccine	
14–16 years	Tet	And every 10 years thereafter

[1] Data from *Report of the Committee on Infectious Diseases* (1974), 17th edn. American Academy of Pediatrics, Evanston, Illinois. (Reproduced from *Immunisation* by G. Dick (1978), Update Books, London, with permission of author and publisher.)

Index

ENT. PM SM

GPTAL AM 8J.

10th IMM. PM. OLD REFECTORY QEC

12th Pharm Circ. PM SM.

14th NEURO. AM SH.